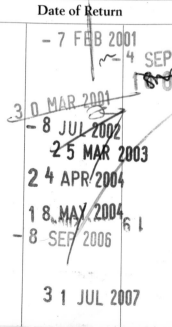

University
Of Dundee

UNIVERSITY LIBRARY

School of Nursing and Midwifery
Fife Campus

Date of Return

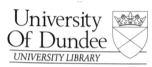

Commissioning Editor: Ellen Green
Project Development Manager: Jim Killgore
Project Manager: Nancy Arnott
Designer: Erik Bigland

Pocket
Neonatology

Terence Stephenson BSc BM BCh DM FRCP FRCPCH

Professor of Child Health and Honorary Consultant Paediatrician, Academic Division of Child Health, School of Human Development, The University of Nottingham, Nottingham, UK

Neil Marlow MB BS DM FRCP FRCPCH

Professor of Neonatal Medicine, Academic Division of Child Health, School of Human Development, University of Nottingham, Nottingham, UK

Sara Watkin MB ChB MD MRCP FRCPCH

Consultant Neonatologist,
Nottingham City Hospital,
Nottingham, UK

Judith Grant MB BCh MRCP DCH FRCPCH

Consultant Neonatologist,
University Hospital,
Nottingham, UK

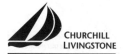

CHURCHILL
LIVINGSTONE

EDINBURGH LONDON NEW YORK PHILADELPHIA
ST LOUIS SYDNEY TORONTO 2000

CHURCHILL LIVINGSTONE
An imprint of Harcourt Publishers Limited

© Harcourt Publishers Limited 2000

 is a registered trademark of Harcourt Publishers Limited

The right of Terrence Stephenson, Neil Marlow, Sara Watkin and
Judith Grant to be identified as authors of this work has been
asserted by them in accordance with the Copyright, Designs and
Patents Act 1988

First published 2000

ISBN 0443 04992 0

British Library Cataloguing in Publication Data
A catalogue record for this book is availble from the British
Library

Library of Congress Cataloging in Publication Data
A catalog record for this book is available from the Library of
Congress

Note
Medical knowledge is constantly changing. As new information
becomes available, changes in treatment, procedures, equipment
and the use of drugs become necessary. The authors and the
publishers have, as far as it is possible, taken care to ensure that
the information given in this text is accurate and up to date.
However, readers are strongly advised to confirm that the
information, especially with regard to drug usage, complies with
the latest legislation and standards of practice.

The
publisher's
policy is to use
**paper manufactured
from sustainable forests**

Printed in China
EPC/01

Preface

Against the success story of perinatal medicine must be set the ever increasing complexity of neonatal intensive care, which is one reason for this book. There are many handbooks of neonatal medicine which are intended to be carried in the coat pocket for ready reference in an emergency. The reality is that no manual currently published fits easily into the pocket. We hope that Pocket Neonatology will fill both the gap in the market and the gap in your pocket. We have tried very hard to place ourselves in the position of the resident on the neonatal unit who requires rapid access to plain information in various emergency and difficult or uncommon management situations. Inevitably, therefore, this pocket book is rather didactic and we would not wish to suggest that the management recommended in this book for a particular problem is the only or even the perfect way to treat that problem, more that this is one way of dealing with this problem which has been tried and tested in the hospitals where we have worked.

Neonatal intensive care is an area of medicine which is changing rapidly and consequently books rapidly become out of date. However, most of these changes relate to the fine tuning of ventilation, the introduction of new modalities such as extra-corporeal membrane oxygenation and nitric oxide, and small adjustments to management policies, for example to parenteral nutrition and the treatment of hypoglycaemia. Fundamental changes in the way newborn infants are managed are unlikely to happen over the next few years and therefore this book will continue to guide practice into the millennium.

Most neonatal units will have developed their own management policies and you may be given these at the start of your post in the form of a handbook. Unfortunately, too often the impression is created that neonatology is some kind of glorifed cookery and there is a recipe for every problem which, if followed to the letter, will result in a happy outcome. Nothing could be further from the truth. Neonatology is firmly rooted as a branch of paediatrics and history and examination are vital before you reach for the nearest recipe book. Part of the excitement of neonatology is that it involves a combination of acute emergencies, requiring rapid decision making and intervention, and long-term follow-up for the 10% or so of infants who have major congenital abnormalities or major handicap. Neonatology is one of the few branches or medicine in which you can continue to be involved in the management of every system (there are very few neonatal cardiologists or neonatal gastro-enterologists - yet!) although you should never hesitate to seek help from anyone who might have more specialist knowledge than you. There are exciting overlaps with antenatal diagnostic techniques and obstetric management and again radiologists, obstetricians and surgeons may be very helpful sources of advice and information.

Finally, whilst there are many other textbooks available, Pocket Neonatology has been written as a 'stand-alone' reference and all the information you need to manage common neonatal problems should be within this book. If you cannot find the answer here, call your consultant.

2000

T.S.
N.M.
S.W.
J.G.

Acknowledgements

We would like to thank the following individuals for their help in preparing this book:

- Philip Baker, Professor of Obstetrics and Gynaecology, University of Nottingham
- Tanya Behrendt, Pharmacist, University Hospital, Nottingham
- Sarah Charlesworth, Senior Pharmacist - Production, Nottingham City Hospital, Nottingham
- Kathy Dilks, Medical Secretary, Children's Directorate, University Hospital, Nottingham
- David James, Professor of Feto-Maternal Medicine, University of Nottingham
- Chris Jarvis, Senior Paediatric Dietitian, Nottingham City Hospital, Nottingham
- Derek Johnston, Consultant Paediatrician, University Hospital, Nottingham
- Eve Knight-Jones, Consultant in Development Paediatrics and Childhood Disability, Nottingham City Hospital, Nottingham.
- Clive Newman, Senior Pharmacist – Paediatrics, University Hospital, Nottingham
- Nick Rutter, Professor of Neonatal Medicine, University of Nottingham
- Julie Stammers, Business Manager, Children's Directorate, University Hospital, Nottingham
- Jean Wardell, Chief Biochemist, Nottingham Hospital, Nottingham
- Gill Wilson and Sue Waring, Divisional Secretaries, Academic Division of Child Health, University of Nottingham

Disclaimer

All management recommended in this pocketbook is believed to be appropriate at the time of going to press. Neither the authors nor the publisher can accept legal responsibility or liability for any errors or omissions that may be made. Most of the drug doses suggested have been used in our neonatal units for over twenty years. The doses have been carefully checked but it is possible that errors have been missed. We recommend that the reader consults the printed instruction issued by manufacturers before administering any drug, especially one with which you are not familiar.

Contents

Abbreviations

αFP	alpha-fetoprotein
ABG	arterial blood gas
ACTH	adrenocorticortrophic hormone
AIDS	acquired immune deficiency syndrome
ALP	alkaline phosphatase
ANNP	advanced neonatal nurse practitioner
Anti-HBe	antibody to hepatitis B e antigen
Anti-HBs	antibody to hepatitis B surface antigen
APTT	activated partial thromboplastin time
AS	aortic stenosis
ASD	atrial septal defect
ATP	alloimmune thrombocytopenia
AVSD	atrial ventricular septal defect
AXR	abdominal X-ray
BCG	bacillus Calmette-Guèrin vaccine
b.d.	twice daily
BE	base excess
BG	blood glucose
BMFs	breast milk fortifiers
BP	blood pressure
BPA	British Paediatric Association (now Royal College of Paediatrics & Child Health)
BPD	bronchopulmonary dysplasia
bpm	beats per minute
Ca^{2+}	calcium
CAH	congenital adrenal hyperplasia
CAM	cystic adenomatous malformation
CBF	cerebral blood flow
CF	cystic fibrosis
CHD	congenital heart disease
Cl^-	chloride
CLD	chronic lung disease
COMV	continuous mandatory ventilation
CMV	cytomegalovirus
CNEP	continuous negative extrathoracic pressure
CNS	central nervous system
CoA	coarctation of the aorta
CPAP	continuous positive airway pressure

CRP	C-reactive protein
CSF	cerebrospinal fluid
CT	computerised tomography
CTG	cardiotocograph
CVP	central venous pressure
CVS	chorionic villous sampling
CXR	chest X-ray
DC	direct current
DCT	direct Coombs' test
DIC	disseminated intravascular coagulation
D-J	duodenal jejunal
DMSA	dimercaptosuccinic acid
DNA	deoxyribose nucleic acid
DoH	Department of Health
DPT	diphtheria, pertussis and tetanus vaccine
DTPA	diethylene-triamine-pentacetic acid
EBM	expressed breast milk
ECG	electrocardiogram
ECM	external cardiac massage
ECMO	extracorporeal membrane oxygenation
EDD	expected date of delivery
EEG	electroencephalogram
EFA	essential fatty acid
ELBW	extremely low birthweight
EM	electron microscopy
ET	endotracheal
ETT	endotracheal tube
FBC	full blood count
FDPs	fibrin degradation products
FFP	fresh frozen plasma
F_iO_2	fractional inspired oxygen concentration
FISH	fluorescent in situ hybridisation
FHR	fetal heart rate
FRC	functional residual capacity
FSH	follicle-stimulating hormone
FTA	fluorescent *Treponema* antibody
GBS	group B *Streptococcus*
GFR	Glomerular filtration rate
GH	growth hormone
GI	gastrointestinal
GOR	gastro-oesophageal reflux
GSD	glycogen storage disease
GTN	glyceryl trinitrate
GU	genitourinary
HAS	human albumin solution
Hb	haemoglobin
HBeAg	hepatitis B e (core) antigen
HbF	fetal haemoglobin
HBsAg	hepatitis B surface antigen

HBV	hepatitis B virus
HCG	human chorionic gonadotrophin
HCO$_3$	bicarbonate
Hct	haematocrit
HFOV	high-frequency oscillatory ventilation
Hib	*Haemophilus influenzae* type B
HIDA	hepatic iminodiactic acid
HIV	human immunodeficiency virus
HNIG	human normal immunoglobulin
HOCM	hypertrophic occlusive cardiomyopathy
HR	heart rate
HSV	herpes simplex virus
HVA	homovanillic acid
HVS	high vaginal swab
IA	intra-arterial
IC	intracardiac
ICP	intracranial pressure
IDM	infant of a diabetic mother
IDDM	insulin dependent diabetes mellitus
IEM	inborn error of metabolism
Ig	immunoglobulin
IM	intramuscular
IMV	intermittent mandatory ventilation
INO	inhaled nitric oxide
IO	intraosseous
IPPV	intermittent positive pressure ventilation
IRT	immune reactive trypsin
ITP	immune thrombocytopenia
IUGR	intrauterine growth restriction
IUT	intrauterine transfusion
IV	intravenous
IVH	intraventricular haemorrhage
IVI	intravenous infusion
IVU	intravenous urography
K$^+$	Potassium
LBW	low birthweight
LCP	long-chain polyunsaturated fatty acid
LFTs	liver function tests
LGA	large for gestational age
LH	luteinising hormone
LP	lumbar puncture
LSE	left sternal edge
LV	left ventricle
LVH	left ventricular hypertrophy
MAG-3	mercapto-acetyl-triglycerine-3
MAP	mean airway pressure
MAS	meconium aspiration syndrome
MBD	metabolic bone disease
MCUG	micturating cystourethrography

MEF	minimal enteral feeding
μg	micrograms
mg	milligrams
Mg^{2+}	magnesium
MIF	Müllerian inhibitory factor
MPH	massive pulmonary haemorrhage
MRI	magnetic resonance imaging
Na^+	sodium
NaCl	sodium chloride
neb	nebulised
NEC	necrotising enterocolitis
ng	nanograms
NGT	nasogastric tube
NIC	neonatal intensive care
NICU	neonatal intensive care unit
NNU	neonatal unit
OFC	occipitofrontal circumference
P_aCO_2	partial arterial carbon dioxide tension
P_aO_2	partial arterial oxygen tension
PCV	packed cell volume
PCR	polymerase chain reaction
PDA	persistent ductus arteriosis
PEEP	peak end-expiratory pressure
PFC	persistent fetal circulation
PIH	prolactin-inhibiting hormone
PIP	peak inspiratory pressure
PKU	phenylketonuria
PO_4^{2+}	phosphate
PO	orally
PPHN	persistent pulmonary hypertension of the newborn
ppm	parts per million
PR	per rectum
PROM	preterm rupture of membranes
PS	pulmonary stenosis
PT	prothrombin time
PTH	parathormone
PTT	partial thromboplastin time
PTV	patient-triggered ventilation
PUJ	pelviureteric junction
PVH	periventricular haemorrhage
PVL	periventricular leucomalacia
q.d.s.	four times per day
RBC	red blood cell
RDS	respiratory distress syndrome
ROP	retinopathy of prematurity
RTA	renal tubular acidosis
RVH	right ventricular hypertrophy
SBR	serum bilirubin
SGA	small for gestational age

SHO	senior house officer
SIDS	sudden infant death syndrome
SIMV	synchronised IMV
SIPPV	synchronised IPPV
SLE	systemic lupus erythematosus
SPA	suprapubic aspiration
SVT	supraventricular tachycardia
T_4	thyroxine
TAPVD	total anomalous pulmonary venous drainage
TB	tuberculosis
T_cO_2	transcutaneous oxygen tension
t.d.s.	three times per day
TF	tetralogy of Fallot
TGA	transpostion of the great arteries
Ti	inspiratory time
TOF	tracheo-oesophageal fistula
TORCH	toxoplasmosis, rubella, cytomegalovirus, herpes + hepatitis B
TPN	total parenteral nutrition
TRH	thyroid-releasing hormone
TSH	thyroid-stimulating hormone
TT	thrombin time
TTN	transient tachpnoea of the newborn
UAC	umbilical artery catheter
UDPTG	uridyl diphosphate glucuronyl transferase
USS	ultrasound scan
UTI	urinary tract infection
UVC	umbilical venous catheter
VACTERL	syndrome with vertebral, anal, cardiac, tracheo-oesophageal, renal, limb defects
VDRL	Venereal Disease Reference Laboratory
VI	ventricular index
VLBW	very low birth weight
VMA	vanillylmandelic acid
VSD	ventricular septal defect
VUJ	vesicoureteric junction
VUR	vesicoureteric reflux
VZV	varicella zoster virus
WBC	white blood cell
WCC	white cell count
WPWS	Wolf–Parkinson–White syndrome
ZIG	zoster immune globulin

ONE

Perinatal care

Introduction

Perinatal care is one of the success stories of modern medicine. Since the 1960s, neonatal mortality in the UK has fallen from around 15 per 1000 live births to the present rate of around 7 per 1000. Early neonatal mortality (deaths in the first week) has fallen dramatically alongside downward trends in other measures of infant mortality (Fig. 1.1). Much of this can be attributed to better obstetric care and maternal health, but for those born very prematurely or who become ill after birth, neonatal intensive care appears to be responsible. Indeed, if lethal congenital malformations are removed from the figures, corrected neonatal mortality may be as low as 2 per 1000 live births, as is demonstrated in our local perinatal mortality data (Table 1.1).

Table 1.1 Nottingham Neonatal Service – perinatal mortality rates 1993–7

	1993	1994	1995	1996	1997
Total births	10 339	10 057	9722	9731	9606
Stillbirth rate (per 1000 total births)	6.3	5.4	6.0	4.4	4.9
Perinatal mortality rate[a] (per 1000 total births)	9.9	10.4	9.3	8.4	7.6
Perinatal mortality rate (per 1000 total births) (excluding antenatal transfers)	9.1	9.5	8.8	7.6	7.0
Neonatal mortality rate[b] (per 1000 live births)	4.7	6.1	4.3	4.2	3.4
Neonatal mortality rate (per 1000 live births) (excluding antenatal transfers and lethal malformations)	3.0	3.6	2.3	2.4	2.2

[a]Stillbirths plus neonatal deaths in the first week.
[b]Deaths among live births before 28 days of age.

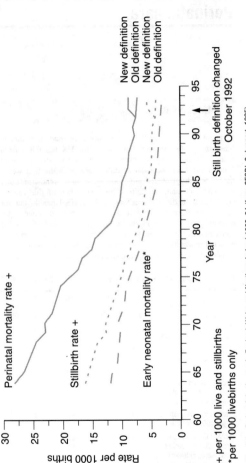

Fig. 1.1 Perinatal death rates in England, Wales and Northern Ireland 1960–94 (from CESDI, 3rd report, 1995).

Consideration of birthweight or gestational age-specific neonatal mortality, however, reveals that mortality for the very small premature survivor remains relatively high. Most data are based upon the number of admissions to a neonatal unit (Fig. 1.2), but this significantly overestimates survival for live births at very low gestations (Fig. 1.3). In addition, very low birthweight (<1501 g) or very preterm babies are at greater risk of developing later disability, primarily from cerebral palsy, perinatally acquired hearing loss, blindness and learning difficulties. For babies born before 26 weeks gestation, the prevalence of major disabling conditions may be as high as 1 in 3 survivors, falling to much lower levels as gestational age advances (Fig. 1.4). Despite this, most very premature and very low birthweight children are free of disability. In Nottingham, we have seen a rise in the number of surviving very tiny babies over the last 15 years, with significant reduction in the rates of disability for this vulnerable group (Fig. 1.5).

The pattern of perinatal illness is changing. For the very preterm baby, simple measures, such as the administration of antenatal steroids to the mother, act to reduce the burden of respiratory illness. Better fetal assessment allows delivery of the hypoxic growth-restricted baby in good condition. Antenatal

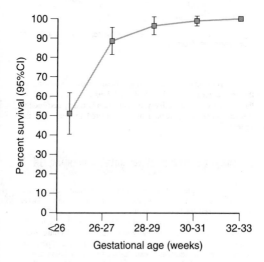

Fig. 1.2 Percentage survival (95% Confidence interval) for babies cared for by the Nottingham Neonatal Service, 1995–97.

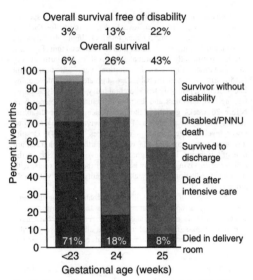

Fig. 1.3   Survival for live births < 26 weeks gestation in the UK and Eire, 1995 (source: the EPICure study 1999).

diagnosis of many malformations means that the option of therapeutic termination for lethal conditions is available, and for those that progress to delivery, the condition is anticipated and the medical team and parents may be prepared to deal with the neonatal consequences.

The organisation of perinatal care in the UK

The UK is unique in that most neonatal intensive care (NIC) occurs at district general hospitals, and not solely in the larger tertiary referral (or 'level 3') units.

Neonatal intensive care developed through the 1970s, usually dependent upon local need and without strategic planning. Most major conurbations will have large neonatal units within perinatal centres where, in addition to care for the local population, the at-risk mother and baby can receive specialist care. Many of these centres have an obstetric fetal medicine specialist to whom women

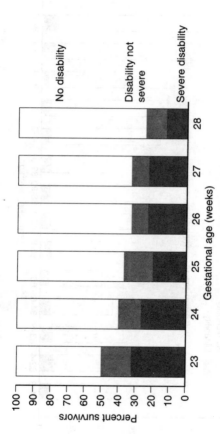

No disability

Disability not severe

Severe disability

Gestational age (weeks)

Percent survivors

Fig. 1.4 Disability rates in very preterm babies (data from published hospital-based reports, 1990–95).

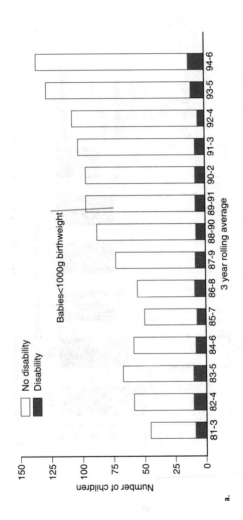

a.

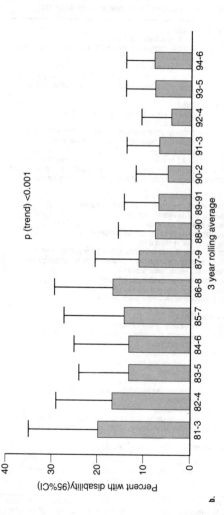

Fig. 1.5 Rates of disability at 18 months of age in Nottingham Neonatal Service graduates of less than 1000 g birthweight, 1980–97 (source: Dr Knight Jones, Nottingham Passport to Health Scheme).

Table 1.2   Clinical categories of neonatal care (BAPM/NNA 1991)

Level 1 Intensive care
Intensive care should be provided for babies:
- Receiving assisted ventilation (including IPPV, IMV and CPAP) and in the first 24 h after its withdrawal
- Of less than 27 weeks gestation for the first 48 h after birth
- With a birthweight of less than 1000 g for the first 48 h after birth
- Who require major emergency surgery — for the preoperative period and postoperatively for 48 h
- On the day of death
- Being transported by a team including medical and nursing staff
- Who require peritoneal dialysis
- Who require exchange transfusions complicated by other disease processes
- With severe respiratory disease in the first 48 h of life requiring $F_iO_2 > 0.6$
- With recurrent apnoea needing frequent intervention, e.g. over five stimulations in 8 h or resuscitation with IPPV two or more times in 24 h
- With significant requirements for circulatory support, e.g. inotropes, three or more infusions of colloid in 24 h, or infusions of prostaglandins

Level 2 High-dependency care
High-dependency care should be provided for babies:
- Requiring total parenteral nutrition
- Who are having convulsions
- Being transported by skilled neonatal nurses alone
- With arterial line or chest drain
- With respiratory disease in the first 48 h of life requiring F_iO_2 of 0.4–0.6
- With recurrent apnoea requiring stimulation up to five times in an 8-h period, or any resuscitation with IPPV
- Who require an exchange transfusion alone
- Who are postoperative and require complex nursing procedures
- With tracheostomy — for the first 2 weeks

Level 3 Special care
Special care should be provided for babies:
- Requiring continuous monitoring of respiration or heart rate, or by transcutaneous transducers
- Receiving additional oxygen
- Being given IV glucose and electrolyte solutions
- Who are being tube-fed
- Who have had minor surgery in the previous 24 h
- Who require terminal care but not on the day of death
- Being barrier-nursed
- Undergoing phototherapy
- Receiving special monitoring (e.g. frequent glucose or bilirubin estimations)
- Needing constant supervision (e.g. babies whose mothers are drug addicts)
- Being treated with antibiotics
- With tracheostomy after the first 2 weeks

Level 4 Normal care
This is usually given by the infant's mother unless the infant has been abandoned or has been placed for adoption.

NB. The term 'transitional care' is sometimes used; within the UK this usually refers to babies with special care needs who are nursed on a postnatal ward with their mother providing most of their care.

may be referred for assessment when there are concerns about fetal anomaly or fetal health and growth (see Ch. 2). Neonatal surgery should only be provided from within a specialist unit.

Smaller centres will provide NIC for their local population and refer more complex cases into these tertiary units. Many units do not offer ongoing NIC but aim to transfer out all high-risk mothers and to stabilise, prior to transfer, sick babies who are born before such transfer can be effected.

Most importantly, babies should be assured of getting the highest quality of NIC, wherever they are cared for. With this aim, the British Association of Perinatal Medicine has defined professional standards for such units (*Standards for Hospitals providing Neonatal Intensive Care*; BAPM, London, 1996). This important publication has been based upon evidence wherever possible, and best professional agreement where not. Because many neonatal units undertake a range of care options from full intensive to special care, these have been defined as follows: level 1, maximal intensive care; level 2, high-dependency intensive care; and level 3, special care (Table 1.2). The nursing establishment of a neonatal unit may be calculated using the formula '1 nurse/shift per 2 intensive care babies or per 4 special care babies', figures which are based upon workload studies and which therefore have validity. The BPAM/NNA levels of care may be used for monitoring unit workload and for commissioning.

The perinatal team

Perinatal care crosses conventional medical disciplines, including midwifery, obstetrics, anaesthetics, radiology, paediatric surgery, neonatology and neonatal nursing. Critical to the functioning of a maternity service is clear communication between these professionals. This applies at all levels and acts to the benefit of both mother and child. Most importantly, the process of delivery is associated with a handing over of care from obstetrician/midwife to neonatal staff. Clear communication of maternal problems and treatments given is important in planning care for the child. Similarly, keeping postnatal ward staff up to date with events in the neonatal unit is equally important. Most good maternity services have established forums for such communication in order to enhance the informal 'hand over' that occurs. Neonatal staff are an essential part of this team and should contribute to this interchange. Increasingly, many of the conventional roles of the junior neonatal medical staff are being supported by nurse practitioners. As permanent members of staff, these individuals have equal responsibility for such teamwork and provide a valuable resource to support training in delivery room and neonatal care.

TWO

Obstetric care

The assessment of the newborn infant demands an understanding of the impact that antenatal events, the results of fetal assessment and perinatal management may have on the fetus and baby. In this chapter we present an outline of antenatal care. For more detail, the reader is advised to consult more specialist texts (see p. 22). Evidence-based perinatal care has been well reviewed in the Cochrane Collaboration, which is found in most medical libraries in either paper or electronic form.

Antenatal care

At booking, women are offered various screening tests for chromosomal anomaly. Biochemical tests are used to infer a risk of abnormality. Chromosomal abnormalities (Ch. 4) can be confirmed with a fetal karyotype, using CVS, amniocentesis or direct fetal blood sampling. These procedures themselves carry a risk of fetal loss and the parents must decide between the risks.

Most women have a fetal anomaly scan at 18–20 weeks gestation, and most have had a dating scan at an earlier point. At best, early assessments are accurate to within ±7 days, but later scans (> 20 weeks) are less accurate and may differ from dates by up to 14 days.

Fetal anomaly

Where fetal anomaly is suspected on a screening examination, a formal assessment, usually by a specialist radiologist or obstetrician, is performed to confirm the presence of abnormality and ensure that no others are present. This assessment will be followed by counselling from the appropriate specialists, which may include a neonatologist, and a plan may be made for the pregnancy and delivery. Despite the involvement of other specialists, it is important to remember that the obstetrician has overall responsibility for the care of both the woman and the fetus until delivery, as other issues, unrelated to the anomaly, may complicate the pregnancy.

- It is important to appreciate that the prognosis for fetuses with serious malformations may not be the same as that determined after birth and information should be sought that is appropriate to your counselling.

Generally, where a baby is to be born with an abnormality, the neonatal (and surgical) team should be aware of the management plan. Where intensive care is likely to be required immediately after birth, delivery should be in a perinatal centre with appropriate (e.g. surgical) facilities. For some women, induction of delivery may not be strictly necessary for that anomaly but, because of the distance to the tertiary unit, induction near term may be undertaken to avoid delivery at the base hospital.

Rhesus haemolytic disease (see Ch. 9)

Oligohydramnios

This is defined as a reduction in amniotic fluid volume, usually measured on USS as part of a semi-quantitative assessment of deepest vertical pool < 3 cm or an amniotic fluid index (AFI) < 5th percentile for GA. Secondary effects of this may be pulmonary hypoplasia and deformation of the limbs (e.g. talipes) and sometimes the face ('Potter's facies'). Most commonly, oligohydramnios follows premature, pre-labour rupture of membranes or IUGR. It also may occur in postmature fetuses. Fetal causes of poor fetal urine output are:

- renal agenesis
- renal dysplasia (usually bilateral if there is oligohydramnios)
- polycystic kidneys
- ureteral or urethral obstruction

A diagnostic amnioinfusion may be helpful in defining fetal anomaly. By the time such fetal anomalies present with reduced liquor volume, renal function (and hence the prognosis) is poor. This relates to both the renal prognosis and the prognosis for survival, which is also impaired because of pulmonary hypoplasia. Occasionally in the presence of an identified obstructive lesion, developing oligohydramnios may be observed. Intrauterine shunting of urine past such obstruction using a 'pig-tail' catheter is possible and may result in preservation of renal and pulmonary function. Such successful cases are rare. Pulmonary hypoplasia is a particular risk if oligohydramnios is present in the middle trimester. Other therapeutic interventions have not been demonstrated to benefit prognosis.

Postnatal renal tract imaging, following careful clinical assessment, is an important part of the neonatal management.

Polyhydramnios

This is defined as an excessive amniotic fluid volume, usually as part of a semi-quantitative assessment of deepest vertical pool ≥ 8 cm or an AFI > 95th percentile for GA. Polyhydramnios occurs most commonly with maternal diabetes mellitus, but a cause is rarely found. *Fetal causes* of polyhydramnios include:

- Obstruction of the passage of fluid through the GI tract:
  - intestinal atresias (oesophageal, duodenal, more common with proximal lesions)
  - oesophageal compression (diaphragmatic hernia, mediastinal masses)
  - choanal atresia.
- Neurological impairment of swallowing:
  - karyotype anomalies (trisomies)
  - neuromuscular lesions (myotonic dystrophy, spinal muscular atrophy, muscular dystrophy)
  - CNS lesions (anencephaly).
- Fetal polyuria:
  - twin–twin transfusion
  - congenital nephrotic syndrome.
- Cardiac failure (usually high output)
  - severe anaemia
  - vascular malformation (AV malformation, sacrococcygeal tumour)
  - chorioangioma.
- Intrauterine infection
  - CMV, syphilis.

The most important issue in antenatal management is the identification of the cause by USS and special investigations. Early delivery is not uncommon, secondary to rupture of the membranes or premature labour. Hence, therapeutic options have been tried. Maternal indomethacin (to reduce fetal urine production) and amnioreduction are the two most popular interventions. For twin–twin transfusion, some success is claimed for laser ablation of placental communicating vessels.

Postnatal assessment of the baby must include a careful clinical examination (especially for dysmorphology and neurological abnormality) and a wide bore catheter should be passed into the stomach and acid secretions demonstrated before feeding to exclude oesophageal atresia.

Hydrops fetalis (see Ch. 14)

Assessment of fetal health

Over the past 10 years, major strides have been made in the assessment of fetal condition before birth. A combination of CTG, real time USS and Doppler evaluation of the umbilical and fetal blood flow velocities identifies children at risk of placental nutrient failure. Such babies are said to suffer intrauterine growth restriction (IUGR). Babies who are thought to be growing poorly are referred for assessment.

- It is important to realise that fetuses may be small for a variety of reasons, including placental nutrient failure, malformation, chromosome abnormalities and intrauterine infection. These latter abnormalities are more likely when the growth failure occurs in early pregnancy.

Formal obstetric assessment will include a fetal anomaly scan, fetal karyotype and maternal serology for CMV, *Toxoplasma gondii* and rubella. In a fetus with trisomy, the clinical picture may mimic that seen in hypertensive disease and fetal growth is impaired. The hypoxic fetus identified before about 28 weeks gestation may be at special perinatal risk, often seen with a reduction in head size as well as body measures, and may develop serious respiratory disease with a high mortality.

In the absence of other fetal anomaly, and the disappearance of umbilical artery diastolic flow velocities, measurement of abdominal circumference and assessment of biophysical profile have produced a system which, in randomised trials, has led to a reduction in neonatal mortality and neonatal encephalopathy. A reduction in diastolic velocities (sometimes confusingly referred to as a raised pulsatility index), followed by a reduction in abdominal circumference and a worsening of the biophysical profile (with reduction in fetal movements, reduction in liquor volume and CTG abnormalities), identifies a group at particular risk (see Table 2.1). These babies are becoming progressively more hypoxic and acidotic.

- Although mild growth restriction seems to be associated with improved neonatal outcome, babies who have a reduction in

Table 2.1   Biophysical profile scoring system

Parameter	Normal behaviour (scores '2')	Abnormal behaviour (scores '0')
Fetal breathing movements	>1 episode of 30 s duration, including intermittent hiccups	Repetitive or continuous breathing without stopping or Absent breathing movements
Gross body and limb movements	4+ discrete body movements in 30 min	< 4 body/limb movements
Fetal tone	Active extension with rapid return to flexion, brisk repositioning/trunk rotation Opening/closing of hand, kicks, etc.	Only low-velocity movements, incomplete return to flexion Abnormal fetal posture No fetal movements
Fetal CTG reactivity	> 2 significant accelerations associated with palpated movement in 20-min CTG	Movements and accelerations uncoupled Too few accelerations or decelerative trace
Amniotic fluid volume	1 pocket of > 3 cm without cord loops More than 1 pocket of > 2 cm Not subjectively reduced	No cord-free pocket of > 2 cm Subjectively reduced

their biophysical assessment (Table 2.1) may be considered to be effectively pre-terminal and have much worse outcomes — they may require resuscitation at birth and the beneficial effect of mild placental insufficiency, in the maturation of fetal systems before birth, is lost.

The clinical significance of more sophisticated measures of fetal blood flow, indicating redistribution of blood flow in the fetus (so called 'brain-sparing' as fetal blood is preferentially distributed to the head with an increase in cerebral blood vessel diastolic Doppler velocities and an increase in resistance to blood flow to other organs), is as yet undetermined.

The decision as to where on this path to deliver is a matter of judgement but, with good antenatal preparation, delivery may be timed to minimise neonatal morbidity from hypoxia at a time when the risk of neonatal morbidity from prematurity may be least (Table 2.2).

Neonatal staff should be present at delivery, which will often be by caesarean section to avoid exposing the sick fetus to the stress of labour.

Table 2.2 Outcome following perinatal hypoxia (adapted from James et al Am J Obstet Gynecol 1992)

	Normal (n=23)	Low AC (n=16)	Abnormal EDFV (n=7)	↓AC+↓EDFV (n=29)	↓AC+↓EDFV+↓BPP (n=28)
Survivors	100%	100%	100%	100%	75%
Neonatal illness	43%	31%	14%	62%	89%
Fetal death	–	–	–	–	7%
Neonatal death	–	–	–	–	18%
Mean GA (r) at delivery	37 (29–40)	38 (35–41)	38 (34–40)	36 (28–40)	32 (26–39)
RDS	9%	6%	–	28%	68%
Ventilation	9%	–	–	10%	29%
CLD	–	–	–	–	11%
Polycythaemia	4%	6%	–	14%	14%
Anaemia	–	–	–	–	11%
Low platelets	–	–	–	7%	11%
IVH	–	–	–	4%	11%
NEC	–	–	–	–	11%
Hypoglycaemia	9%	–	14%	17%	18%

AC, abdominal circumference; EDFV, end-diastolic flow velocities (Doppler); BPP; biophysical profile.

Pre-labour preterm rupture of the membranes (PPROM)

One of the commonest obstetric complications is PPROM. Most women will deliver within 24–48 h of this and traditionally there is thought to be a linear relationship between the duration of ruptured membranes and risk of chorioamnionitis and fetal infection. Some women, however, will remain out of labour without signs of infection for some time. Important aspects are:

- Where PPROM occurs before 24 weeks gestation, there is an increased risk of lung hypoplasia due to oligohydramnios; this should be anticipated at delivery.
- Women should be monitored for infection; high vaginal swabs may identify pathogens.
- There appears to be some benefit from antibiotics administered to mothers before birth (for neonatal implications, see Ch. 13).
- Despite weak evidence of benefit, antenatal steroids should be given and have not been associated with increased risk of infection.

Preterm labour

For many women, the first indication of preterm delivery is the onset of preterm labour. Trials of antibiotic prophylaxis are underway as infection has been implicated in the onset of premature labour. There may be a benefit in delaying labour for 24 h to allow antenatal steroids (see below) to have maximal effect, but trials of tocolysis have not been convincing in terms of fetal benefit and ß2-agonists in particular are associated with significant maternal risks.

Pre-eclampsia

Hypertensive disease is the commonest disorder of pregnancy (1–2% of pregnancies). Where hypertension is associated with proteinuria, it is part of the multisystem disease called pre-eclampsia and a common indication for early delivery. Two major groups are apparent:

- Women who present with fetal IUGR, where the major indications for delivery are fetal
- Women with pre-eclampsia or eclampsia where the major indications are maternal.

The spectrum of maternal illness is wide and encompasses eclampsia, HELLP (hypertension, elevated liver enzymes, low platelets), acute fatty liver and a variety of other multisystem disorders. Often these women are very ill and require intensive care themselves — a sick fetus may also be anticipated. Delivery in this scenario is indicated primarily to reverse the maternal disease process. Where possible, antenatal steroids will be given. The eclamptic or pre–eclamptic mother may have received large doses of medication which may cause depression of the baby at birth and for some time afterwards (e.g. alfentanil, diazepam). Make sure you are aware of these.

Other maternal illnesses

Many maternal conditions have implications for the fetus and careful history is essential. The major effects of some common conditions are described in Table 2.3.

Preparation for preterm birth

Prematurity is an infrequent obstetric event but it is responsible for 7 out of 8 neonatal deaths, which are mainly in the highest risk categories, below 30 weeks gestation. Alongside advances in obstetric care, the recognition that antenatal administration of corticosteroids to women expecting a very preterm birth may reduce mortality and morbidity has been the most important advance. Other antenatal interventions (e.g. TRH) have not been shown to confer additional benefit.

Two doses of 12 mg beta- or dexamethasone (12 h apart) produce measurable benefit for the newborn infant born between 12 h and 7 days later, producing a 40% reduction in mortality and similarly reduced rates and severity of respiratory distress syndrome, through the induction of lung surfactant and anti-oxidant production. The role of repeated courses of steroids is not as yet clear and results of randomised trials are awaited.

There are probably no contraindications to antenatal steroids, but caution is advised in the face of overt infection and diabetes, and steroids are likely to be less effective where lung maturation may occur through normal pathophysiological conditions (prolonged rupture of membranes, IUGR). Steroids appear to have a smaller but measurable effect if given as late as 6 h before delivery or in pregnancies earlier than 28 weeks gestation and should be given to all mothers in whom preterm delivery is anticipated. Target rates for steroid

Table 2.3 Effects of common maternal conditions on the fetus and newborn

Condition	Fetal/neonatal effect
Diabetes mellitus	Increased risk of congenital anomaly Fetal macrosomia — i.e. large-for-dates Increased perinatal mortality Range of neonatal problems (see Ch. 3)
Hypertensive disease	IUGR (see text) Effects of maternal drug treatment usually minimal and does not interfere with breast feeding — occasionally lowers neonatal BP and may cause hypoglycaemia. Associated with neonatal leucopenia and thrombocytopenia
Renal disease	As for hypertension Perinatal mortality raised in renal failure; usually good following successful transplant and immunosuppression
Cardiac disease	Mothers with cardiac disease usually have good prognosis but need intensive cardiovascular monitoring during delivery. May be on thromboprophylaxis (see below) Increased rate of heart problems in infants
Anticoagulant therapy	Heparin is preferred to warfarin during pregnancy, especially in the first trimester, when a dysmorphic syndrome (fetal warfarin syndrome), stillbirth and abortion may occur. There is a risk of fetal bleeding before birth during warfarin therapy
Hyperthyroidism	Neonatal thyrotoxicosis (from transplacental thyroid stimulating IgG) rare (see Ch. 11). Radioactive iodine contraindicated in pregnancy Drug treatment with carbimazole or propothiouracil may cross into breast milk in small amounts, but allow to feed and monitor neonatal TSH levels
Thrombocytopenia	May be due to: • *Immune thrombocytopenia* — even if the maternal platelet count is normal, this maternal antibody-mediated disease may present as neonatal thrombocytopenia. A history of maternal splenectomy worsens the prognosis (see Ch. 14) • *Alloimmune thrombocytopenia* — due to maternal-fetal platelet discordance for the PIA1 antigen. May cause intrapartum or antenatal fetal bleeding and is a more serious condition (see Ch. 14)
SLE	High fetal loss rate (antiphospholipin syndrome) Early delivery because of hypertensive/renal disease Anti-Ro antibody secretors may present with fetal bradycardia due to heart block (see Ch. 7)
Myasthenia gravis	Antibody-mediated neonatal myasthenia may present with neurological depression after birth, but presentation may be delayed for some time. Generally self-limiting (see Ch. 12)

administration are 70–80% of women delivering before 34 weeks gestation.

● Neonatal staff should ensure that obstetric staff give steroids to all women in this group.

Fetal health in labour

Continuous fetal monitoring is undertaken in at risk pregnancies. In low-risk situations intermittent monitoring using a Pinard stethoscope has not been shown to be worse than continuous. Fetal condition may be inferred from continuous CTG traces, scalp pH measurements and the presence of meconium (Table 2.4). It must be appreciated that, profound prolonged terminal bradycardia apart, very few of the abnormalities described have even a reasonable predictive value for neonatal problems.

Table 2.4 Monitoring for fetal distress

I — Interpretation of the fetal heart rate in the 1st stage of labour (i.e. from onset of labour to full cervical dilatation)

Pattern	Description	Action
Normal	FHR 120-160 bpm; no significant change in FHR during contractions Baseline variability ('beat to beat variability') >5 bpm	None
Acceleration pattern	FHR increases at start of contraction, returning to baseline during or at the end of the contraction; normal pattern	None
Loss of baseline variability	Baseline variability <5 bpm ('flat trace'); commonly indicates fetal hypoxia	Check fetal pH
Baseline bradycardia	FHR <120 bpm; abnormal only if accompanied by loss of baseline variability ± decelerations	Turn patient on her side; check fetal pH
Baseline tachycardia	FHR >160 bpm; abnormal only if persistent or accompanied by loss of baseline variability ± decelerations	
Early deceleration (type 1 dip)	Deceleration begins with the onset of contraction; returns to baseline by the end of contraction (dips by >15 bpm for >15 s) Deceleration is usually <40 bpm; it may be due to head compression or may be an early sign of hypoxia	None

Table 2.4 *cont'd*

Later deceleration (type 2 dip)	Deceleration with the lowest point beyond the peak of the contraction; the later the deceleration, the more serious its significance, especially if accompanied by loss of baseline variability ± tachycardia	Check fetal pH immediately
Variable deceleration	Deceleration of irregular shape and large amplitude (>50 bpm) appearing at a variable time during the contraction; if this occurs with each contraction, it suggests developing fetal hypoxia	Check fetal pH
Normal uterine contractions	3–4 contractions every 10 min; duration <75 s (uterine catheter: baseline 5–12 mmHg, peak 30–60 mmHg)	None

II — Interpretation of fetal blood pH from scalp or buttock samples

pH	Interpretation	Action
> 7.3	Normal	None needed (provided there is no other evidence of fetal distress. Infants, particularly those small-for-dates, may be hypoxic in the absence of significant fetal acidosis)
7.25–7.29	Borderline	Repeat in 1 hour or if CTG is abnormal
7.20–7.24	Abnormal	Expedite delivery (consider caesarean section or forceps delivery)
<7.2	Very abnormal	Immediate delivery

III — Meconium stained liquor

This is neither sensitive nor specific for fetal distress. Approximately 50% of term infants with meconium stained liquor will have other evidence of fetal distress or require some resuscitation at delivery, but 50% will need no assistance whatsoever. Meconium staining is very rarely seen in preterm deliveries.

Perinatal hypoxia

The terms fetal, birth or perinatal asphyxia are poorly defined and should not be used. Many babies are erroneously classified as having suffered 'asphyxia' when in fact they turn out to have a variety of conditions, such as major malformations, intracranial haemorrhage, perinatal infection and chromosomal disorders. It is wise for neonatal staff not to prejudge aetiology, as this may close their minds to other aetiologies besides causing distress to parents and obstetric staff. Antepartum factors are thought to play a major part in 70% of neonatal encephalopathies.

Acute intrapartum hypoxia can occur in:

- cord accidents (prolapsed umbilical cord)
- antepartum haemorrhage (placenta praevia, placental abruption)
- sudden onset of bradycardia during labour — often idiopathic.

Less acute hypoxia may occur in a variety of situations, often in the presence of risk factors such as IUGR, and this is reflected in changes in the CTG pattern, fetal scalp pH or the passage of meconium (Table 2.4), although none are good predictors of outcome by themselves.

Prompt resuscitation should be available for all babies in whom acute or subacute intrapartum hypoxia is anticipated. Condition at birth is a poor predictor of outcome, except at extremes of state, and good early neonatal care is mandatory. Even taking the extreme case of the unexpected apparent stillbirth, although mortality is high at 40%, more than 50% long term survivors are free of severe disability.

In utero transfer

Most authorities agree that transfer to a perinatal centre for delivery is the ideal situation when resources at the base hospital are inadequate to provide ongoing care for the baby. In utero transfer is, however, not always optimal and neither the mother nor her fetus should be put at risk by the rush to transfer for delivery. Situations in which transfer is undesirable include:

- Where there is a risk to the woman's life (e.g. severe pre-eclampsia where there is a risk of eclampsia)
- Where either woman or fetus is placed at risk (e.g. antepartum haemorrhage which poses threat to mother and child)
- Scenarios where the fetus may deliver en route (established preterm labour) — it is *never* necessary for neonatal staff to accompany an in utero transfer, which places mother, fetus and the neonatal team at risk.

In utero transfer must be discussed with the obstetric and neonatal teams at the receiving hospital as there are issues relating to the woman's care and to the baby's potential care that should be discussed. The scenario should also be agreed with the woman and her partner and back transfer accepted without delay once the need for the transfer is resolved.

For audit purposes, hospitals must keep a record of those situations where requests for transfer are declined and the reasons for doing so.

The old fashioned obstetric 'flying squad' system has now been abandoned. Paramedic teams can attend emergencies much faster and undertake transfer to a suitable obstetric centre more quickly than a hospital based team.

FURTHER REFERENCE

James DK, Steer PJ, Weiner CP, Gonik B. High risk pregnancy – management options. 2nd edn. London: WB Saunders; 1999.

Cochrane Pregnancy and Childbirth Group. Cochrane Database of Systematic Reviews. Issue 4. Oxford: Update Software; 1999.

THREE

Early care

Resuscitation of the newborn

PHYSIOLOGY OF RESUSCITATION

In response to the physiological hypoxia which occurs when the umbilical cord is clamped or obstructed, a healthy term baby usually takes the first breath within 60 s. Respiratory efforts are also provoked by physical stimuli such as the release of the chest wall as it is delivered and the change in environmental temperature. The first breath generates a negative pressure of -40 to -100 cmH$_2$O (10–15 times larger than subsequent breaths) to overcome:

- surface tension of collapsed alveoli
- viscosity of fluid filled lungs
- elastic recoil and compliance of lungs and chest wall.

Once a functional residual capacity is achieved, tidal breathing begins — usually within 90 s.

Surfactant reduces surface tension within the alveoli, preventing collapse at end-expiration, thus reducing the work of breathing. Its production is reduced by acidosis (pH < 7.25), hypoxia and hypothermia (< 35°C).

The transition from fetal to neonatal circulation is described in Chapter 7.

RESPONSE OF THE FETUS/NEWBORN INFANT TO HYPOXIA

In response to hypoxia, there may be an initial transient increase in breathing rate and heart rate. Subsequently apnoea, gasping and bradycardia occur, followed by apnoea and asystole (Fig. 3.1).

Additionally, hypoxia in the term infant causes relaxation of the anal sphincters, gut peristalsis and the passage of meconium in utero. The infant is at risk of aspirating meconium in utero if gasping respirations have taken place or with the onset of

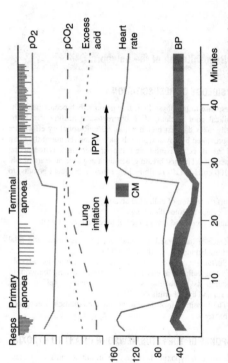

Fig. 3.1 Physiological changes during acute hypoxia and resuscitation. (Reproduced with permission from *Principles of Resuscitation at Birth*, 6th edn, Northern Neonatal Network.)

respiration following delivery. Meconium may block terminal bronchi causing alveolar collapse or act as a ball valve and cause alveolar overdistension.

INFANTS REQUIRING RESUSCITATION AT BIRTH/ATTENDANCE AT DELIVERY (see also Ch. 2)

Two-thirds of all babies requiring resuscitation at birth will have one or more risk factors (Table 3.1). A member of the neonatal team trained and experienced in advanced resuscitation of the newborn, including ET intubation, must be present at every delivery where fetal compromise is anticipated. Where major resuscitation is anticipated (congenital anomaly, severe hypoxia, extreme prematurity), a middle grade or consultant neonatologist should also be present. For multiple births < 33 weeks there should be one individual trained in advanced neonatal resuscitation per baby.

Up to one-third of babies needing support will have no risk factors for resuscitation. It is therefore essential that one person in attendance at every delivery is able to perform adequate basic neonatal resuscitation, including bag and mask ventilation.

The obstetric or midwifery staff are responsible for calling neonatal staff, but good neonatal staff will be aware of potential problems and have made contingency arrangements. When you are on call for the delivery suite, make sure you are in regular contact.

Table 3.2 lists a number of conditions which the neonatal SHO or ANNP should be aware of, but not necessarily requiring attendance at the delivery.

Table 3.1 Those deliveries which a neonatal SHO or ANNP should always attend

- Fetal distress (as assessed by the obstetrician/midwife, e.g. pathological CTG, pH on FBS < 7.2)
- Meconium staining of the liquor
- Emergency caesarean section
- Elective caesarean section under general anaesthesia or for placenta praevia, multiple births or where admission to the neonatal unit is likely
- Vaginal breech delivery
- Multiple pregnancy
- Rotational forceps (i.e. Kielland's forceps) delivery
- Preterm delivery at less than 34 weeks gestation
- Severe intrauterine growth restriction
- Maternal insulin-dependent diabetes
- Maternal myasthenia gravis
- Known serious fetal abnormality, e.g. diaphragmatic hernia, hydrops fetalis
- Severe rhesus disease likely to require neonatal intensive care

Table 3.2   Conditions which a neonatal SHO or ANNP should be informed of (but not necessarily requiring attendance at the delivery)

- Low birthweight infants (<2500 g)
- Preterm infants (< 37 weeks)
- Prolonged rupture of membranes (>48 h), offensive purulent liquor or maternal pyrexia (see Ch. 13)
- Babies born to mothers colonised with group B *Streptococcus*
- Congenital abnormalities — consideration must be given to admitting babies with serious abnormalities to the neonatal unit. Minor abnormalities, e.g. talipes, do not require a paediatrician at delivery but the infant should be checked for other abnormalities
- Polyhydramnios — a large-bore NG tube should be passed and an acid reaction obtained to exclude the diagnosis of oesophageal atresia
- Siblings of previous abnormal infant or perinatal death
- Any illness in the mother which may cause problems in the baby, e.g. idiopathic thrombocytopenic purpura, hyperparathyroidism, thyrotoxicosis
- History of maternal opiate abuse
- Maternal hepatitis B carriage (see Ch. 13)

EQUIPMENT REQUIRED FOR RESUSCITATION

- Resuscitation surface with:
  - overhead radiant heat source
  - oxygen/air supply with variable regulated flow rate and adjustable pressure relief valve
  - stop clock
- Warm towels
- Gloves
- Neonatal stethoscope
- Y-piece or 500 mL self-inflating resuscitation bag with reservoir bag available if required
- Face masks size 0, 1 and 2
- Straight-bladed laryngoscopes × 2
- ETTs — 2.5 mm × 2; 3.0 mm × 2; 3.5 mm × 2
- ETT connectors
- ETT introducers if required
- Magill's forceps if infants to be nasally intubated
- Suction catheters — FG6 × 5; FG8 × 5; FG10 × 5
- NG tubes — FG6 × 2; FG8 × 2
- UVC pack or equipment:
  - UVCs: FG5 or 6 × 2
  - linen ligature
  - scalpel blade
  - three-way tap
  - artery forceps × 2
  - fine artery dilator × 1
  - suture
- IV cannulae — 22FG × 3; 24FG × 3

- IV butterfly needles — 21FG × 2; 23FG × 2; 25FG × 2
- IV needles — 21FG × 3; 23FG × 3; 25FG × 3
- IO needle — 18FG × 1 (optional)
- Syringes — 1 mL × 2; 2 mL × 2; 5 mL × 2; 10 mL × 2
- Alcohol swabs
- Resuscitation drugs box containing:
  — 10 mL of 1:10 000 epinephrine (adrenaline)
  — 20 mL of 0.9% saline
  — 20 mL of 4.2% sodium bicarbonate
  — 4 mL of neonatal naloxone (20 µg/mL) or 2 mL of adult naloxone (400 µg/mL)
- 100 mL 4.5% HAS
- 500 mL bag 10% dextrose
- Checklist

PROCEDURES PRIOR TO DELIVERY

1. Liaise with obstetricians and/or midwives.
2. Obtain obstetric history.
3. Call for senior assistance if the infant is < 30 weeks gestation or there is loss of fetal heartbeat prior to or after delivery.
4. Check resuscitaire:
   — Is the heater switched on?
   — Is the delivery room warm enough (25°C)?
   — Is the oxygen supply switched on and working? Set flow rate at 5 L/min
   — Is the pressure-limiting valve set at 30 cmH$_2$O?
   — Is the suction working? (In general the maximum negative pressure used should be no more than 100 mmHg. Occasionally, with thick meconium, the pressures may need to be increased to a maximum of 200 mmHg).
   — Are endotracheal tubes available?
   — Is the laryngoscope illuminating effectively?
   — Are there some dry, warm towels to wrap the baby in?

PROCEDURE AT DELIVERY

1. Start the clock.
2. Transfer baby to resuscitaire.
3. Dry baby off, remove wet towels and wrap in warm towel. Ensure that the head is covered (use hat or wrap within towel). These procedures must be done, however sick the infant, to prevent rapid cooling.
4. Immediately assess the condition of the infant and decide on the intervention required. This primary assessment should be based on the infant's breathing, colour and heart rate. Heart rate may be assessed during this primary assessment by compressing the umbilical cord. Colour is assessed by looking at the baby's trunk and not the peripheries.

5. Having assessed the baby, assign the condition to one of four groups (see below). As always, resuscitation should proceed in the following order: **A** — airway, **B** — breathing, **C** — circulation, **D** — drugs.

PRIMARY ASSESSMENT AND MANAGEMENT

Breathing/crying, HR ≥100, centrally pink. Dry infant and give to mother. Ideally these babies should be delivered directly onto their mother's abdomen and dried with a towel. Temperature is then maintained by direct skin to skin contact.

Blue, apnoeic/gasping respirations, heart rate ≥100. Stimulate, e.g. rub back with towel or gently tap feet. Open the airway by placing head and neck in neutral position and performing chin lift. If obstructed with secretions, clear airway with gentle oral followed by nasal suction. Give facial oxygen. If no response is shown by 1 min of age, i.e. HR is falling or the baby remains cyanosed, then bag and mask or mask and Y-piece ventilation should be commenced. It is essential that IPPV tries to mimic the physiology of the infant's first breath. The first five breaths should be given at 30 cmH₂O and be held for 2 s if using a mask and Y-piece or by compressing the bag slowly for 1–2 s if using a bag, valve, mask system. Following the first 5 breaths, the pressure can be reduced to 15–20 cmH₂O and a rate of 30–40 ventilations/minute used. If, despite effective mask ventilation, HR falls to less than 100, intubation should be performed.

Blue/pale, apnoeic, HR <100. Bag and mask or mask and Y-piece ventilation should be commenced immediately. If there is no increase in heart rate within 2 min, intubation should be undertaken.

White, apnoeic, HR <60. Full cardiopulmonary resuscitation is required (Fig. 3.2). Intubate immediately and commence IPPV. If there is no-one immediately available who is experienced at intubation, or it is technically difficult, then mask ventilation should be commenced until help arrives. After 30 s, reassess HR by auscultation. If HR <60, commence ECM.

 The commonest reason for failure of the HR to improve is ineffective lung inflation. Check this is correct before commencing ECM.

 If there is no response to IPPV and ECM, then a UVC should be inserted. If this is not possible, obtain intraosseous (IO) access. In extreme cases where attempts at UVC and IO access have been unsuccessful, the intracardiac (IC) route can be used for giving drugs. A baseline blood gas, blood sugar and FBC should be obtained and resuscitation drugs given (Table 3.3 and Fig. 3.2).

Table 3.3 Resuscitation drugs

Approx. gestation	Drug doses (mL)							
	23	27	30	33	35	37	39	42
Weight (kg)	0.5	1	1.5	2	2.5	3	3.5	4
Epinephrine (adrenaline) (mL of 1:10 000) Initial dose								
via IV			0.1	0.15	0.2	0.25	0.3	0.35	0.4
via ETT			0.2	0.3	0.4	0.5	0.6	0.7	0.8
Subsequent (IV/IO/IC)			1.0	1.5	2.0	2.5	3.0	3.5	4.0
Sodium bicarbonate (mL of 4.2%) IV/IO/IC			2	3	4	5	6	7	8
Neonatal naloxone (mL of 20 µg/mL) IM/IV	0.25	0.5	0.75	1.0	1.25	1.5	1.75	2.0
Human albumin solution 4.5% (mL) IV/IO	5	10	15	20	25	30	35	40
Glucose 10% (mL of 10%) IV/IO	2.5	5	7.5	10	12.5	15	17.5	20

Notes:
1. IV, intravenous including via UVC.
2. IV/IO access should always be used in preference to ET access.
3. All drugs should be checked before giving and a record of drug administration kept.
4. Some units use adult naloxone (400 µg/mL) in a dose of 100 µg/kg IM in view of its prolonged duration of action.
5. Do not use epinephrine (adrenaline) in babies < 26 weeks gestation (see text).

RESUSCITATION TECHNIQUES

The techniques of airway opening, suction, bag and mask ventilation, mask and Y-piece ventilation, intubation, ECM, UVC insertion, intraosseous access and intracardiac access are discussed in detail in Chapter 21.

FAILURE TO RESPOND TO RESUSCITATION AT DELIVERY

If mask ventilation is being performed:
- Is the face mask of the correct size?
- Is there a good seal?
- Is the neck position correct?
- Are oral secretions present?

If baby is intubated and there is poor or absent chest movement:
- Is the ETT in the oesophagus? Air entry will be better over the stomach than over the lung fields.

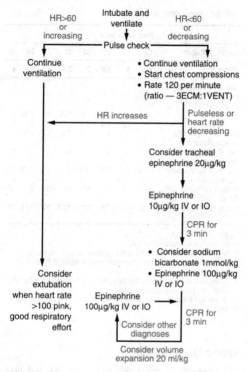

Fig. 3.2 Advanced Neonatal Life Support.

1. All drugs should be followed by a 0.5–1.0 mL flush of 0.9% saline.
2. If there is likely to be a delay in establishing IV access, then epinephrine (adrenaline) should be given via the ETT. This should be given rapidly down a catheter placed to lie just beyond the end of the ETT and followed by a 0.5–1.0 mL normal saline flush and five rapid inflations. This route should only be used whilst IV access is being established. It must not be used in preference to IV access.
3. This dose of sodium bicarbonate is not intended to correct the metabolic acidosis but to increase the pH within the coronary arteries and hopefully increase the action of the subsequent epinephrine (adrenaline).
4. During the process of prolonged resuscitation, hypoglycaemia (i.e. whole BG <2.6 mmol/L) should be sought and treated, if present, with 10% glucose 5 ml IV.

All drugs should be checked before giving and a record of drug administration kept.

- Is the ETT down the right main bronchus? Consider this if there is asymmetry of breath sounds and chest wall movement. Inflation and air entry will improve as the tube is withdrawn.
- Is the inflation pressure adequate? If the ETT appears to be in the correct position. i.e. breath sounds present and symmetrical but poor chest wall movement, then the most likely problem is that the baby is receiving insufficient pressure to open up the lungs. Therefore:
  — Check the PIP on the pressure manometer and increase to 30–40 cmH$_2$O.
  — Check oxygen flow rate. This should be set on the resuscitaire at 5–8 L/min for mask ventilation, and 3–5 L/min for ET IPPV.
  — If, on increasing inspiratory pressure, there is still poor or absent chest movement, consider increasing the inspiratory time.
- Does the baby have lung pathology? For example:
  — Pneumothorax
  — Diaphragmatic hernia (Is there a scaphoid abdomen? Is the apex beat displaced?)
  — Hypoplastic lungs (Does the child have signs of Potter's syndrome?)
  — Pleural effusions
  — Evolving lung disease such as severe respiratory distress syndrome
  — Thoracic dystrophy (the baby may benefit from having the peak inspiratory pressure reduced.)

If in any doubt, reintubate.

If there is good chest movement:
- Has there been fetal haemorrhage? Suspect if mother has had large antepartum haemorrhage or abruption.
  If hypovolaemia due to fetal blood is suspected, then plasma, uncross-matched O-negative blood or blood cross-matched against mother should be given in a volume of 10–20 mL/kg, repeated as necessary.
- Is there severe birth asphyxia?
- Does the baby have severe cyanotic congenital heart disease?

SPECIAL SITUATIONS

Mothers who have received opiate pain relief

If with mask ventilation the baby becomes pink and has a good HR but does not breathe spontaneously and if the mother has received opiate analgesia more frequently than 3 hourly or within 4 h pre-delivery, then naloxone may be given (Table 3.4). Bag and mask ventilation must not be stopped whilst naloxone is being administered. *Naloxone must not be given to the infant of an opiate dependent mother as it can cause acute withdrawal.*

Thick/particulate meconium-stained liquor

- Thin meconium staining does not require intervention.
- When the child is vigorous or cries immediately at birth
  - oral suction only
  - do not attempt direct laryngoscopy
- In *all* other situations proceed as described in Figure 3.3.

The preterm infant

Resuscitation of the preterm infant should follow the principles described above. Remember the surfactant deficient infant often requires an increased peak airway pressure when receiving IPPV. We do not recommend the use of cardiac drugs in the resuscitation of infants less than 26 weeks gestation.

Resuscitation of babies at the limit of viability

When a mother is likely to deliver at or before the limits of viability, a doctor experienced in neonatology should see the parents pre-delivery. Having gathered together all the relevant information about the baby's true gestational age, the doctor should talk with the parents about the survival of babies at that gestational age (Figs 1.2–1.5). The parents' feelings and responses to that information should be carefully listened to.

An experienced doctor should be present at the delivery as well as the neonatal SHO. At birth, assess the baby's size, gestational characteristics, including fusion of the eyelids, bruising (which is known to be a critical determinant of outcome) and respiratory effort. Babies who are considered pre-viable are likely to be 23 weeks of gestation or less, although some may be 24 weeks. Usually, the pre-viable baby will be white, flaccid and not making breathing movements. In this case the parents will usually want to hold the baby. If the baby is clearly making efforts to establish respiration, this should be supported, either with mask or endotracheal positive pressure ventilation. Respiratory support with ventilation/oxygenation in a viable baby will always result in establishment of a good HR. Extraordinary measures, e.g. cardiac massage and epinephrine (adrenaline), should not be used at extreme gestations (below 26 weeks).

If as an SHO you are called unexpectedly to such a delivery and if there is any doubt about the viability of the baby then always initiate resuscitation until the arrival of a more experienced paediatrician.

Higher-order births

Higher-order multiple births (triplets, quadruplets or more) are becoming more common as a result of the more frequent use of assisted reproduction techniques. The risk of prematurity is very high and the simultaneous delivery of several infants below 30 weeks gestation can stretch neonatal resources to the limit.

Higher-order multiple pregnancies are usually diagnosed early. The neonatal unit must be aware of these, particularly after

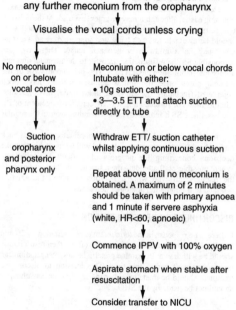

Suction the baby's head on the perineum using a
10g (black) suction catheter

↓

Following delivery, transfer the baby to the
resuscitaire and, using direct laryngoscopy, suction
any further meconium from the oropharynx

↓

Visualise the vocal cords unless crying

**No meconium
on or below
vocal cords**

Suction
oropharynx
and posterior
pharynx only

Meconium on or below vocal chords
Intubate with either:
• 10g suction catheter
• 3—3.5 ETT and attach suction
directly to tube

↓

Withdraw ETT/ suction catheter
whilst applying continuous suction

↓

Repeat above until no meconium is
obtained. A maximum of 2 minutes
should be taken with primary apnoea
and 1 minute if servere asphyxia
(white, HR<60, apnoeic)

↓

Commence IPPV with 100% oxygen

↓

Aspirate stomach when stable after
resuscitation

↓

Consider transfer to NICU

Fig. 3.3 Management of the baby with thick or particulate meconium stained liquor.

24 weeks gestation. Close cooperation between the obstetric and neonatal staff is necessary to ensure that sufficient resources are available for intensive care, especially when delivery seems likely under 34 weeks. Antenatal transfer may be desirable if too few spaces are available or if there are not enough high-quality neonatal staff. The neonatologist should meet the parents before delivery and explain what is likely to happen at and after birth; the parents should be offered the opportunity to visit the neonatal unit. A standard dose of antenatal steroids should always be given, even if delivery seems imminent.

If transfer is impossible, postnatal transfer of selected infants may be necessary, even though this means splitting the babies up, as the babies and those already in the neonatal unit should not be put at risk by inadequate resources to care for them. Whilst this is undesirable, finding an intensive care cot for each baby who needs it is the first priority.

Delivery is usually by caesarean section, which makes planning easier, although it may be urgent even so. At the delivery one resuscitaire and one trained member of the neonatal staff should be available for each baby, and supported by an assistant who may be a midwife or neonatal nurse. These two are responsible for the resuscitation, transfer to the neonatal unit and admission/stabilisation of each baby. This pair should write up the clinical notes once the initial admission tasks have been completed (including the siting of lines, initial investigations, administration of surfactant, first CXR, initial management of BP and baseline USS if indicated) prior to handing over to the regular staff.

A consultant should be designated coordinator and act as back up for the difficult resuscitation. He/she will be available to make decisions concerning the progress of difficult resuscitations. Where possible, staff attending the resuscitation should be extra to the regular staff who will be required to attend the existing neonatal unit population and other deliveries.

DISCONTINUATION OF RESUSCITATION

If there is no response in the term infant to resuscitation by 20 min (i.e. the infant has no HR or respiratory effort) then resuscitation should be withdrawn. In extreme preterm babies, resuscitation can be stopped well before this time. The decision to discontinue treatment should be made by either the registrar or consultant: it should not be made by the SHO.

APGAR SCORE (Table 3.4)

This is not a substitute for good note-keeping or a good predictor of neurodevelopmental outcome.

Care of the infant requiring neonatal intensive care in the first hour after birth

Table 3.5 outlines the indications we use for admission of infants to a NICU. These indications will vary to some extent between hospitals depending on the transitional care facilities available.

Table 3.4 Apgar score

	0	1	2
HR	None	<100	>100
Respirations[a]	None	Slow, irregular, gasping	Good, crying
Muscle tone	Limp	Some flexion	Active motion
Reflex irritability (to nasopharyngeal suction)	No response	Grimace	Cough or sneeze
Colour (of trunk)	White	Blue	Pink

[a]This should reflect the baby's underlying respiratory effort if receiving IPPV.

Table 3.5 Indications for admitting a baby to the NICU

Babies requiring immediate admission to the neonatal unit from the labour suite or immediately after delivery elsewhere
- Infants <1800 g or < 34 weeks gestation
- Infants who appear unstable and cause concern/require intensive care
- Suspected significant perinatal asphyxia
- Respiratory problems — if a baby has any two of the following respiratory signs between 1 and 4 h of age, it should be admitted for further investigation:
  - tachypnoea >70 bpm
  - grunting
  - central cyanosis
  - recession
- Congenital abnormalities — where intensive care is anticipated or diagnosis of multiple anomalies is in doubt
- Haemolytic disease where exchange transfusion is likely
- Consider admitting where there is unexplained death of sibling in first week of life
- Chorioamnionitis, i.e. presence of maternal pyrexia, purulent liquor and prolonged rupture of membranes

Admit from postnatal wards
- Convulsions, apnoeic or cyanotic attacks
- Respiratory distress (including grunting) at or beyond 4 h of age
- Hypoglycaemia not responding to regular 3-hourly feeds of breast milk or formula milk at a total volume of 90 mL/kg per day (see hypoglycaemia guideline)
- Spontaneous bleeding
- Jaundice requiring exchange transfusion
- Major feeding problem and/or vomiting
- Any bile-stained vomit
- Low temperature (<36°C) not responding to measures available on postnatal ward

TRANSFER FROM LABOUR WARD

- Inform neonatal staff of baby's imminent transfer.
- Make sure baby is wrapped in warm towels and the head is covered.

- Confirm that there are two correct name labels.
- Transfer on **resuscitaire**:
  - Check there is sufficient cylinder oxygen.
  - Change from wall to cylinder oxygen supply and unplug electrical supply to resuscitaire.
- Transfer in **neonatal transport incubator**:
  - Attach appropriate monitoring leads, e.g. ECG and pulse oximeter.
  - Check transport incubator is warm and that ventilator settings and/or oxygen concentration are appropriate.
  - Transfer baby to incubator and attach ventilator and monitors.
- Show baby to parents.
- Transfer calmly and promptly to NICU.

MANAGEMENT OF THE SICK NEWBORN INFANT ON ADMISSION TO THE NEONATAL UNIT

Both sick and preterm babies benefit from minimal handling. The aim should be to undertake all nursing and medical procedures as quickly and with as little disturbance to the baby as possible, usually within 1 h of admission, and then to allow the baby to rest.

1. Weigh baby.
2. Transfer to incubator or radiant heater.
3. Attach to ventilator if intubated. See Chapter 6 and Table 3.6 for initial ventilator settings.
4. Allow nursing staff 5 min to:
   - take infant's temperature
   - attach temperature probe, cardiac, respiratory and transcutaneous oxygen ± carbon dioxide monitors. A transcutaneous oxygen monitor should be used in preference to a pulse oximeter, especially in preterm babies at risk of hyperoxaemia.
   - give vitamin K: 1 mg IM if = 1.5 kg; 0.5 mg IM if <1.5 kg
   - take Polaroid photographs for parents.

Table 3.6 Initial ventilator settings

	Non-compliant stiff lungs	Compliant normal lungs
Rate	60/min	40/min
Ti	0.4s	0.3–0.4 s
PIP	Increase from 18 cmH$_2$O until adequate chest wall movement	14 cmH$_2$O
PEEP	4 cmH$_2$O	3 cmH$_2$O
F_i0$_2$	As required to maintain oxygenation	As required to maintain oxygenation

Preterm infant ventilated for respiratory distress

● Give surfactant (Ch. 6) — observe clinical effect and adjust ventilator settings accordingly.
● Obtain venous access either peripherally or, in the extremely preterm baby <26 weeks, via a UVC. Obtain a blood glucose (BG) reading and send blood for FBC, blood group, DCT and blood culture.
● Commence IV fluids of 10% dextrose at 60 mL/kg.
● Give IV antibiotics where indicated. Our practice is to give antibiotics, to cover risk of GBS, to all babies with respiratory distress for 48 h until blood cultures are known to be negative.
● Commence pain relief/sedation with either morphine or diamorphine.
● If the baby is requiring > 40% oxygen and obtain, arterial access preferably via the umbilical artery (Ch. 21). In infants > 30 weeks gestation where early enteral feeding is likely, some neonatologists prefer peripheral arterial access.
● Complete examination of baby (see below). This should include gestational assessment if there is any doubt of the baby's gestational age (Fig. 3.4).
● CXR at 4 h. Include AXR if either UAC or UVC inserted

Fig. 3.4 Ballard assessment of gestational age. (Reproduced with permission from Ballard JL, Khoury JC, Wedig K, Wang L, Eilers-Walsman BL, Lip, R, 1991 New Ballard score, expanded to include extremely premature infants. Journal of Pediatrics; 119: 417–423.)

Notes on neurological assessment
Posture. Observed with infant quiet and in a supine position.
Square window. The hand is flexed on the forearm between the examiner's thumb and index finger. Apply enough pressure to obtain as full flexion as possible. Measure the angle between the hypothenar eminence and the ventral aspect of the forearm.
Arm recoil. With the infant in the supine position, flex the forearms for 5 s, then fully extend by pulling on the infant's hands, and then release.
Popliteal angle. With the infant supine and the pelvis flat on the mattress, the thigh is held in the knee-chest position by the examiner's left index finger and thumb supporting the knee. The leg is then extended by gentle pressure from the examiner's right index finger behind the ankle and the popliteal angle is measured.
Scarf sign. With the infant supine, take the hand and try to put it around the neck and as far posteriorly as possible around the opposite shoulder. Assist this manoeuvre by lifting the elbow across the body. See how far the elbow will go across the chest.
Heel to ear. With the infant supine, position the foot as near to the head as it will go without forcing it. Observe the distance between the head and the foot as well as the degree of extension at the knee.

Notes on physical assessment
Plantar length. Measured from the tip of the great toe to the back of the heel.
Eyelid separation. Loosely fused is defined as closed but with one or both lids to be partly separated by gentle traction. Tightly fused is defined as bilaterally inseparable by gentle traction.

Neuromuscular Maturity

	-1	0	1	2	3	4	5
Posture							
Square window (wrist)	>90°	90°	60°	45°	30°	0°	
Arm recoil		180°	140°-180°	110°-140°	90°-110°	>90°	
Popliteal Angle	180°	160°	140°	120°	100°	90°	>90°
Scarf sign							
Heel to ear							

(For notes see p. 37)

Physical maturity

	-1	0	1	2	3	4	5
Skin	Sticky friable transparent	Gelatinous red, translucent	Smooth pink visible veins	Superficial peeling and/or rash, few veins	Cracking pale areas rare veins	Parchment deep cracking no vessels	leathery cracked wrinkled
Lanugo	None	Sparse	Abundant	Thinning	Bald areas	Mostly bald	
Planter surface	heel-toe 40-50mm: -1 <40mm: -2	>50mm no crease	faint red marks	anterior transverse crease only	creases ant. 2/3	Creases over entire sole	
Breast	Imperceptible	Barely perceptible	Flat areola no bud	Stippled areola 1-2mm bud	Raised areola 3-4mm bud	Full areola 5-10mm bud	
Eye/Ear	Lids fused Loosely: -1 tightly: -2	Lids open pinna flat stays folded	Sl. curved pinna;soft; slow recoil	Well-curved pinna; soft but ready recoil	Formed and firm instant recoil	Thick cartilage ear still	
Genitals male	Scrotum flat, smooth	Scrotum empty faint rugae	Testes in upper canal rare rugae	Testes descending few rugae	Testes down good rugae	Testes pendulous deep rugae	
Genitals female	Clitoris prominent labia flat	Prominent clitoris small labia minora	Prominent clitoris enlarging minora	Majora and minora equally prominent	Majora large minora small	Majora cover clitoris and minora	

Maturity rating

Score	Weeks
-10	20
-5	22
0	24
5	26
10	28
15	30
20	32
25	34
30	36
35	38
40	40
45	42
50	44

- Inform consultant of all admissions < 26 weeks gestation or where there is a major congenital malformation.
- Explain to both parents the reason for admission and the care the baby is receiving.

Infant with suspected perinatal hypoxia (see Ch. 12)

PROBLEMS RELATED TO SIZE AND MATURITY (Tables 3.7–3.9)

Definitions of prematurity, LBW and SGA are given in Table 3.7. With early fetal USS, the gestational age is often reliably known. If doubt exists, a gestational assessment should be performed (Fig. 3.4). Unfortunately, these scores are only accurate to within ± 2 weeks.

SGA babies may be proportional or asymmetrical (i.e. normal head circumference and length with low weight). Proportional SGA suggests early-onset IUGR, e.g. chromosomal abnormality, congenital infection, early placental insufficiency or severe maternal disease (renal failure, CF.) Asymmetrical SGA suggests late onset of IUGR, e.g. placental insufficiency, maternal cigarette smoking, maternal drug abuse, placental insufficiency and pre-eclampsia (Table 3.8).

LGA babies are frequently infants of diabetic mothers. Problems associated with LGA babies are shown in Table 3.9.

Table 3.7 Definitions of size and gestation

Term	Definition
LBW	Birthweight <2500 g irrespective of gestation
VLBW	Birthweight <1500 g irrespective of gestation
ELBW	Birthweight <1000 g irrespective of gestation
Preterm	Born at < 37 weeks gestation
Post-term	Born at > 42 weeks gestation
SGA	Birthweight below 10th centile for gestation
LGA	Birthweight above 90th centile for gestation

Table 3.8 Problems associated with preterm and SGA babies

Preterm babies
- Respiratory
  — RDS
  — apnoea
- Hypothermia
  — immature control
  — high surface area:body ratio
  — thin skin – high transepidermal water loss
- Infection
  — reduced maternal antibodies
  — thin, delicate skin
  — immunologically incompetent
  — invasive procedures

Table 3.8 *cont'd*

- Metabolic — jaundice of prematurity
- Feeding problems
  - poor suck and swallow
  - functional ileus
  - necrotising enterocolitis
- CVS — PDA
- Renal
  - immaturity: poor conservation of sodium and water
- CNS
  - periventricular haemorrhage
  - periventricular leukomalacia
- Retinopathy of prematurity
- Late anaemia

SGA
- Respiratory
  - perinatal asphyxia
  - meconium aspiration
  - pulmonary haemorrhage
- Hypothermia — large surface area:body ratio
- Infections in utero
  - toxoplasma
  - rubella
  - CMV
- Metabolic — symptomatic hypoglycaemia: poor glycogen stores
- Congenital anomalies

Table 3.9 Problems of LGA infants

Risks to all LGA infants
- Shoulder dystocia, fractured clavicle, Erb's palsy
- Perinatal asphyxia
- Birth injury

Additional problems in infants of diabetic mothers
- Congenital abnormalities
- Hypoglycaemia
- Respiratory distress
- Jaundice
- Polycythaemia
- Cardiomyopathy
- Small left colon syndrome
- Renal vein thrombosis

TEMPERATURE CONTROL

Babies lose heat via convection, evaporation and radiation. Only minimal amounts of heat are lost by conduction. If babies are allowed to become cold they may develop several problems:

- increased oxygen consumption — acidosis, hypoxia
- increased energy expenditure — hypoglycaemia, poor weight gain/increased weight loss
- decreased surfactant production — increased severity of RDS
- increased risk of sepsis
- increased risk of IVH
- cold stress — non-shivering themogenesis (metabolism of brown fat), vasoconstriction, increased activity, flexed posture
- decreased survival.

Overheating of babies is less common but is especially likely to occur during the summer months if the baby is left near a window in direct sunlight. It is also associated with significant adverse effects, as follows:

- increased apnoea in preterm infants
- shock
- convulsions
- DIC
- renal failure
- hypernatraemic dehydration
- SIDS
- heat stress — sweating (term infants and preterm infants > 2 weeks postnatal age), vasodilation, extended posture, decreased activity/sleepy.

The thermoneutral range is the zone of environmental temperature within which an infant's heat production is at a minimum, the body temperature is normal and there is no sweating. Core temperature is a poor indicator of whether larger infants are feeling hot or cold.

Significant thermal stresses are required to increase or decrease body temperature outside the normal range. Babies less than 30 weeks gestation behave as if they are poikilothermic, i.e. their body temperature alters directly with the environmental temperature. Body temperature is therefore a good indicator of the thermal environment in this group.

Measurement of temperature

Rectal, axilla and between-skin and mattress temperatures all correlate well with core temperature. The normal range, for all gestations, for rectal temperature is 36.5–37.5°C and for axilla temperature is 35.6–37.3°C. For skin temperature, the range is 35.5–36.5°C for term infants and 36.2–37.2°C for preterm infants.

Heat loss

Heat loss from convection depends on the difference in temperature between the infant and the surrounding air. It is also affected by air speed, increasing if there is a draft. It is increased by the large surface area to volume ratio of the newborn infant.

Loss by radiation is proportional to the difference in temperature between the baby and the surrounding surfaces. Preterm babies have very high transepidermal water loss (TEWL), and therefore evaporative heat loss, because the stratum corneum of the skin is thin and poorly keratinised. By 2 weeks of age, the TEWL of an extreme preterm infant is similar to a term infant. Use of radiant warmers and phototherapy increase evaporative heat loss. Conductive heat loss depends on the difference in temperature between the infant and the objects (e.g. bedding) he is in contact with and the conductance of those objects.

Table 3.10 Appropriate environmental temperatures

Healthy clothed newborn babies in the neonatal period

>2 kg — nurse clothed, with bedding at a room temperature of 25°C

1.5–2 kg — nurse clothed, with a hat and bedding at a room temperature of 26°C

<1.5 kg — nurse clothed, with a hat, in an incubator at 30–32°C

- Do not nurse infant naked unless frequent observation is needed
- Naked babies will require nursing in a much warmer environment

Healthy naked babies in a double-walled incubator on the first day

1.0–1.5 kg	35°C
1.5–2.5 kg	34°C
>2.5 kg	33°C

Abdominal skin temperature settings for infants nursed under a radiant heater or in servo-mode incubators

<1 kg	36.9°C
1.0–1.5 kg	36.7°C
1.5–2.0 kg	36.5°C
2.0–2.5 kg	36.3°C
>2.5 kg	36.0°C

Prevention of heat loss in the preterm infant is as follows:
Appropriate environmental temperatures are given in Table 3.10.

- Convection
  — nurse in incubator
  — heat air/oxygen surrounding baby
  — reduce draughts/air flow
  — heat ventilator gases.
- Evaporation
  — dry skin at resuscitation
  — humidify air/oxygen surrounding baby (<1 kg birthweight in first week)
  — nurse in an incubator rather than under a radiant heater
  — humidify ventilator gases
  — cover in bubble blanket.

- Radiation
  - dress especially with a hat
  - wrap in blankets (especially in delivery suite)
  - nurse in a double-walled incubator or under a heater
  - maintain temperature of nursery at 24–25°C.
- Conduction
  - heat all bedding, clothes and surfaces before baby comes into contact with them
  - dress baby especially with a hat.

The type of heat source used often depends on the unit's preference. The disadvantage of radiant heaters is that significant amounts of heat are lost via evaporation. They are therefore best reserved for use in large term infants where evaporative heat loss is low or for initial stabilisation of infants and insertion of lines prior to transfer to an incubator. Using an incubator in air mode (i.e. air temperature set to a desired level) as opposed to servo mode (i.e. heater output dependent on baby's temperature) reduces fluctuations in air temperature and prevents the provision of an inappropriately low environmental temperature in the febrile infant.

Humidity

Humidification of the incubator reduces evaporative heat loss and helps to maintain normal temperatures. It should be used routinely in infants <30 weeks and/or <1000 g in the first week. The maximum humidity possible should be given. Condensation is reduced by using double-walled incubators and high room temperatures.

MINIMAL HANDLING

Sick newborn infants tolerate handling extremely badly and this should be kept to a minimum. The monitors should be used to provide observation of the infant and an arterial line inserted if frequent blood gas measurements are required. Painful procedures should be kept to a minimum and, during them, babies should be observed constantly for hypoxaemia. Suctioning is not routinely required during the first 48 h of RDS. After 48 h, the frequency of suctioning is tailored to the baby's individual requirements. All babies should be turned at least 6-hourly to prevent skin damage.

FLYING SQUAD TRANSFER

Ideally all babies who are likely to require NIC should be born in a maternity unit where this is possible and transfer in utero undertaken if facilities are not available locally.

Organisation/management pre-transfer

- Criteria for transferring babies vary from hospital to hospital and will depend on the level of equipment and expertise available locally.
- Always inform the paediatric consultant before arranging transfer of a baby.
- Never transfer a baby without close liaison with the receiving hospital or before a neonatal cot has been found.
- Specific arrangements for postnatal transfer vary around the country, but it is best performed by a dedicated and trained team. The information which the receiving hospital will require is found in Table 3.11. This allows the retrieval team to:
  — assess the urgency of the request
  — assess the amount of equipment required
  — provide guidance on management until their arrival.
- The transport system should always be fully equipped and ready to undertake a transfer:
  — check daily
  — restock immediately following any transport
  — batteries, e.g. in monitors, syringe pumps and the mobile phone, should be fully charged
  — leave heater on standby

Table 3.11   Information needed by receiving hospital

From referring hospital
- Baby's name
- Gestation
- Birthweight
- Date and time of birth
- Date and time of transfer request
- Doctor requesting transfer
- Baby's paediatric consultant
- Name of referring hospital
- Contact number
- Provisional diagnosis/reason for transfer
- Respiratory
  — oxygen/CPAP/IPPV: F_iO_2, PIP, PEEP/CPAP, rate, inspiratory time
  — blood gas art/cap: pH, P_aO_2, P_aCO_2, base excess
- Circulation — BP, perfusion, plasma/inotropes
- Temperature
- Blood sugar
- Drugs and infusions
- Other information

From own neonatal unit
- Number of intensive care cots available
- Number of nursing staff available
- Predicted demand 'in house' for intensive care cots in next few hours

- Always consider the baby's potential needs before leaving the base unit and confirm that all drugs and equipment which may be necessary for the baby are available, e.g. sedating and paralysing agents, sufficient infusion pumps.

Stabilisation prior to transfer

Intervention during transfer carries considerable risk. This can be reduced by fully stabilising the baby prior to transfer, as follows (this may take several hours):

Airway

- Should the baby be intubated prior to transfer? Yes if: unstable, $F_iO_2 > 50\%$, rising P_aCO_2, recurrent apnoea, < 30 weeks gestation.
- If already intubated, is the ETT in the correct position, patent and secure?

Breathing

- Does respiration need supporting? Is respiratory support adequate?
- Are the blood gases stable and satisfactory?
- Is arterial access required?
- Is surfactant required? Always allow ventilator parameters to stabilise post treatment.
- Is there a pnemothorax? If present, insert drain and attach to a Heimlich flutter valve.
- Are appropriate monitors of ventilation in place, e.g. respiratory monitor, T_cO_2, continuous P_aO_2 or pulse oximeter with pulse waveform trace?

Circulation

- Are tissue perfusion and BP optimal?
- Is adequate support with colloid and inotropes being given?
- Is arterial access required?
- Is continuous IA monitoring of BP required during transfer?
- Are IV and IA lines and catheters correctly positioned and secure enough for transfer?

Temperature

- Is the baby's temperature 36.2–37.2°C?
- Does the temperature need further support?

Blood glucose

- Is the baby normoglycaemic?
- Is the IV glucose infusion secure?

Nasogastric tube

- Is there a nasogastric tube in situ?
- Has it been aspirated and placed on free drainage to prevent gastric aspiration during transfer?

Infection
- Has the possibility of infection been considered?
- Has antibiotic treatment been commenced?

Documentation
- Are the notes complete and do they include results of investigations?
- Are the X-rays available?

Parents
- Have plans for transfer been discussed with parents?
- Have parents been given written information which includes contact numbers for the referral unit?
- Do parents have Polaroid photographs of their baby?
- Has a contact number for parents been obtained?
- Has surgical consent been obtained if required ?
- Has a sample of maternal blood been obtained to cross-match blood for the baby at the receiving unit?

Very occasionally a baby cannot be stabilised. Transfer should only go ahead in this situation if a treatment modality which may help the baby, e.g. ECMO, HFOV or INO, is available in the receiving centre.

Transfer into transport system
Poor temperature control during transport has been shown to be associated with an adverse outcome. Most heat is lost during transfer into the transport incubator. To prevent this, no more than 15 s should be allowed from disconnection to reconnection of heat and oxygen therapy. Do not open the transport system door more than momentarily.

Management during transfer
- Once the baby is in the transport incubator, confirm that all monitoring devices and pumps are working correctly and that the baby's vital signs remain stable.
- Use the ambulance's battery power source and oxygen supply.
- Monitor baby's vital signs constantly and document every 15 min.
- Check infusions, ventilator settings and gas supplies at regular intervals.
- Keep the ambulance warm, minimise drafts and avoid opening the incubator portholes.
- Babies do not tolerate high speed ambulance rides with their associated episodes of sudden breaking or swerving. As long as the traffic is moving, it is far better to go with the flow. Occasionally a police escort or police support to alter traffic lights can be of help.

The normal newborn

SKIN AND UMBILICAL CORD CARE (see Ch. 18)

VITAMIN K

Prevention of vitamin K deficiency bleeding (haemorrhagic disease of the newborn) is discussed in Chapter 15.

NEWBORN EXAMINATION

All infants should be examined at least once in the neonatal period, irrespective of the presence of symptoms or signs. This should be within 24–48 h of birth and in the presence of the mother so that a history can be obtained, her questions can be answered and any anxieties about feeding or neonatal care discussed.

As a minimum history, the doctor should have ascertained the name of the mother and her baby, the sex of the baby and the mother's obstetric and family history before the examination is undertaken. A checklist of all of the items of maternal and perinatal history which may be relevant, depending on whether the infant is well or ill and on which systems are involved, is given in Table 3.12 but for many healthy term infants this information is not required. Much of this information should be available from the obstetric notes, or the mother may be asked directly.

There is little evidence that a second neonatal screening examination prior to discharge identifies new problems. However, if the baby has spent a long period of time in hospital, a further full examination at the time of discharge is entirely appropriate and will answer further maternal questions.

Table 3.12   Important aspects of maternal and perinatal history

Family history
Inherited diseases, e.g.:
 Metabolic disorders
 Haemophilia
 Cystic fibrosis
 Polycystic kidneys
 Perinatal death

Maternal history
Age
Blood type, transfusions, blood group sensitisation
Chronic maternal illness, e.g.:
 Hypertension
 Renal disease
 Cardiac disease
 Bleeding disorders
 Diabetes

Table 3.12 *cont'd*

Sexually transmitted disease
Infertility
Recent infection, exposure to infection, vaginal discharge, flu-like illnesses

Previous pregnancies — problems and outcomes
Abortions, fetal deaths, neonatal deaths
Prematurity, postmaturity
Malformations
RDS
Jaundice
Apnoea

Drug history
Medications
Drug abuse
Alcohol
Cigarettes

Current pregnancy
Gestational age (dates/scan)
Results of fetal testing:
  CVS
  Amniocentesis
  Ultrasound
  αFP (alpha-fetoprotein)
  Down's screeening
Pre-eclampsia
Bleeding
Trauma
Infection
Surgery
Poly/oligohydramnios
Antenatal steroids

Labour and delivery
Presentation, e.g. cephalic, breech
Onset of labour
Rupture of membranes
Duration of labour
Fever
Fetal monitoring
Meconium-stained liquor
Analgesia
Anaesthesia
Method of delivery
Initial assessment
Apgar scores at 1, 5 and 10 min
Resuscitation
Placental examination
Birthweight and sex

Neonatal period
Has the infant passed urine?
Has the infant passed meconium?
Are there any concerns with feeding?

Physical examination

During the newborn period, more information is obtained from 'inspection' than from 'palpation, percussion and auscultation'. Certain aspects of the examination of the older children (e.g. percussion of the chest) are irrelevant to the newborn and other parts of the examination are difficult once the infant is crying. It is therefore best to try to obtain as much information as possible from inspection of the fully clothed infant, particularly if he or she is asleep, and only then to proceed to undress the infant, leaving the most unpleasant parts of the examination until last. With experience, the examination becomes more rapid and most experienced examiners take only 5 min or so. Formal gestational assessment (see Fig. 3.4) takes longer.

General examination

Before undressing the baby, try to assess:
- colour
- respiration
- HR
- the head, face and neck.

Colour. The infant may be:
- pink and well
- obviously centrally cyanosed (see Chs 6 and 7)
- jaundiced (see Ch. 9)
- pink but with cyanosis of the hands and feet (common in term infants and requires no action)
- initially apparently cyanosed but in fact there is contusion of the lips and bruising of the face as a result of trauma — again no action is required
- pale — the most common cause is anaemia due to fetoplacental haemorrhage at the time of delivery.

Respiration can usually be counted by observing movement of the abdomen (infants are predominantly abdominal breathers rather than chest breathers). The normal neonatal respiratory rate is 40–60 breaths/min. Note that many newborn infants have periodic breathing (alternating periods of very obvious respiratory effort and periods of shallow breaths); there may even be pauses between breaths, which are of no consequence provided they are of less than 10 s duration.

Signs of respiratory distress may be more obvious when the infant is undressed, but listen for an expiratory grunt (expiration against a partially closed glottis which is only heard in infants with respiratory disease) and observe for flaring of the ala nasae.

Heart rate. Gently palpate the radial pulse in a sleeping term infant and count the HR (much more reliable than trying to count when the infant has been undressed and crying). The normal neonatal heart rate is 100–160 bpm.

Head, face and neck
- *Skull* — examine for moulding, caput, cephalohaematoma; check that there are only two fontanelles (a third fontanelle is often palpable in Down's syndrome and other trisomies)
- *Anterior fontanelle* — best assessed with the infant sitting later in the examination when it should be soft and slightly concave with easily palpable margins
- *Face* — look at it carefully and try to list any definite abnormalities or asymmetry rather than simply describing the infant as 'funny looking'.
- *Ears* — look at the size and shape of the ears and decide whether they are low-set.
- *Eyes* — this part of the examination should be left until the end.
- *Nose* — if there is any question of the infant having choanal atresia, a NG tube should be passed via both nostrils.
- *Mouth and palate* — feeling the palate with the volar surface of the pulp of your little finger will only detect a cleft of the hard palate. To exclude a cleft of the soft palate, it is necessary to examine the baby's mouth with a pen-torch and, usually, a tongue depressor. Epstein's pearls (small white inclusion cysts in the midline between hard and soft palate) are a normal finding and neonatal teeth (Ch. 4) may be seen.
- *Neck* — look for fractured clavicles.

Now undress the baby — doing this tells you quite a lot about the infant's tone and state of alertness, besides your own manual dexterity!

The chest
- Shape
- Respiratory pattern
- Indices of respiratory distress syndrome (intercostal recession, sternal recession, increased abdominal excursion). **NB.** Unless there is severe CNS disease, significant respiratory disease in the absence of tachypnoea is rare
- Auscultation of the chest is rarely of much help in the newborn except for the asymmetry of breath sounds noted with pneumothorax, congenital diaphragmatic hernia etc.
- Gynaecomastia is common in both sexes and milk can often be expressed from the nipples.

The cardiovascular system
- Check that both brachial pulses are present (for femorals see below).
- Check that the apex beat is on the left side.

- Auscultate the precordium for HR (unless measured above), first and second heart sounds, any murmurs.

Cardiac murmurs are common in the newborn period (see Ch. 7). If the infant is crying, a nipple, bottle or dummy should be offered (depending on the parent's preference) as it is impossible to hear heart sounds in a crying infant.

The abdomen
- Palpate the abdomen for liver, spleen, kidneys, bladder and any abnormal masses. The newborn infant does not have strong abdominal muscles and the borders of the liver, spleen or bowel can often be seen through the thin abdominal wall, especially in preterm infants or before the first feed.
- Check the umbilical cord stump for signs of infection, and also check the number of cord vessels. The presence of a single umbilical artery indicates you should look hard for other dysmorphic signs or for renal masses; in their absence it is of no significance.
- Look for umbilical and inguinal herniae.
- Check whether the genitalia are obviously male or female or ambiguous (see Ch. 11). The scrotum of the male infant is often quite large and hydroceles are not uncommon but usually disappear in time spontaneously. Hydroceles and inguinal herniae never occur together. Check that there is no hypospadias (in which case circumcision is contraindicated). A normal term female infant has prominent labia majora, and a creamy-white vaginal discharge is common. Vaginal bleeding (from withdrawal of maternal hormones) is not uncommon.
- Check that the anus is present and patent.
- Turn the infant over and look at the back. Examine skin abnormalities and naevi (see Chs 12 and 18).
- Palpate the femoral pulses and assess any radiofemoral delay if the child is quiet.
- Check that both testes are descended.

The hands and feet
- Count the numbers of fingers and toes and look at the palmar and plantar creases.
- A single palmar (Simian) crease extends from the radial to the ulnar border of the palm and is commonly found in Down's syndrome, but may often be an incidental finding of no significance.
- A wide 'sandal' gap between the great and second toes is equally difficult to assess in the absence of other dysmorphic features.
- Erb's palsy (brachial plexus injury) will be apparent by a lack of motion of the affected arm and the arm will lie by the side rather than being flexed with the fist near the mouth (see Ch. 5).

The central nervous system. This is the most difficult part of the examination to do well and demands practice (see Ch. 12).

Information about tone is obtained while undressing the infant. Whilst examining the other parts of the body, the examiner should assess symmetry of movement and posturing, alertness and the infant's response to being handled and disturbed (i.e. crying appropriately and quieting appropriately when cuddled or fed).

Facial nerve weakness is more apparent when the infant is crying. This is often blamed on forceps deliveries but is more probably due to pressure of the ischial spines on the face during labour which is progressing slowly and which results in a forceps delivery (see Ch. 12).

Much has been written about the large number of newborn reflexes and detailed neuromuscular assessment, but a simple screening approach to neurological examination of the newborn is as follows:

- Observe general tone, posture, alertness and consolability as above.
- Put your index finger in the infant's palm and obtain the palmar grasp reflex.
- With the infant grasping your fingers, pull him to a sitting position — note the normal traction response as the shoulders tense and the amount of head lag.
- The Moro response is often now performed but will cause a normal infant to cry as part of the reflex; hence it is best left out unless you are concerned about neurological depression. It is performed by placing one palm behind the infant's head, supporting it and then allowing your palm to drop suddenly, allowing the head to fall backwards about 1–2 cm. This will test the Moro reflex when the infant should rapidly and symmetrically extend arms and legs, with a slow recovery and a cry.
- Check that the infant has a sucking and rooting reflex by stroking the cheek near the mouth with your fingertip. Then insert your little finger, fingernail downwards, into the infants mouth and press against the hard palate.
- Parents often like to see the stepping reflex demonstrated. Hold the infant upright under the arms with the feet on a hard surface and usually the infant will start a slow alternate stepping action; extending the neck may help to bring out the response.
- If you remain concerned about the baby's condition, use a simple structured assessment, such as the neurological part of the gestational assessment (Fig. 3.4 and Ch. 12).

A number of newborn reflexes give clues as to the infant's gestational age; these are shown in Table 3.13.

Finally, complete the parts of the check that are most likely to disturb the baby:

Table 3.13 Newborn reflexes and gestational age

Reflex	Stimulus	Positive response	Gestation if reflex absent (weeks)	Gestation if reflex present (weeks)
Pupil reaction	Light	Pupil constriction	≤31	≥29
Glabellar tap	Tap on glabellar	Blink	≤34	≥32
Traction response	Pull up by wrists from supine	Flexion of neck or arm	≤36	≥33
Neck righting	Rotation of head	Trunk follows	≤37	≥34

The eyes (see Ch. 17)
- Check that two eyes are present.
- Use an ophthalmoscope to elicit a red reflex in both eyes. Absence of red reflex indicates presence of cataract.
- Glaucoma is indicated by a large cloudy cornea and a corneal diameter greater than 11 mm. The baby may be irritable (due to pain), there may be photophobia and the eyes are noted to be large or bulging.
- Other ocular abnormalities which may be detected in the newborn period are conjunctivitis (often chlamydial but Gonococcus should be considered) and colobomata (this may affect only the iris but perhaps also the eyeball and retina).
- Strabismus is very rarely detected in the newborn period except due to ophthalmoplegia as part of a syndrome.

The head circumference
Measure the maximum OFC. Use a disposable paper tape measure and take the largest of three readings, not the average. There are no defined anatomical landmarks; the maximum OFC is just that, the largest measurement you can make. If there is any concern about the OFC, plot this measurement on a centile chart appropriate to the infant's sex and gestation.

Test for dislocation of the hips (see Ch. 19)
- Look for asymmetry of the thighs or skin creases.
- Gently test for limited abduction of the hips.
- Perform the two provocation manoeuvres:
  — *Barlow's test.* Baby is placed supine and the examiner grasps the baby's thighs with the middle finger over the greater trochanter (i.e. the lateral aspect of the upper thigh) and the thumb around the distal medial femur. This is probably done most easily if both hips are examined at the same time. Both hips and knees are placed at 90° of flexion,

and with the thighs in the adducted position (i.e. legs together) the femur is pushed gently downwards towards the surface on which the infant is lying. If the femoral head can be pushed backwards out of the acetabulum, the hip is dislocatable and Barlow's test is positive.

— *Ortolani's test* follows Barlow's test. The legs are held in the same way, with the knees and thighs still in 90° of flexion. The hips are then abducted. There will be a 'clunk' as the hip returns from its dislocated position into the acetabulum. The is called a positive Ortolani's sign.

These tests are perhaps best remembered by this mnemonic; during Barlow's test, the head of the femur is pushed Backwards; during Ortolani's test, the femur is abducted Outwards. As the infant becomes older, if congenital dislocation of the hip has been missed, it becomes more difficult to reduce the femoral head back into the acetabulum and the Ortolani's test may become negative. With the child lying supine and the knees flexed, the knees will not be at the same levels (a positive 'Galeazzi' sign).

When you have completed the examination, reassure the mother about your findings and record them accurately in the clinical notes, *remembering to sign and date the entry*. If you have elicited any abnormal signs, be open about them and contact your superior to discuss management. Do not try to make diagnoses unless you are confident about them and do not reassure parents unless you feel honestly able to do so.

FOUR

Congenital anomalies

Up to 5% of all newborn infants will have some form of anomaly, however trivial. Many of these will be obvious at birth or will be picked up by the parent. A few will be identified de novo by the neonatal screening examination (Ch.3) and some will not become apparent until physiological changes allow them to declare themselves later in the neonatal period or the first year. In this section we wish to provide a guide through the assessment and investigation of such anomalies and to introduce the means by which parents may be counselled as to the import of these conditions.

A congenital anomaly is a morphological defect present at birth and may arise through:

- **Malformation** — a developmental planning defect, e.g. oesophageal atresia, transposition of the great vessels, spina bifida
- **Deformation** — an induced alteration to a previously normal structure consequent on the intrauterine environment or an underlying condition, e.g. talipes equinovarus secondary to oligohydramnios or spina bifida
- **Disruption** — a disturbance in the normal sequence of structural development, e.g. amniotic bands.

The frequencies of some major anomalies are shown in Table 4.1.

Table 4.1   Approximate incidence of some common anomalies in the UK

Malformation	Rate per 1000 live births
Club foot (idiopathic talipes)	1.0
Cleft lip/palate	2.0
Congenital hip dislocation	5.0
Down's syndrome	1.6
Congenital heart malformation	6.0

Clinical assessment

Detailed clinical evaluation of the child with overt or suspected malformation is critical to establishing an accurate diagnosis.

FAMILY HISTORY

This may provide valuable clues as to the origin of the anomaly:

• Pregnancy history, including fetal growth and health assessments, amniotic fluid volume, the quality of fetal movements, etc.
• History of infertility or recurrent miscarriage (may imply a chromosomal translocation or sex linked dominant — see below)
• Consanguinity (may imply a recessive disorder)
• Any stillbirth or explained or unexplained neonatal/infant deaths
• Maternal medical and drug history, e.g. anticonvulsants, alcohol, cocaine (all of which may produce dysmorphism)
• Disorders in other children
• Similar features in close family members.

CLINICAL EXAMINATION

Always completely undress the baby and follow a structured approach, recording abnormal findings accurately in the clinical record. Pay particular attention to definite or 'hard' clinical signs, such as coloboma (radial defect in the iris) or polydactyly, but also record the presence of other minor signs which may help to confirm a diagnosis, such as:

• Facial appearance, skull shape, presence of an extra third fontanelle
• Eyes — palpebral fissures, angulation and spacing
• Ears — position, rotation, formation and ear lobe creases, ear pits and skin tags
• Mouth — shape, philtrum
• Nose — nasal bridge, anteversion of nares
• Neck — webbing
• Chest — nipple number and spacing
• Hand — shape [e.g. clinodactyly (incurving fifth finger, may have missing middle phalanx), short fingers relative to hand (brachydactyly)] and palmar creases
• Foot — shape, sandal gap and plantar creases.

Always record length, weight and maximal OFC on an appropriate chart. Clinical geneticists will often make other measures, e.g. palpebral length or eye spacing, but such detailed assessments are best left to the specialists as the measurement error may be great for the inexperienced. Charts for the normal ranges of some of these are found in the back of commonly used dysmorphology texts (see 'Further reading', p. 68).

FURTHER INVESTIGATIONS

X-rays are essential for the diagnosis of skeletal dysplasias but may also be of value in other conditions. X-ray the spine and long bones to assess vertebral shape and epiphyseal and metaphyseal status, respectively. The classic X-ray changes of many conditions are not present at birth and specialist assessment is necessary. X-rays later in the first year may be more helpful. Intracranial calcification may be seen on skull X-ray, although USS is equally sensitive.

Other imaging. USS and, increasingly, MRI may be indicated. Facial and neurological abnormality may indicate a likely intracranial developmental abnormality (e.g. hypertelorism and holoprosencephaly). Renal tract and cardiac abnormalities are associated with other conditions which may present early, e.g. oesophageal atresia when part of the VATER syndrome. Routine USS in the presence of other marker anomalies (e.g. oesophageal atresia, diaphragmatic hernia) is usually undertaken. Imaging for unusual conditions is best discussed with a paediatric radiologist.

Photographs may be of great value as a record, for comparison with published examples and for discussion between colleagues.

Karyotype. Most chromosomal disorders are expressed as dysmorphic features and may have multiple structural malformations. Beware of accepting a 'normal' antenatal karyotype, which will have simply involved looking for major karyotypic abnormalities. Where detailed karyotype assessment is required, it is best to discuss with the cytogenetics department the advisability of repeating the evaluation, especially where, for example, the antenatal sample was from CVS or only assessed for chromosome number. An ever increasing range of submicroscopic chromosomal rearrangements have been described. These may be detected by techniques such as FISH. The most common of these are the 22q11.2 microdeletion found in children with heart, cleft palate and parathyroid/thymic abnormalities; the 15q11 microdeletion in Prader–Willi/Angelman complex; and the triplet replication on chromosome 19q13.3 in myotonic dystrophy. Some disorders have a more complex genetic basis and may require the culture of chromosomes from other sources, such as skin fibroblasts, but you will be advised on this by your clinical geneticist. Always discuss with the parents your reasons for doing this investigation and emphasise that for many of the specialist investigations, a delay of several weeks is likely.

Screening or targetted investigations for inborn errors of metabolism may be required (see Ch. 11) and serological and urine testing for intrauterine infections are often usefully performed (see Ch. 13). Do not simply ask for a 'TORCH screen' as you are leaving the laboratory to decide which tests to do. It is better to refine which infections you think are likely to have caused the features you see (e.g. punctate intracranial calcification) and specify what organism you think is likely to have caused it (e.g. *Toxoplasma gondii*). On all request forms, if you have not discussed the scenario with your local laboratory put all the relevant clinical information — 'dysmorphic infant – TORCH' will not suffice!

Refining your diagnosis. All neonatal units should carry an up-to-date edition of a dysmorphology atlas; many carry several and some have access to computerised databases. Use hard findings (e.g. coloboma) rather than more subjective ones (e.g. small mouth) as 'handles' to search these texts for conditions which include them. Cross-referencing with more than one such handle will assist your search. Don't forget that the newborn may not show established external features of conditions represented by photographs of older children. Your clinical geneticist will also have access to the major genetic journals and computerised databases, and may be able to present the specific features of the child to colleagues in an attempt to refine prognosis where this may be in doubt.

Always seek help from your consultant and other experts before embarking on disclosure of diagnosis. If it is not obvious, time is a good investigation. Arrange expert review later in the first year and explain this to the parents.

GENETIC COUNSELLING

This is always better undertaken by a clinical geneticist — *much harm may be done by inexpert handling of genetic recurrence data*. The process comprises the following:

1. Obtain a precise diagnosis, including the autopsy report if one has been performed — without these the process cannot be informed. Do not set about explaining risk to parents until you are certain of the diagnosis.
2. Construct a family tree, including details of consanguinity (you will need to ask this question directly).
3. Learn about the condition — literature searches and discussions with colleagues will often be necessary before the prognosis can be refined.

4. Learn about potential for antenatal diagnosis — whether there are biochemical or genetic tests available (e.g. galactosaemia or CF) or whether there are typical USS appearances which may guide diagnosis. Many conditions are rapidly becoming detectable by antenatal genetic investigation and up to date information must be obtained from the laboratory.

5. Calculate the risk. This is straightforward if simple Mendelian inheritance is anticipated (Table 4.2). Where this is not the case, risk assessment may be based on:

- empirical evidence from population studies of similar cases (e.g. spina bifida) — consult empirical risk tables in dysmorphology texts
- modified risk, where clinical or laboratory information alters the background risk, e.g. maternal age and risk of trisomy (Table 4.3), Huntington's chorea and male age. Some conditions differ in expression when the copies of a chromosome are both inherited from the same parent (uniparental disomy e.g. in some children with Prader–Willi syndrome) and some appear to be matrilinear, being inherited as a mutation in mitochondrial DNA passed via the oocyte (e.g. Leigh's encephalopathy)
- composite risk, where different variants of conditions are inherited in different ways and not determinable from the present clinical information (e.g. osteogenesis imperfecta).

6. Communicate the prognosis and recurrence risk to parents—this is a skilled process, in which the parents must feel informed and able, if necessary, to take decisions about the future without being directed down a particular path. It may be helpful to give some comparative risks (Table 4.4) or to have other professionals with more experience of the condition or aspects of care (e.g. obstetrics), present.

Chromosomal abnormalities

These are much rarer incidental findings in the neonatal period due to the accuracy of fetal screening with serological and ultrasound screening.

TRISOMY 21 (DOWN SYNDROME)

This is the commonest chromosomal disorder, due to trisomy 21 in 95% cases (the remainder of children with Down syndrome have a translocation of chromosome 21 material, with a different and higher recurrence risk for some translocation and parent combinations — seek help in allocating risk). Screening for trisomy 21 in fetal life may be performed using a combination

Table 4.2 Mendelian inheritance patterns

Pattern/features	Examples
Autosomal dominant	
• Largely or completely expressed as heterozygote	Adult polycystic kidney disease
• Risk in affected heterozygote offspring is 1:2 (50%)	Huntington's chorea
• Homozygotes tend to be rare and more severe (risk 1:1 (100%))	Achondroplasia Ectrodactyly
• Complicated by variable onset or penetrance in heterozygous state which may lead to erroneous belief that a child has a new mutation	Osteogenesis imperfecta (type 1)
Autosomal recessive	
• Often single enzyme defects	Most IEFS
• May be difficult to determine except from pedigree	CF
• Confirmed recessive has 1:4 recurrence risk for siblings	Thalassaemia
• Antenatal diagnosis frequently possible	
X-linked disorders	
• No serious disorders carried on the Y chromosome	
• Over 100 X-linked disorders are known	
• X-linked dominance (XLD) is difficult to assess because of expression in heterozygote state dependent on activation of only 1 X chromosome (at random)	XLD – incontinentia pigmenti
• Some X-linked dominants are lethal in males	
• X-linked recessives (XLR) are the most common group	XLR::
— male–male transmission never occurs	Ocular albinism
— affected male passes gene to all daughters	Nephrogenic diabetes insipidus
— unaffected males do not transmit condition	Anhydrotic ectodermal dysplasia
— female carriers pass to 50% of sons, and 50% of daughters are carriers	Haemophilia A and B
— female homozygote is very rare	Ornithine transcarbamylase deficiency

Table 4.3 Recurrence risk of trisomy 21 in relation to maternal age

Maternal age (years)	Prior risk	Recurrence risk[a]
15	1:1578	1:200
20	1:1528	1:200
25	1:1351	1:200
30	1:909	1:200
35	1:384	1:192
40	1:112	1:56
45	1:28	1:14
50	1:6	1:3

[a]The risk of any chromosomal abnormality in a pregnancy following an affected child is twice this value.

Table 4.4   Approximate UK reproductive risks for comparison

Outcome	Risk
Spontaneous miscarriage	1:6
Any congenital anomaly in a baby	1:30
Perinatal death	1:100
Baby with severe disability	1:50
Post neonatal infant death	1:150

of serological (the 'triple test') or ultrasound markers. At best these indicate the potential risk of trisomy 21 and not its presence or absence: occasional babies with trisomy 21 will not have been allocated a high risk and parents and carers will have been given a false sense of security. The risk rises with maternal age (Table 4.3). As is the case with all trisomies, some children may show mosaicism for the trisomy, i.e. some cells are trisomic and others normal. The outlook for such children is unclear and variable.

Clinical features include hypotonia, brachycephaly (skull flattening in the anteroposterior axis) with crowded mid-face and relative macroglossia, upward slant to palpebral fissures, epicanthic folds, Brushfield spots (a ring of light coloured spots on the iris), brachydactyly, clinodactyly, simian crease, proximal migration of axial tri-radius and wide sandal gap. The diagnosis can usually be made clinically immediately after birth when the commonest presenting features are (at least four are present in all babies and more than six in 89%):

- Hypotonia — 80% of newborns
- Poor Moro response — 85%
- Hyperflexibility of joints — 80%
- Excess skin on back of neck — 80%
- Flat facial profile — 90%
- Slanted palpebral fissures — 80%
- Anomalous auricles — 60%
- Dysplasia of pelvis (on X-ray) — 70%
- Dysplasia of mid-phalanx of fifth finger — 60%
- Simian crease — 45%

Every junior SHO should be familiar with the classical features of this condition. In 40% there is an associated cardiac defect (usually AVSD) and routine cardiac USS is indicated. In 12%, a GI tract anomaly (oesophageal atresia, duodenal atresia, Hirschsprung's disease, exomphalos) occurs. A small proportion will develop a neonatal leukaemoid reaction or frank leukaemia. Almost all children will have severe learning difficulties, although social performance is often misleadingly good.

Where the diagnosis is unanticipated and suspected after inspection, it is important that a senior paediatrician reviews the child as soon as possible. Parents rapidly know if clinical staff suspect a problem and it is better to be open and honest with them. Take blood for karyotype and let the cytogenetic laboratory know your suspicions so that the sample may be processed as fast as possible (usually a result is available in 48–72 h). Following a cardiac USS, even in the absence of early symptoms, counselling should be arranged with the team(s) who will provide ongoing care. Let the obstetric team know of the diagnosis so that their screening arrangements can be reviewed, if necessary.

TRISOMY 18 (EDWARDS SYNDROME)

As in the case of trisomy 21, there is a wide potential spectrum of abnormalities which may be found in babies with trisomy 18. The incidence rises with maternal age, and mosaicism, partial trisomy and translocation are found in small proportions. Where children show partial trisomy, the outlook is variable, depending on whether it is of the short arm (good outlook) or long arm (indistinguishable from full trisomy 18). Recurrence risk for trisomy 18 is probably very low, but it is known that many fetuses with trisomy 18 die in early fetal life.

Classically, babies with trisomy 18 show the following features:

- hypotonia
- SGA
- typical low set malformed (almost 'trumpet-like') ears, a prominent occiput, small mouth and jaw
- typical clenched hands with overlapping index finger and hypoplastic nails
- a short sternum and abdominal herniae, cryptorchism
- 'rocker-bottom' feet
- CHD
- diaphragmatic hernia
- renal tract anomalies.

Most babies with this condition die soon after birth and all longer-term survivors (5–10% survive the first year) have severe developmental retardation.

TRISOMY 13 (PATAU SYNDROME)

This is usually considered a lethal anomaly as most children die rapidly after birth, only occasional children surviving the first month. All long-term survivors appear severely developmentally retarded. The range of chromosomal arrangements may be found but the majority are complete trisomy 13. These children have:

- severe hypotonia, often with CNS malformations such as holoprosencephaly
- microcephaly

- microphthalmos, colobomata
- cleft lip and palate
- abnormal auricle development
- capillary haemangiomata and parieto-occipital scalp defects
- overlapping index finger, polydactyly, flexion deformities of hands (camptodactyly) with simian crease
- 'rocker-bottom' feet
- cryptorchism
- complex CHD
- diaphragmatic hernia.

TURNER SYNDROME (XO)

Most XO fetuses die early in gestation. Antenatal diagnosis may be suggested by increased nuchal skin folds. Neonatal identification, where unsuspected, may be relatively difficult, but XO often presents as a female infant with a relatively broad ('shield') chest and congenital lymphoedema (80%), manifest as puffy hands and feet. Webbing of the neck and hypoplastic wide-spaced nipples may be found. Thirty per cent have a bicuspid aortic valve and 10% coarctation of the aorta, and thus routine cardiac USS is indicated following neonatal diagnosis. The longer-term problems with reduced cognitive scores, short stature and infertility mean that expert counselling is recommended and long term follow-up undertaken. Egg donation programmes have enabled XO females to give birth.

PRADER–WILLI AND ANGELMAN SYNDROMES (15q11 MICRODELETION)

These two syndromes present with the same microdeletion. Prader–Willi syndrome may present as a hypotonic newborn with typical almond shaped eyes and oval face, whereas symptoms of Angelman syndrome ('happy puppet') do not present until early childhood. Children with Prader–Willi will show hypogonadism and obesity with a compulsive eating disorder and learning difficulties in later childhood. The microdeletion in this condition tends to affect the paternally derived chromosome, whereas it is the maternal chromosome that is affected in children with Angelman syndrome. Some cases arise from uniparental disomy.

DIGEORGE/SHPRINTZEN SYNDROME (22q11.21–q11.23 MICRODELETION)

These two syndromes are also examples of one important microdeletion, which is usually only detectable by FISH. The DiGeorge sequence follows abnormal development of the fourth branchial arch and the third and fourth branchial pouch derivatives, with anomalies in thymic and parathyroid development in association with aortic arch anomalies (and some minor facial dysmorphisms). The same genetic defect also appears to cause a more pervasive disorder, Shprintzen syndrome (velocardiofacial syndrome), in which anomalies outside the branchial arch/pouch structures are found and, importantly, include learning disabilities and short stature with a typical phenotype. Specific investigation for the microdeletion should be undertaken in all aortic arch anomalies and parents should be investigated for Shprintzen syndrome in all cases where this is positive.

Other anomalies

Congenital anomalies relating to the following systems are found in their appropriate chapters. Skin (Ch. 18); CNS (Ch. 12); eye (Ch. 17); GI system (Ch. 9); cardiovascular system (Ch. 7); respiratory system (Ch. 6); renal and urinary systems (Ch. 10); congenital hip dislocation and talipes (Ch. 19).

CRANIOSTENOSIS

This is premature fusion of the bones of the skull which may lead to characteristic and progressive skull deformity. It must be distinguished from postural plagiocephaly, a postnatal deformity caused by moulding of the head consequent on a preferred position. This is usually occipital and due to back-lying. In craniostenosis, the suture lines may be ridged and the deformity is progressive, whereas in postural plagiocephaly the sutures are flat and the condition resolves over the latter half of the first year. Craniostenosis is found in several syndromes, some of which are genetically determined and have other marker anomalies. Radiological confirmation of the synostosis is required and surgical intervention necessary, the best results coming from procedures carried out in the first few months after birth.

CHOANAL ATRESIA

A bony or membranous obstruction to the posterior nares may present with signs of respiratory obstruction at birth, as babies are obligate nasal breathers (rapidly overcome with an oropharyngeal airway). Aspiration of the anterior nares often produces a typical jelly-like mucous cast. Unilateral lesions may present later. After failing to pass a nasal catheter, the lesion should be confirmed by X-ray; MRI and CT may give clearer views — discuss investigation with a paediatric radiologist. Surgical correction is undertaken.

CLEFT LIP AND PALATE

Cleft lip may occur as a unilateral or bilateral defect, with or without an associated palatal defect. Isolated palatal defects also occur. In 10%, other anomalies are found. Polygenetic inheritance is likely and a family history should be sought, in which case the recurrence risk rises to about 1:20 (see Ch. 16).

PIERRE–ROBIN SEQUENCE

In this anomaly, a small jaw (micrognathia) results in posterior placement of the tongue root and failure of palatal development, with a superiorly angulated tongue and a typical rounded posterior palatal defect. It may be associated with other anomalies, particularly of the heart. It may present with respiratory obstruction at birth, and may be ameliorated by prone positioning which may allow the tongue to fall out of the airway. Intubation is difficult and the placement of an oral airway must be done with care to ensure it is over the obstructing tongue. Management is as for cleft lip and palate but, for a proportion of children, the respiratory obstruction is a major issue and may lead to life-threatening obstructive episodes, hypoxia and cor pulmonale. Management includes oxygen saturation monitoring, careful positioning and the use of an airway which may impede feeding. The small jaw tends to grow out over the first 2 years.

THE TONGUE AND MOUTH

Neonatal teeth, usually lower incisors, are not infrequently present at birth. They require a dental opinion and removal if loose or supernumerary. Primary dentition erupts normally.

Macroglossia may be relative to a small mouth (Down syndrome) or real (Beckwith syndrome) and in time require surgical attention, although it tends to reduce in size with age.

Retention cysts under the tongue are sometimes found (ranula or epulis) and require surgical removal.

Tongue ties are not uncommon and, despite folklore to the contrary, may require surgical freeing if interfering with feeding or speech.

MALFORMATIONS OF THE EXTERNAL EAR

Absence of the external ear, poor pinnal development, the presence of ear pits or skin tags may all occur. More major lesions may be part of a syndrome (Goldenhaar, Treacher–Collins) and have associated anomalies. It is important that hearing is carefully assessed and imaging may be necessary to define internal structure, especially if the external auditory meatus is absent. Refer early for specialist plastic surgery/ENT help if a major lesion is found. Ear tags should be removed surgically.

CYSTIC HYGROMA

These are sporadic multicystic lymphangiomas which are commonly found in the neck or axilla. They may cause respiratory embarrassment and surgical removal may be necessary and extremely difficult. On the limbs, as with haemangiomas, they may be associated with limb overgrowth.

THE VATER (VACTERL) ASSOCIATION

This is a non-random association of **V**ertebral defects, **A**norectal anomaly, **T**racheo-**E**sophageal fistula and oesophageal atresia and **R**enal anomalies, with which **C**ardiac defects and **L**imb abnormalities are often found (VACTERL) and occasionally genital anomalies and a single umbilical artery. Although early development may be slightly delayed, long-term cognitive outcome is usually normal unless it occurs as part of a wider spectrum disease (e.g. trisomy 18). The association occurs sporadically.

POTTER SEQUENCE

This is the compressed appearance which is found in association with oligohydramnios or renal agenesis (Potter syndrome). There is a flattened face and ears with limb deformations. Such children usually have severe pulmonary hypoplasia and will not survive the neonatal period. The sequence may also occur in other causes of urinary obstruction. Where it is secondary to oligohydramnios due to non-renal tract causes, the pulmonary hypoplasia may not be as severe and outcome is less compromised.

LIMB ANOMALIES

Limbs may be absent (amelia), hypoplastic or show defects of the proximal segment (phocomelia), the distal segment (hemimelia) or a lateral segment (radial hypoplasia). Radial defects may be associated with cardiac, renal or platelet disorders.

Digit anomalies are not uncommon. Polydactyly is usually manifest as a rudimentary digit attached to the ulnar surface of the hand, which should be removed surgically. In Afro-Caribbean families there may be a dominant inheritance. More substantial extra digits and syndactyly may be associated with other syndromes (e.g. Apert syndrome: coronal synostosis and syndactyly).

Arthrogryposis (multiple joint contractures) may be the end result of a variety of different aetiologies, ranging from muscular disorders (myotonic dystrophy), neurological disorders (severe spinal muscular atrophy or meningomyelocele), abnormal joints or fetal constraint (e.g. Potter sequence), although many cases appear idiopathic. Precise diagnosis is important for counselling and management. Arthrogryposis due to neuromuscular disorders has a poor prognosis, but where oligohydramnios and fetal compression have occurred, steady improvement may occur.

DWARFISM

The differential diagnosis of extremely short babies with abnormal body proportions may be very difficult and the causation ranges over a variety of conditions, in some of whom the prognosis is reasonable (e.g. achondroplasia). Some present with pulmonary hypoplasia and do not survive the neonatal period (Table 4.5). Precise diagnosis is again critical for counselling and often rests on expert assessment of a skeletal survey.

Table 4.5 Frequently lethal neonatal bone dysplasias presenting as dwarfism

Condition	Inheritance
Achondrogenesis	Recessive
Chondroectodermal dysplasia	Recessive
Jeune's type thoracic dystrophy	Recessive
Majewski and other short rib-polydactyly syndromes	Recessive
Metatrophic dwarfism	Recessive
Severe type hypophosphatasia	Recessive
Thanatotrophic dwarfism	Usually sporadic
Osteogenesis imperfecta congenita	Uncertain (some recessive)
Camptomelic dwarfism	Uncertain (some females are XY)

FURTHER REFERENCE

Gorlin R J, Cohen M M, Levin L S (1990) Syndromes of the head and neck. New York: Oxford University Press.

Harper P S (1993) Practical genetic counselling, 4th edn. London: Wright.

Jones K L (1997) Smith's recognizable patterns of human malformation, 5th edn. Philadelphia: WB Saunders.

OMIM(TM): Online Mendelian Inheritance in Man (2000). McKusick-Nathans Institute for Genetic Medicine, John Hopkins University (Baltimore, MD) and National Centre for Biotechnology Information, NLM (Bethesda, MD). URL: http://www.ncbi.nlm.nih.gov/OMIM/

Smith D W (1981) Recognizable patterns of human deformation. Philadelphia: WB Saunders.

FIVE

Birth injuries

Obstetric trauma is much less common than was previously the case, but it remains a significant cause of early neonatal morbidity. Risk factors are:

- surgical delivery (forceps, vacuum, caesarean section)
- malpresentation (face, brow, arm)
- preterm delivery
- dystocia
- breech delivery.

Where birth injuries are considered iatrogenic, it is prudent to photograph superficial lesions (e.g. laceration from scalpel incisions during caesarean sections) and to X-ray suspected fractures. It is important to explain the nature of the lesion carefully to parents and to inform the delivery suite staff of the findings and action taken.

The scalp

Oedema of the presenting part (caput succedaneum) usually settles rapidly over 1–2 days without problems.

Oedema following vacuum extraction ('Chignon'):
- usually settles rapidly
- may be associated with local skin trauma requiring attention or occasionally with local haemorrhage
- very occasionally scars.

Direct trauma to the skin may follow the application of forceps, scalp electrodes or scalp pH sampling.

- These injuries rarely cause major long-term problems.
- Sometimes injuries are followed by fat necrosis (small firm moveable masses usually over the mandible or zygoma that persist for 4–6 weeks and resolve).

- Pressure necrosis may evolve over the first few days following birth and be mistaken for a parietal skull fracture (see also aplasia cutis Ch. 18).

SUBAPONEUROTIC HAEMORRHAGE

- This is extensive bleeding into the space beneath the epicranial aponeurosis.
- Often there are few local signs, but occasionally one finds a boggy generalised swelling.
- Systemic effects may be immediate (shock) or delayed (jaundice, anaemia) but these are unusual.
- Management of acute symptoms is as for acute haemorrhage.

CEPHALHAEMATOMA

- This is a common injury.
- Bleeding occurs into the subperiosteal space usually over the parietal (or sometimes occipital) bones.
- The diagnosis is made when the non-pitting swelling is limited by the suture margins.
- The swelling is maximal usually on the second postnatal day.
- Over time, the margins of the haematoma calcify, producing a hard ridge.
- Complications are rare and no action is usually required (aspiration is not indicated).
- Once the swelling has reduced over 1–2 weeks, the parietal rim may take several months to settle. This should not be confused with a fractured skull.

The face

Facial 'cyanosis', bruising or petechiae are not uncommon following local pressure around the neck from the cord or birth canal. The cyanosis in this situation is confined to the face; peripheral cyanosis is not present in the nail beds and no action is usually indicated.

Superficial injuries are common and usually settle rapidly — e.g. subconjunctival haemorrhages, swelling, bruising.

FACIAL NERVE PALSY

- This is usually unilateral.
- It is thought to result following pressure from the ischial spine on the side of the face during descent of the head; as this

indicates some degree of disproportion, these children are often also delivered using forceps (which are erroneously blamed).

- Asymmetry of the face occurs during crying — the eye on the affected side remains open and the mouth is drawn to the opposite (normal) side.
- No specific action is required unless the eye remains open and the conjunctiva seems at risk, when methylcellulose eye drops should be used and antibiotic cream prescribed as indicated by the clinical appearances.
- Recovery usually occurs over the first 1–2 weeks.
- If it persists, consider congenital syndromes, e.g. Moebius syndrome, especially if bilateral.
- Occasionally nerve grafts are needed.

Brachial plexus injury

The brachial plexus may become injured during stretching of the neck during difficult delivery, which is usually complicated by shoulder dystocia. Such injuries may also be associated with fracture of the clavicle, and rarely other fractures, dislocation or injuries.

UPPER PLEXUS LESION (ERB'S PALSY)

- This is the commonest lesion, involving C5–C6 roots.
- The arm is held in limp extension with forearm pronation, and the presence of unopposed wrist flexion produces the typical waiter's tip posture.
- X-ray of the spine and chest are required to rule out bone injury, if suspected.
- Passive gentle physiotherapy may be taught to the parents, in order to discourage contractures, and is usually the only treatment required.
- Referral for nerve or tendon transfer should be made within the first 6 weeks, particularly if there is no sign of recovery in biceps tone. Referral for nerve conduction studies may also be helpful in assessment.
- Recovery usually occurs within 6 weeks but is complete in only two thirds of cases.

OTHERS

Complete brachial plexus palsy

- Second commonest.
- Involves C5–T1 roots and presents with a flaccid arm.

Lower plexus lesion (Klumpke's paralysis)

- Rare.
- This involves C8–T1 roots (and therefore may be associated with a Horner's syndrome).
- Affects the small muscles of the hand and the flexors of the wrist, producing the typical 'claw hand' deformity.

Most of these lesions also recover and management is as for Erb's palsy.

Fractures

SKULL FRACTURES

These are not uncommon and usually require no treatment. Depressed fractures are very rare and surgical advice is indicated.

CLAVICLE

- Fractures of the clavicle are most commonly seen following either shoulder dystocia or trauma to the arms during a breech delivery.
- They occasionally present with clinical signs (break ± crepitus) or 'pseudo-paralysis' of the arm on the same side as the fracture.
- The diagnosis should be confirmed by X-ray (such fractures are often found incidentally when a CXR is taken for other reasons). NB. In any suspected fracture, where none is found suspect osteomyelitis.
- An accurate diagnosis is important as this encourages gentle handling with analgesia if necessary.
- If the child is thought to be in pain (this is unusual), support from a typical 'figure-of-eight' bandage may be helpful.

CERVICAL SPINE

- A rare but usually very severe injury.
- Associated with breech extraction or abnormal in utero posture ('deflexed' head/extended neck).
- It has a predilection for the C6–C8 region, although other vertebrae are occasionally involved.
- Presentation:
  — apnoea and flaccid paralysis, often with facial sparing
  — phrenic nerve injuries are apparent in the acute phase but often recover subsequently
  — urinary retention should be sought and managed appropriately.
- Permanent quadriplegia is likely.

LONG BONES

- Long bone fractures are sometimes found following difficult or breech deliveries.
- These are usually midshaft or result from avulsion of the lower femoral or tibial epiphyses.
- If suspected from clinical examination, X-ray (angulation, shortening, pseudo-paralysis, swelling).
- Simple splinting is usually all that is required and most bones heal very satisfactorily with rapid remodelling.
- An orthopaedic referral is prudent.

Soft tissue trauma

Visceral trauma may follow manipulation of the abdomen during breech delivery or caesarean section, but is very *rare*. Subcapsular haematoma of the liver or rupture of the spleen may present as life-threatening conditions requiring urgent treatment for haemorrhagic shock.

Breech delivery may also be associated with extensive skin, testicular and muscle haemorrhage. In these situations, jaundice may be troublesome but it is rare that a coagulopathy coexists, even with quite extensive bruising (either as a primary/secondary event).

Torsion of the testes may present as an old (hard enlargement, painless) or fresh (soft swelling, painful) lesion (see Ch. 16).

SIX

Cardiorespiratory care

Causes of respiratory distress

Many very different conditions present with 'respiratory distress' — the combination of raised respiratory rate, chest wall recession with or without cyanosis. The commoner causes are shown in Table 6.1. Although it may appear easy to determine the cause of a baby's respiratory symptoms on clinical grounds, precise diagnosis, including chest X-ray, is critical to facilitate planned management.

RESPIRATORY DISTRESS SYNDROME (RDS)

This is the commonest cause of respiratory symptoms in the premature newborn and occasionally occurs in more mature babies. The frequency is increased with increasing prematurity, maternal diabetes, acute perinatal hypoxia and caesarean section and is decreased where there has been prolonged rupture of membranes, mild growth restriction and maternal opiate addiction. The most important underlying cause is the inability of the lung epithelium to secrete sufficient surfactant to replace losses after birth. Other contributory factors include delayed clearance of lung fluid, inadequate lung inflation (because of hypotonicity and a soft rib cage) and pulmonary arterial constriction. The clinical picture of RDS is worse if the baby becomes cold, acidotic or hypoxic, if there is congenital bacterial infection or if the child fails to develop an adequate FRC after birth, and therefore care must be directed to optimising the child's condition as soon as possible (see Ch. 3).

Prevention

Corticosteroids. The administration of two doses of beta- or dexamethasone 12–24 h apart between 1 and 7 days before birth has been shown in randomised trials to reduce the frequency of RDS by 40% and also to improve mortality and other neonatal outcomes. Shorter periods before, and delay in, delivery have reduced effects. Antenatal steroids encourage surfactant

Table 6.1 Causes of respiratory distress in the newborn

Early onset (<4 h age)	Later onset
Common respiratory causes	
RDS	Pneumonia
Transient tachypnoea	Collapse/consolidation
'Congenital' pneumonia	Pulmonary haemorrhage
MAS	Pneumothorax, other air leaks
Pneumothorax	Pulmonary hypertension
Pulmonary hypertension	Aspiration of milk
	Congestive cardiac failure
	(PDA, CHD, fluid overload)
	CLD
Systemic illness	
Anaemia	Anaemia
Hypothermia	Sepsis/meningitis
Mild encephalopathy	Acidosis
Hyperviscosity syndrome	Myocarditis
Acidosis	
Aspiration of milk (consider	
possibility of oesophageal atresia)	
Aspiration of blood, amniotic fluid	
Malformations	
Pulmonary hypoplasia	Congenital diaphragmatic hernia
Congenital diaphragmatic hernia	CAM
CAM	Congenital lobar emphysema
Congenital lobar emphysema	
Mediastinal duplication cysts	
Upper airway obstruction (choanal	
atresia/Pierre–Robin sequence)	

production and have other fetal effects (e.g. mature lung antioxidant systems). There appears to be no increased risk of infection or other significant side effects, although steroids may be less effective in situations where the risk of RDS is reduced. The use of multiple weekly or fortnightly doses of steroids in at risk women has not been systematically studied. Other antenatal interventions have not been shown to be effective (e.g. maternal TRH administration).

Delivery room care. Good delivery room care may reduce the severity of later lung disease. In one study of very preterm babies, prior to the use of steroids or surfactant, intubation at birth was associated with decreased mortality, rates of RDS and other neonatal complications, presumably by the establishment of a more optimal FRC than the baby can develop itself. Although routine intubation is not generally recommended, staff should maintain a low threshold for intervention for very preterm babies (see Ch. 3).

Presentation and treatment after birth

- Tachypnoea, chest wall recession, grunting, flaring of the ala nasae and cyanosis commence within the first 4 h of birth (usually <1 h).
- CXR shows typical reticulogranular pattern ('ground glass' appearance) with air bronchograms and usually reduced lung volume.
- The illness worsens progressively over the first 48–72 h and regresses after about 96 h as endogenous surfactant secretion is induced.
- Management is aimed at optimising the baby's condition until endogenous improvement commences.

Surfactant replacement therapy has been available since the early 1990's. Four preparations are currently available in the UK (Table 6.2). 'Natural' surfactants have a more rapid onset of action than do artificial products. All are more effective if given very early in the illness and, unless the practice in your unit is to administer in the delivery suite, should be given to all babies ventilated for presumed RDS who need >30% oxygen as soon as possible after intubation, with a second dose 8–12 h later if the illness persists. Later ('rescue') therapy for severe disease is less effective.

Table 6.2   Commercially available surfactants (UK 1999)

	Source of product	Dosage	Volume	No. of doses
Colfosceril palmitate (Exosurf Neonatal)	Artificial	67.5 mg/kg	5 mL	2–3
Pumactant (ALEC)	Artificial	100 mg/kg	2 mL	2–3
Poractant alfa (Curosurf)	Natural derived (porcine)	100 mg/kg	1 mL	2–3
Beractant (Survanta)	Natural derived (calf)	100 mg/kg	4 mL	1–4

Notes
1. Surfactant is best administered as a bolus injection into the ETT. With the larger-volume preparations, this is often done as two aliquots.
2. The practice of varying the posture of the baby during the instillation has little evidence base.
3. Practice varies widely but instillation of surfactant is usually followed by a period of bag ventilation before reconnection. Some units use various ventilator tubing ports to administer the drug while continuing ventilation.
4. A second dose after 8–12 h is usually dependent upon response; where F_IO_2 has reduced to <0.3, we do not give a further dose.
5. There is little evidence to support the practice of routinely giving two doses to extremely immature babies.

For some children, three or four doses may be required. Usually, this is where other complications are present which tend to inhibit surfactant activity, such as infection or meconium in the airways. Pulmonary haemorrhage occurs in about 6–8% of children following surfactant therapy.

Outcome following RDS

Most children recover well from this condition and have few directly attributable long term consequences. A proportion who are the sickest and most immature will develop chronic lung disease (CLD formerly known as bronchopulmonary dysplasia). The reasons for this are poorly understood, but barotrauma, volume trauma and oxygen toxicity are candidate aetiologies.

CLD is defined by oxygen requirement and typical CXR changes at 28 days of age. In practice this is not useful as treatment needs to be commenced earlier than 28 days to minimise longer-term problems and the most immature babies are almost always receiving oxygen at 28 days. As an outcome measure, CLD is now usually reported at 36 weeks gestation-equivalent age, defined by need for oxygen and CXR appearances.

About 18% of babies ventilated for RDS have CLD defined at 28 postnatal days, but only 4–6% at 36 weeks post-conceptional age.

WET LUNG (TRANSIENT TACHYPNOEA OF THE NEWBORN, TTN)

- Respiratory symptoms occurring usually after term birth due to delayed clearance of lung fluid.
- Particularly common following elective caesarean section; symptoms come on over the first 4 h.
- Tachypnoea is usually the most predominant sign, with grunting and cyanosis.
- CXR shows streaky changes, fluid in the horizontal fissure and often air-trapping.
- Oxygen requirement is usually mild (30–40%) and settles rapidly.
- A small proportion develop persisting pulmonary vasoconstriction and take 3–4 days to settle.
- This is always a diagnosis of exclusion and it is frequently impossible to differentiate this benign condition from bacterial infection in the initial phase.

CONGENITAL PNEUMONIA

- This may occur at any gestation and is often indistinguishable from other causes of respiratory distress.

- Associated with prolonged rupture of the membranes and colonisation of the birth canal with group B (β-haemolytic streptococcus, *E. coli* and *Listeria*, among other organisms.
- May present as septicaemia with secondary RDS or as a primary pulmonary pathology.
- Onset as for RDS (sometimes delayed for up to 24 h) with often identical CXR appearances. Beware the asymmetrical CXR or the 'RDS pattern' that is not homogenous.
- Associated with early-onset apnoea, shock and hypotension. Good respiratory and circulatory support is critical to survival.
- Treatment initially is with broad-spectrum antibiotics (commonly penicillin and gentamicin) following culture of blood, tracheal aspirates and CSF if appropriate.

MECONIUM ASPIRATION

This occurs in about 5% of babies born with meconium stained liquor, usually identified at birth with particulate meconium in the airway. Good delivery room care is essential (see Ch. 3). The presence of meconium in the airway may cause mechanical obstruction, chemical pneumonitis and inhibition of surfactant. Associated pulmonary vasoconstriction may be severe and predominate. Of all indications, this is the one most effectively treated by ECMO (see below).

- Presents soon after delivery, often with severe respiratory distress and cyanosis.
- CXR shows overinflation with patchy consolidation. Air leaks are common.

ACQUIRED CONDITIONS

Pulmonary air leaks (see p. 97)

Pulmonary haemorrhage (see p. 99)

Pleural effusion

This may accompany or cause hydrops fetalis. Aetiology also includes chylothorax, pneumonia, cardiac failure and infection. CXR shows opacity which may differ from the adult picture because the child is usually supine leading to small collections of fluid behind the lung, and sometimes may be more easily seen using a lateral decubitus or shoot though lateral X-ray. May be treated by aspiration or formal drainage if symptomatic.

Pulmonary consolidation/collapse

During mechanical ventilation, or occasionally following birth, areas of collapse and consolidation are found which may be difficult to differentiate from infection. Plugging of large airways should be treated with physiotherapy and tracheal toilet (see Ch. 20), with antibiotic cover as appropriate. Only rarely is bronchoscopy helpful.

Lobar emphysema

This may complicate recovery from RDS. It is usually right-sided and follows pulmonary interstitial emphysema; the CXR is diagnostic, showing hyperinflation and cystic changes in one lobe. Bronchoscopy may be of value in diagnosis and lavage. Selective intubation of the contralateral bronchus or balloon dilatation of a narrowed bronchus may be required, but open surgical procedures are rarely needed. External drainage is unnecessary and dangerous.

CONGENITAL

Pulmonary hypoplasia

This is associated with oligohydramnios, fetal pleural effusion, neuromuscular disorders and diaphragmatic hernia, usually presenting during the second trimester or earlier. Respiratory failure may be severe and air leak and pulmonary vasoconstriction are common complications.

Diaphragmatic hernia

Now frequently diagnosed antenatally, these occasionally present after birth, usually immediately but may be delayed for 24 h (see Ch. 16).

- Respiratory distress is variable, but may be severe and inhibit resuscitation.
- Clinical signs of mediastinal shift (usually to the right) and scaphoid abdomen.
- X-ray is diagnostic, with air-filled loops of bowel in the chest; it is occasionally difficult if the gas pattern is not established or if the abdomen is not included on the film.
- Survival is dependent upon the degree of associated pulmonary hypoplasia and/or other associated abnormalities.

Lung malformations

Cystic adenomatous malformation (CAM) usually presents as a one-sided cystic mass which may be confused with a diaphragmatic hernia. Associated with preterm delivery and hydrops fetalis. Three types are described, classified by cyst size. Antenatally diagnosed lesions may resolve spontaneously; postnatally, treatment is by lobectomy.

Congenital lobar emphysema. This is characterised by overexpansion of one part of the lung due to bronchial obstruction (stenosis, plugs, mucosal folds) or external bronchial compression (cysts, aberrant vessels, tumours). Usually a single lobe is involved (50% left upper, 28% right middle, 20% right upper). Classic appearance occurs following aeration, which may be delayed. Treatment is usually by surgical removal of the affected lobe/segment.

Early management of the infant with respiratory symptoms

SCENARIO 1: THE ANTICIPATED DELIVERY OF A VERY PRETERM INFANT (<30 WEEKS) (see also Ch. 3)

- An experienced resuscitator should be present. Following delivery and attention to thermal care, a careful assessment of the infant is made.
- For births below 30 weeks gestation, there should be a low threshold for intubation and ventilation as it is likely that this will better establish FRC and minimise the initial illness.
- The use of 100% oxygen should be avoided if possible (may cause cerebral and retinal vasoconstriction). It is preferable to use air/low-concentration oxygen unless cyanosis persists despite adequate ventilation.
- Once intubated (unless the baby is very vigorous), maintain gentle IPPV until assessed in the neonatal unit.
- Administer surfactant if intubated and requires >30% oxygen to remain pink.
- Ventilator and supportive care as below.

SCENARIO 2: THE NEWBORN INFANT WHO DEVELOPS RESPIRATORY DISTRESS AFTER BIRTH

- Many infants remain tachypnoeic for 1–4 h after delivery, during the period of early adaptation. Infants who have been allowed to get cold may grunt, and therefore close attention to thermal control will avoid unnecessary admission to the neonatal unit and separation from the family.
- Children with major signs of respiratory problems should be admitted to the neonatal unit for assessment — (recession ± grunting, cyanosis, poor peripheral circulation). Children with tachypnoea alone and who are not cyanosed may be reassessed after a short period (<1 h), as should children at high risk of respiratory illness (e.g. following meconium aspiration from

trachea). Admit babies whose tachypnoea or grunting does not settle over the first 4 h or in whom symptoms seem to be worsening. Do not wait 4 h if the child is ill, as this may be the first presentation of bacterial infection.

- The differential diagnosis of the infant's symptoms must include infection, and appropriate cultures should be taken and broad-spectrum antibiotics commenced.
- In an ill child who is not responding to simple measures, the first CXR should not be delayed until 4 h.

Respiratory support

HEADBOX OXYGEN

The cyanosed infant should be given oxygen by an appropriate route without delay, in increasing concentration to abolish central cyanosis. Some newer incubators may provide humidification and oxygen directly into the circulating gas and have servocontrol mechanisms for maintaining a stable concentration; for other situations this is supplied via a headbox.

In the child who seems to require oxygen concentrations over 30%:

- apply a transcutaneous or saturation oxygen monitor
- obtain a blood gas
- order a CXR — the optimal time for this is > 4 h after birth (most fetal lung fluid cleared by this time)
- insert an arterial catheter early in the course and monitor blood pressure, correct hypotension or poor perfusion as necessary
- consider the precise diagnosis
- if infection is in the differential diagnosis (usual situation) take appropriate samples and commence broad-spectrum antibiotics (e.g. penicillin and gentamicin).

Consider the need for respiratory support:

- CPAP is suitable for RDS if the main issue is oxygenation and inspired oxygen concentrations are over 40–50%.
- Intubation and ventilation if:
  — P_aO_2 <6.0 kPa (45 mmHg) and inspired oxygen concentration >80%
  — P_aCO_2 >8.0 kPa (60 mmHg), or >7.5 kPa (55 mmHg) and pH <7.15
  — apnoeic/collapsed.
- Do not leave the extremely immature baby struggling in increasing concentrations of oxygen in the first 24 h; intubate early (if inspired oxygen concentration >40%).

CPAP

Indications
- RDS — (start if inspired oxygen concentration >40% and P_aO_2 <6.5 kPa (50 mmHg). There is evidence that even small infants may be successfully managed using CPAP without continuing to IPPV.
- Weaning from mechanical ventilation for small infants — by prevention of post extubation atelectasis, may reduce need for re-ventilation.
- Recurrent apnoea — by increasing respiratory drive, may reduce periodicity of breathing.

Methods of application
- Double nasal prongs attached to a CPAP valve/ventilator circuit
- Single nasal prong (shortened ETT cut to length of palate — measure from lips to tragus of ear) providing nasopharyngeal CPAP attached to a ventilator circuit
- The EME Infant Flow Driver system — dedicated venturi-driven CPAP system with monitor.

Other methods, e.g. using a face mask or ETT (rarely indicated as it increases the work of breathing by extending dead space), have largely fallen into disuse. CPAP is usually well tolerated by very small infants but often not by larger babies.

Procedure
1. Start at a CPAP of 5–6 cmH$_2$O, with a similar F_iO_2 to that in the headbox.
2. Place a gastric tube on free drainage to reduce gastric distension.
3. Increase F_iO_2 as appropriate, using monitoring and blood gases (take first blood gas sample 30 min after establishing CPAP).
4. CPAP may be temporarily increased to 7–8 cmH$_2$O in RDS if hypoxia not resolving.
5. Note that where CPAP improves lung inflation by preventing atelectasis, the P_aCO_2 will fall, whereas applying CPAP to well inflated lungs may reduce CO$_2$ elimination.
6. As the child's condition improves, wean first the F_iO_2, then decrease the CPAP in 1 cmH$_2$O steps to 3 cmH$_2$O before removing prongs.
7. If inspired oxygen concentrations increase >80% (P_aO_2 <6.0 kPa [45 mmHg]) or P_aCO_2 >8.0 kPa (60 mmHg), abandon CPAP, intubate and ventilate.

Although CPAP is generally well tolerated, watch for sudden deterioration because of pneumothorax. Take care in positioning prongs over long periods of time, as nasal distortion and even septal necrosis may occur.

There have been reports of successful prophylaxis against apnoea using IMV or even SIMV via nasopharyngeal tubes. Take care not to increase the ventilator rate over 10–15 breaths/min (prefer 5–10) as this may actually impede respiration (use a longer inspiratory time, e.g. 0.5 s, and low pressure (15 cmH$_2$O).

MECHANICAL VENTILATION

Although it is usually clear if a baby requires ventilation, it is important to intervene early if a baby is deteriorating — intubation should be an elective procedure (see Ch. 20); avoid emergency intubation and the need for resuscitation.

Indications for intubation and ventilation

- P_aO$_2$ <6.0 kPa (45 mmHg) and inspired oxygen concentration >80% (despite CPAP if appropriate)
- P_aCO$_2$ >8.0 kPa (60 mmHg), or >7.5 kPa (55 mmHg) and pH <7.15 (note that higher P_aCO$_2$ values may be tolerated in the face of CLD or a compensated respiratory acidosis)
- Apnoeic/collapsed.

Types and modes of ventilation

Conventional ventilators. Most neonatal ventilators in current use are time-cycled, pressure-limited machines which provide ventilation at a range of rates from 1 to >100/min. Several have a variety of modes (see Fig. 6.1). In addition, new volume-limited and hybrid machines are becoming available but, as their role is not as yet established, these are not discussed further.

High-frequency oscillatory ventilators. High-frequency ventilation is currently popular for babies whose respiratory disease is refractory to conventional treatment and in some centres for the primary treatment of RDS in very preterm children, although experimental evidence of effectiveness for this last indication is awaited.

HFOV is a method of mechanical ventilation which employs supraphysiological breathing rates and tidal volumes which are frequently less than dead space. This method aims to avoid large pressure and volume swings at bronchiolar/alveolar level and thus to minimise the risk of complications such as air leaks and later CLD. The strategy of HFOV depends on:

- inflation of the lungs and recruitment of lung volume by the application of distending pressure (MAP)
- alveolar ventilation and CO$_2$ removal by the imposition of an oscillating pressure waveform on the MAP.

Negative pressure ventilators. Negative pressure ventilation has been advocated for a range of conditions, including RDS and

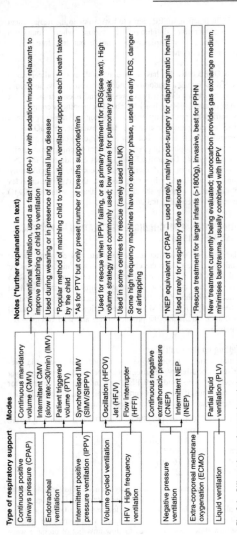

Fig. 6.1 Different forms of neonatal respiratory support.

Type of respiratory support	Modes	Notes (*further explanation in text)
Continuous positive airways pressure (CPAP)		
Endotracheal ventilation	Continuous mandatory volume (CMV)	*Conventional ventilation, used as fast rate (60+) or with sedation/muscle relaxants to improve matching of child to ventilation
	Intermittent CMV (slow rate: <30/min) (IMV)	Used during weaning or in presence of minimal lung disease
	Patient triggered volume (PTV)	*Popular method of matching child to ventilation, ventilator supports each breath taken by the child
Intermittent positive pressure ventilation (IPPV)	Synchronised IMV (SIMV/SIPPV)	*As for PTV but only preset number of breaths supported/min
Volume cycled ventilation	Oscillation (HFOV)	*Used for rescue when IPPV failing, or as primary treatment for RDS(see text). High volume strategy most commonly used; low volume for pulmonary airleak
HFV High frequency ventilation	Jet (HFJV)	Used in some centres for rescue (rarely used in UK)
	Flow interrupter (HFFI)	Some high frequency machines have no expiratory phase, useful in early RDS, danger of airtrapping
Negative pressure ventilation	Continuous negative extrathoracic pressure (CNEP)	*NEP equivalent of CPAP — used rarely, mainly post-surgery for diaphragmatic hernia
	Intermittent NEP (INEP)	Used rarely for respiratory drive disorders
Extra-corporeal membrane oxygenation (ECMO)		*Rescue treatment for larger infants (>1800g), invasive, best for PPHN
Liquid ventilation	Partial liquid ventilation (PLV)	New treatment currently being evaluated; fluorocarbon provides gas exchange medium, minimises barotrauma, usually combined with IPPV

CLD. In practice, CNEP seems to have value in the management of postoperative diaphragmatic hernia, where long-term ventilation is contemplated (>7 days), but has found little application elsewhere.

ECMO. Recently this has become available at several centres in the UK following a randomised study. It is an invasive technique requiring cannulation of major vessels and is only indicated for larger infants (>1800 g body weight). For conditions complicated by refractory pulmonary vasoconstriction, in association with MAS or congenital pneumonia, for example, ECMO seems particularly effective, but for conditions complicated by pulmonary hypoplasia (e.g. with congenital diaphragmatic hernia) this is less clear. Generally, ECMO is not considered if the CNS prognosis is poor or if there is an uncorrected coagulopathy. Consider in refractory hypoxia, calculate the oxygenation index (often used to quantify the shunt) and discuss with the ECMO centre early (see Table 6.3).

CONVENTIONAL MECHANICAL VENTILATION — PRACTICAL CONSIDERATIONS

The goals of ventilation are to facilitate gas exchange whilst minimising the risk to the child from complications such as air leak and CLD. Most neonatal ventilation is applied to treat RDS and, for this indication, the pressure-limited system is most efficient. Within this conventional practice, oxygenation is determined by F_iO_2 and MAP and ventilation (or CO_2 elimination) by minute ventilation (the product of rate and tidal volume – see Fig. 6.2).

Setting up the ventilator

Initial settings depend upon the clinical indication and pre-existing ventilatory requirements. For RDS, generally long inspiratory times and high PEEP are indicated; in contrast, for normal lungs, meconium aspiration or air leak, these settings are inappropriate. Suggested initial settings are:

F_iO_2:	0.4–0.5 (40–50%) — or 10% more than F_iO_2 before ventilation
Ti:	0.4 (0.3–0.6) s
Rate:	60 (50–70) /min
PIP:	18 (16–20) cmH₂O
PEEP:	4 cmH₂O

The inspiratory pressures may then be adjusted to produce gentle movement of the chest wall, and the F_iO_2 adjusted to abolish cyanosis. With variable flow rate ventilators and lungs without intrinsic lung disease (e.g. when ventilating for apnoea), use low flow rates (5 L/min) to slow upswing of pressure wave

Table 6.3 Pulmonary gas calculations

Alveolar air equation and derived measures
The calculation required to work out alveolar oxygen tension (P_AO_2) is:
$$P_AO_2 = P_IO_2 - [(P_ACO_2/R) + (P_ACO_2 \times F_IO_2 (1-R)/R)]$$
The *alveolar air equation* may be approximated as:
$$P_AO_2 = P_IO_2 - P_ACO_2$$
and *inspired oxygen tension* (P_IO_2) as:
$$P_IO_2 = F_IO_2 \times (B - \text{water vapour pressure})$$
or
$$P_IO_2 = F_IO_2 \times (760 - 47)$$

a:A ratio
The ratio between arterial and alveolar oxygen tensions:
$$P_aO_2 : P_AO_2$$

A:aDO_2
The alveolar arterial oxygen difference:
$$P_AO_2 - P_aO_2$$
This is the most frequently used measure: the bigger the value, the larger the intrapulmonary shunt:
- Adults: usually 10–20 mmHg (1.3–2.7 kPa)
- Newborns after birth: 40–50 mmHg (5.3–6.7 kPa)
- Newborns first few days: 20–40 mmHg (2.7–5.3 kPa)

In severe RDS it may rise to 600 mmHg (80 kPa).

Oxygenation index (OI)
This is a measure of arterial oxygenation by ventilation and inspired oxygen:
$$OI = \frac{MAP \times F_IO_2}{P_aO_2} \times 100$$
This is often used by ECMO centres to give some idea of the severity of lung disease and therapy. Levels >10 are associated with moderate disease and >25 with severe disease (approx. 50% mortality).

P_AO_2, alveolar oxygen tension (mmHg); P_IO_2, inspired oxygen tension (mmHg); P_ACO_2, alveolar CO_2 tension (effectively equates to arterial CO_2 tension (mmHg)); R, respiratory quotient (usually approximates to 0.8); B, barometric pressure (mmHg); MAP, mean airway pressure (cmH$_2$O); F_IO_2, fractional inspired oxygen (0.21–1.0); P_aO_2, arterial oxygen tension (mmHg) — should be a post-ductal sample.

(using fixed flow machines, switch to round wave mode), slow rates (15–20/min) and lower pressures of 12–14/3–4 cmH$_2$O. Volume-limited ventilation may be more appropriate for such applications.

Adjusting the ventilator
Measure blood gases 30 min after each ventilation change, noting the settings on oxygen and CO_2 monitors if used. Adjust the MAP and ventilation (Fig. 6.2) to maintain blood gases in the ranges shown in Table 6.4.

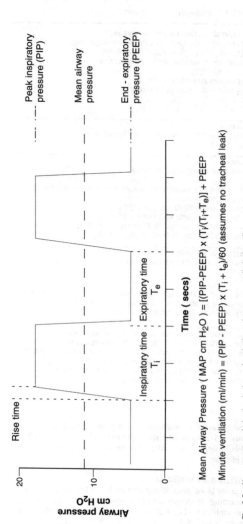

Mean Airway Pressure (MAP cm H_2O) = $[(PIP-PEEP) \times (T_i/(T_i+T_e)] + PEEP$

Minute ventilation (ml/min) = $(PIP - PEEP) \times (T_i + t_e)/60$ (assumes no tracheal leak)

Fig. 6.2 Airway pressure during inspiration and expiration using a pressure-limited ventilator system.

Table 6.4 Blood gas measurements to be aimed for in conventional mechanical ventilation

Parameter	Range	Notes
P_aO_2	6.5–10 kPa (50–80 mmHg)	In the extremely preterm baby, aim for slightly lower levels of oxygen (5.8–7 kPa) to minimise risk of retinal vasospasm with high oxygen tensions. In the term baby with pulmonary hypertension, aim for the higher end of the range to maximise its pulmonary vasodilator effect; use higher levels in the presence of CLD (see p. 105)
P_aCO_2	4.5–6.5 kPa (35–50 mmHg)	Overventilation (using low P_aCO_2 values) is associated with an increased risk of CLD and cerebral ischaemia — in the presence of good perfusion it is preferable to allow these levels to rise slightly to 7 kPa rather than to pursue vigorous ventilation.
pH	7.25–7.35 (first few days, 7.3–7.4 thereafter)	Accept a mild degree of acidosis in the first few days and concentrate on maintaining perfusion. In extremely preterm babies, renal bicarbonate loss may produce acidosis with alkaline urine (pH >6); parenteral nutrition may also induce acidosis unless buffered using metabolisable base.

The general principles of ventilation centre around minimising the effect of barotrauma by ventilating with the minimal pressure to achieve adequate (not necessarily normal) blood gases. It is important to observe the child carefully — there should be synchronous respiratory activity and only gentle movement of the chest. The use of continuous oxygen and CO_2 monitors may be helpful in fine tuning ventilation, avoiding frequent blood gases. In small infants, saturation monitors are not helpful and may be dangerous as they will underestimate hyperoxia (Fig. 6.3).

To remove more CO_2, consider the following options:
• increase ventilator rate
• increase the size of each breath ($\uparrow$ PIP or $\downarrow$ PEEP)
• ensure that the inspiration:expiration (I:E) ratio allows sufficient time for expiration (at high rates, should not be >1:1)
• observe respiratory activity carefully — is the baby fighting the ventilator or is the chest wall moving with inspiration? (see below).

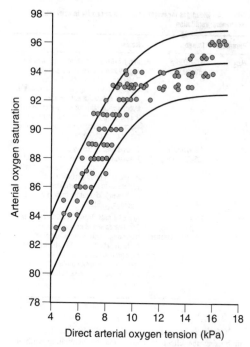

Fig. 6.3 Comparison of transcutaneous SaO₂ with arterial oxygen tension in vivo. (Adapted from Wasana A, Whitelaw AGL 1987 Arch Dis Child 62: 957–971.)

To improve oxygenation, consider the following options:
- Increase F_iO_2
- Increase the MAP by one of the following changes:
  — ↑ I:E ratio (i.e. ↑ Ti)
  — ↑ PIP
  — ↑ PEEP
  — ↓ inspiratory rise time (variable flow ventilators only) by increasing ventilator gas flow rate — check PIP and PEEP after this change
- Observe respiratory activity carefully — is the baby fighting the ventilator or is the chest wall moving with inspiration? (see below).

- Does the baby need a dose of surfactant?
- Is there a suspicion of PPHN (see below)?

Troubleshooting

Acute clinical deterioration — sudden onset of hypoxaemia ± hypercarbia ± peripheral circulatory failure.

Action. Disconnect from ventilator and ventilate using a self-inflating bag.

Response.
- Condition improves — rectify ventilator fault
- Condition remains poor
  — has the child extubated?
  — assess airway (ETT position and patency)
  — consider possibility of pneumothorax.

Slow clinical deterioration — slow worsening of condition ± hypercarbia.

Action. Assess airway and interaction with ventilator:
- Is the chest still inflating?
- Is the respiratory disease getting worse?
- Consider disconnection and bag ventilation
- Assess non-respiratory systems.

Strategies to minimise interaction

For the ventilation of non-compliant, atelectatic, surfactant-deficient lungs, this system functions well. However, babies often appear unsettled during conventional mechanical ventilation and various strategies have been developed to entrain the baby's respiratory drive in order to minimise interaction or asynchrony, such as:

- *'Fast rate' ventilation* — in this scenario the ventilator rate is adjusted to be faster than the child's spontaneous respiratory rate, in order to minimise interaction and suppress spontaneous activity.
- *Use of muscle relaxants* — the infant's interaction is abolished during paralysis; however, ventilator pressures often need to be increased and fluid balance problems are common. Over the past 5 years, their use in small infants has fallen out of favour, although they are of great value in the term baby ventilated for many indications. Note that pancuronium and gentamicin should not be used together as they potentiate each other's effects. We use atracurium, which is short-acting and does not accumulate during infusion.
- *Use of analgesics and sedatives* — the intention here is to sedate the infant to minimise activity against the ventilator;

however, available sedatives are not good at suppressing spontaneous respiration unless large doses are used (associated with cardiovascular side effects), and other methods of entraining the child's ventilation should be considered. Intubated infants should generally receive analgesics on humanitarian grounds, unless being prepared for extubation.

- *Synchronised ventilation using trigger systems* — this has the promise of maximising the use of the child's spontaneous respiratory activity and minimising the additional support provided by the ventilator. Results of trials of this style of ventilation paradoxically suggest higher rates of pneumothorax.

Weaning

The management of a sick ventilated infant demands accurate diagnosis so that predictions can be made about the likely response to treatment — expect a very preterm infant with RDS to have increasing ventilator requirements for longer than a child ventilated prior to surgery. Once the condition is stable, weaning may commence. A good principle is that, once you feel that the child is (or should be) improving, an alteration should be made with each blood gas result — do not allow a child to remain on the same ventilator settings with normal blood gases unless a positive decision has been made to do so for other reasons. Leaving a child on high ventilator pressures as the lung compliance is improving following RDS runs the risk of pneumothorax.

Weaning may be accomplished using PTV or SIMV (see below). If weaning during conventional mechanical ventilation is desired:

- reduce PIP in steps of 2 cmH$_2$O to 16 cmH$_2$O.
- reduce rate in steps of 10 breaths/min to 30 breaths/min and then in steps of 5 to 10 breaths/min.
- extubate into headbox or onto nasal CPAP if very preterm.

Patient-triggered ventilation (PTV)

Theoretically if the ventilator could be used to support the baby's own breath, adverse interaction would not occur and lung injury may be reduced, although this benefit has not been supported by large-scale randomised trials. Two modes of triggered ventilation are used:

- *PTV.* Ventilation rate is determined by the baby's own rate. Breaths are detected by an airway flow or pressure sensor (occasionally via impedance electrodes or abdominal sensor); the ventilator responds to each sensed breath but has a variable operator-set back-up rate if the trigger mechanism fails.
- *SIMV/SIPPV.* The ventilator delivers a preset number of breaths which are synchronised with the infant's breath but

which will also be delivered even if breaths are not sensed (useful in weaning).

Apart from the very smallest infants, most babies will trigger modern ventilators satisfactorily. The use of large doses of sedatives or of muscle relaxants will prevent this. A useful strategy is to try to use PTV during the early phase of the disease, except in the smallest infants, watching the baby carefully to confirm that the triggering is effective. Once settled on PTV, the disease process follows its normal course. Weaning is possible using a progressive reduction in inspiratory pressure or by switching to SIMV (see below).

Critical to the success of PTV is the ability of the ventilator to sense a breath, to respond rapidly to it and to complete its inspiratory support phase before or soon after expiration has commenced. Hence, when setting up PTV:

- reduce the Ti to 0.28–0.35 s.
- set a back-up rate of about 50% of the spontaneous respiratory rate.
- switch to PTV, observing the baby's response.
- Adjust the sensitivity of the trigger system and reduce the Ti if necessary until every breath is supported.
- watch the child for several minutes to confirm that the triggering is functioning well.
- measure blood gas within 30 min and adjust settings as required.

Note that to increase MAP or ventilation, the PIP must be increased.

Weaning via PTV. Gradually reduce the PIP to 12 cmH$_2$O or lower prior to extubation.

Weaning via SIMV. Change to SIMV at a rate equivalent to half of the child's spontaneous rate (usually <40/min); wean by progressively reducing SIMV rate to 5–10 /min prior to extubation; leave PIP ≥16 cmH$_2$O.

HIGH-FREQUENCY OSCILLATORY VENTILATION

Types of ventilator

Three ventilators are available in the UK at the time of writing:

Sensormedics 3100A. Oscillation is provided by a heavy duty 'loudspeaker' diaphragm placed in the inspiratory limb, producing oscillation in airway pressure with both positive and negative pressure components. It is a dedicated oscillator, but has restrictions in the positioning of infants during its use and is noisy.

However, it is the most powerful machine available and will ventilate children well into the PICU age range (~ 30 kg).

SLE 2000HFO. Oscillation is provided by a rotating jet in the expiratory line, which can be combined with conventional ventilation, although the value of these combinations is uncertain. This ventilator is useful for babies up to about 4.0 kg, depending on pulmonary compliance.

Drager Babylog 8000. Oscillation is provided by a small diaphragm and negative pressure induced using a venturi device. Oscillation may be combined with other modalities. This ventilator is only useful for small infants (approx. 2000 g or less) in oscillation mode.

Principles of HFOV

In its usual 'high volume' application, lung inflation is provided by a continuous distending pressure, which is usually 2–6 cmH$_2$O higher than the MAP during conventional ventilation. This optimises the lung surface area available for gas exchange. Mechanical forces act to minimise pulmonary vascular resistance and the combination maximises ventilation–perfusion matching. Because this technique reduces alveolar collapse and the need for reinflation, it should preserve endogenous surfactant and minimise traction forces on the alveolar–bronchiolar interface, which may contribute to the development of CLD. The major danger of this strategy lies in overdistension of the airways. In addition to local lung injury and risk of air leak, high airway pressure compresses the alveolar vessels, increasing pulmonary vascular resistance, and will reduce venous return to the heart and reduce cardiac output. Optimal oxygenation is achieved, therefore, by gradually increasing MAP to recruit lung volume while monitoring arterial oxygenation and lung volume using regular X-rays.

Ventilation, in contrast, is provided by varying the airway pressure around the MAP. Although the amplitude of each 'breath' appears large by comparison to conventional ventilation pressures, the attenuation of oscillation through the ETT and the respiratory tree means that the transmitted amplitude at the level of the alveolus is very small. CO$_2$ elimination is still dependent on tidal volume, but, with increasing ventilator frequency, lung impedance and airway resistance increase, so the tidal volume delivered to the alveoli decreases. This leads to the apparent paradox that increasing ventilator frequency may reduce CO$_2$ elimination, leading to raised P_aCO$_2$. Rate is measured in Hertz (10 Hz = 600 breaths/min) and ventilator pressure is measured using the difference between the peak and trough of the oscillation, measured at the T-piece, termed amplitude or dP (ΔP) and measured in cmH$_2$O.

In animal experiments, HFOV causes less lung trauma than does conventional ventilation, and human experiments to determine the place of HFOV in the early treatment of RDS are underway; early results from recent trials seem promising. HFOV has an established place as a rescue therapy where respiratory failure has supervened and may be used in conjunction with nitric oxide therapy in scenarios where previously referral for ECMO was the only option. In trials in the USA, HFOV/INO has been shown to reduce the need for ECMO.

All children are initially placed on a high volume strategy, using the principles outlined above but for children with air leak, a low-volume/high F_iO_2 strategy is preferred in the longer term.

Indications

- RDS unresponsive to, or deteriorating despite, surfactant therapy
- MAS
- Pulmonary interstitial emphysema (low-volume, high F_iO_2 strategy)
- RDS plus TOF
- Persistent pulmonary hypertension
- Pneumonia
- Congenital diaphragmatic hernia
- Pulmonary hypoplasia.

Adjusting the oscillator

- When commencing HFOV, start with the MAP at 2 cmH$_2$O above that on conventional mechanical ventilation; if commencing HFOV de novo for RDS, commence at 8 cmH$_2$O.
- Set the frequency to 10 Hz and amplitude (ΔP) to 20 cmH$_2$O; increase amplitude until oscillation is gently visible over the whole precordium.
- Increase MAP slowly (1 cmH$_2$O/10–20 min) until oxygenation starts to improve. In treating RDS, the target is to reduce inspired oxygen to at least 25–35%. Less ambitious targets are usually accepted during rescue therapy.
- CXR at 1 h after commencing HFOV will allow the estimation of lung volume — about eight ribs should be visible posteriorly. Intercostal bulging, air under the cardiac shadow and flattened diaphragms are ancillary signs of overdistension and should lead to a reduction in MAP.
- Beware of increasingly bad gases despite turning the MAP up — consider overdistension or hypovolaemia (a low circulating blood volume may be unmasked during oscillation and it is wise to ensure good circulatory filling before commencing HFOV; hypovolaemia may be revealed if manual pressure over the liver — to increase venous return — rapidly results in improvement in blood gases).

- Once stable, MAP and amplitude should be reduced steadily depending upon the results of blood gas analysis and X-ray. MAP can be reduced to 6–7 cmH$_2$O before extubation.

GENERAL SUPPORTIVE CARE DURING VENTILATION

Thermal control. Manage in an incubator, set skin temperature to 36.5°C if using servo control.

Blood pressure and perfusion. Assess perfusion regularly and monitor BP through an indwelling arterial line if regular blood gas monitoring is required. Most early metabolic acidaemia is related to perfusion; acidosis and hypotension exacerbate pulmonary vasoconstriction — early use of volume expansion and inotropes is encouraged.

Minimal handling. The widespread availability of reliable remote sensors and indwelling arterial lines means that the handling of the child can be minimised. Most children deteriorate during periods of handling and positive action should be taken to avoid unnecessary intervention.

Comfort. In adult or paediatric practice there is no discussion as to whether sedatives or analgesics are necessary; we recommend low- to medium-dose opiate infusions to facilitate comfort during ventilation. Additional analgesia is still necessary during painful or unpleasant procedures (e.g. chest drain insertion or intubation). The immediate environment may be adjusted to enhance comfort, and prevent deformation of the soft newborn skeleton, and the child may be clothed once the initial illness has settled.

Fluids are managed as discussed in Chapter 8. It is prudent to be cautious with fluids until a good urine output is established. Enteral feeds are usually delayed until there is circulatory stability (12–24 h). Subsequently, small quantities of milk, preferably the infant's own mother's colostrum, may be given to enhance gut activity. These may be increased slowly over the first few days. The presence of an indwelling UAC does not constitute a barrier to increasing feeds, which if tolerated have beneficial effects in terms of gut adaptation, nutrition and comfort.

Investigations. Serial haematology, glucose and electrolyte/renal function investigations should be monitored daily during the initial phase, the latter until urine output is established. Maintain haemoglobin at 12 g/dL or above during early intensive care. Monitor bilirubin levels if jaundiced — remember that lower levels for phototherapy and exchange transfusion are recommended for ill babies.

PROBLEMS ARISING DURING VENTILATION

Air leak

Extra-alveolar air may track into any of the chest structures — pleura (pneumothorax), interstitium, mediastinum, pericardium — and into the neck and abdomen. Small amounts of extra-alveolar air cause little problem and resolve rapidly, but if under tension they may severely compromise the child, causing collapse and death. Pneumothorax and pneumopericardium respond well to drainage if symptomatic (Ch. 21).

Pneumothorax

- Suspect whenever a baby's condition worsens during respiratory support:
  — clinical evaluation of the chest may reveal displacement of mediastinum, asymmetric expansion or breath sounds
  — size of ECG complex on monitor may have decreased suddenly (as the heart moves away from the ECG leads)
  — diagnosis of pneumothorax in small babies is easily achieved by transillumination with a cold-light source; darken the room or use suitable incubator cover — beware larger infants (false negatives are common) and hydrops fetalis (false positives)
  — do not use needle aspiration to diagnose air leak, as you may convert a manageable situation into a crisis by causing an air leak.
- CXR will identify all significant air leaks, a horizontal beam film may be helpful if in doubt, but X-ray not necessary if transillumination identifies a pneumothorax.
- Mature, unventilated infants with pneumothorax who have minimal symptoms and no evidence of mediastinal shift on CXR may be nursed in high inspired oxygen concentrations — the nitrogen in the pleural space is absorbed into the blood, encouraging resolution.
- In an emergency, following diagnosis, needle aspiration may be helpful whilst preparing for formal chest drain — the treatment of choice (see Ch. 21).
- Beware pleural air following chest surgery — aspiration of the normally present air following repair of a diaphragmatic hernia may cause mediastinal shift and severely compromise the baby.

Pulmonary interstitial emphysema

- Suspect if ventilation becomes more difficult. There are no localising signs. CXR is diagnostic, with honeycomb pattern of air (probably in lymphatics). Differentiate from distended bronchioles seen during high-pressure ventilation.

- This condition is very difficult to treat and many manoeuvres will not have the desired effect. The goal should be to reduce MAP as much as possible, even if this means allowing the F_iO_2 to rise — to achieve this, increase rate and shorten Ti.
- Where unilateral, an experienced clinician may consider selective intubation of the other lung.
- HFOV (low-volume strategy) may be helpful.

Pneumomediastinum

- This rarely needs intervention by itself.
- May occasionally lead to surgical emphysema in the neck and free abdominal air.
- Maintain low-pressure strategy.

Pneumopericardium

- This is a rare complication, which presents as tamponade.
- Drainage by needle aspiration may be attempted by an experienced clinician.

Persisting arterial duct (PDA)

A clinically apparent PDA is found in the majority of extremely preterm babies undergoing ventilation, particularly the sick or hypoxic child. In more mature children, this prevalence falls off rapidly. Doppler studies show that the duct is frequently open even if clinically 'silent' and may still compromise respiratory care. In the non-ventilated very preterm child, the decision to intervene becomes more difficult. The PDA in most asymptomatic well preterm infants will close spontaneously by 46 weeks postconceptional age. Early use of indomethacin on empirical or echocardiographic grounds (without symptoms) is currently being studied.

Regular assessment for signs of a PDA is necessary during ventilator care. These include:

- bounding, high-volume peripheral pulses
- active precordial impulse
- cardiac murmur — usually systolic, maximal upper left sternal border, radiates to back, only occasionally continuous machinery murmur
- cardiomegaly and pulmonary plethora on CXR.

Management

- The role of fluid restriction is debatable; conventionally restrict to 75% requirement.
- Diuretics: Furosemide (frusemide) 1–2 mg/kg 12-hourly.
- If the above methods do not result in reduction in symptoms within 24 h, consider indomethacin therapy.
- If indomethacin fails after two courses, or is contraindicated, consider surgical ligation.

Indomethacin. Prostaglandin synthetase inhibitors (indomethacin, ibuprofen) alter the balance of prostaglandins acting on the smooth muscle of the arterial duct and encourage constriction. Indomethacin is the widest used and most studied to date; initial results using ibuprofen are encouraging.

Several dose regimes are in current use (total dose 0.6 mg/kg):

- 0.2 mg/kg IV or oral 12–24 hourly for three doses
- 0.1 mg/kg IV or oral daily for six doses
- 0.2 mg/kg IV followed by 0.1 mg/kg daily for four doses.

Side-effects are common with indomethacin — transient oliguria, hyponatraemia, GI bleeding (reduced platelet aggregation), reduced CBF and displacement of bound bilirubin. Re-opening rates and side-effects are less with the longer low-dose course; closure rates appear similar. Occasionally the higher-dose regime is given with concurrent frusemide.

Caution is neccessary if there is:

- active bleeding or thrombocytopenia (platelet count $<100 \times 10^9$/L)
- high creatinine (>110 mmol/L)
- high bilirubin (close to exchange level; see Ch. 9).

Surgical ligation is occasionally performed in the neonatal nursery, with minimum disturbance for the child. Postoperative pulmonary vasospasm may occur.

Pulmonary haemorrhage

Massive pulmonary haemorrhage (MPH — haemorrhagic pulmonary oedema) is a life-threatening condition, associated with asphyxia, hypothermia, surfactant and tolazoline therapy and coagulopathies. Acute haemorrhage (trauma, coagulopathy) into the airway may be difficult to differentiate. MPH tends to occur during weaning from ventilation and is recognisable by a dramatic deterioration in condition associated with copious volumes of bloodstained fluid which well up from the ETT.

Action (in addition to general supportive care)
- Try not to remove ETT if in situ, unless blocked — it may be difficult to replace!
- Increase PEEP by 2–3 cmH$_2$O
- Give diuretics: Furosemide (frusemide) 1–2 mg/kg stat.
- Send sample for coagulation screen; meanwhile give FFP 10 mL/kg, consider a further dose of vitamin K and transfuse if blood loss is high
- Consider HFOV and, paradoxically, further doses of surfactant in the very sick child, as blood inhibits surfactant activity.

Infection

Intercurrent infection may complicate ventilator therapy. Usually this will be systemic infection due to colonisation of lines. Suspect respiratory infection if:

- increase and changed nature of secretions from ETT
- patchy changes on CXR
- generalised signs of sepsis or change in sepsis indicators (CRP, WCC, etc.; Ch. 13).

Take samples for culture (include ET secretions) and commence on broad-spectrum antibiotics.

Persisting hypoxaemia

If the P_aO_2 remains consistently below 5.5 kPa (40–45 mmHg) in the face of adequate ventilation (ie normal P_aCO_2):

- Is the baby fighting the ventilator?
- Is there increased intrapulmonary shunting through unventilated sections of lung?
- Is there persistent pulmonary hypertension and extra-pulmonary shunting?

Consider:

- increasing the ventilator rate > spontaneous (70–80 breaths/min)
- the use of sedatives/muscle relaxants (see above — paralysis may worsen ventilation)
- PTV
- HFOV
- the use of pulmonary vasodilators (see PPHN, below).

Persistent pulmonary hypertension of the newborn (PPHN)

PPHN may occur as a primary condition or complicate several neonatal scenarios, such as RDS, MAS, polycythaemia and pulmonary hypoplasia. It may be induced by hypoxia, acidosis and cold injury and following collapse with pneumothorax. Several vasodilators are currently available:

- Nitric Oxide (INO) — (inhalation)
- Prostacycline — (infusion, case reports of successful nebulisation)
- Tolazoline — (bolus and infusion, case reports of successful intratracheal instillation)
- Magnesium sulphate — infusion
- Sodium nitroprusside — infusion
- Glyceryl trinitrate (GTN) — infusion.

INO has recently become available and has been the subject of much research. It is probably the most effective of the above and its use is attended with minimal side effects (see below). Intratracheal administration of tolazoline or prostacycline may avoid many of the systemic side-effects noted below, but as yet their use via this route remains experimental. Concerns remain about long-term effects of INO, but the same caveat applies to all of the above drugs.

Systemic administration of vasodilators other than INO is attended with major cardiovascular side-effects, as none are specific pulmonary vasodilators. Prostacycline and GTN infusion (the latter is an NO donor) are particularly useful as, if hypotension occurs, the infusion may be stopped and the short drug half-life ensures rapid reversal of effect. Tolazoline must be used with great caution as the hypotensive effects may be profound. Magnesium infusion has only been studied in a few infants but its effect is delayed compared with the other preparations. It may also cause hypotension in addition to sedation and a reduction in respiratory drive. GTN and INO work via the same route but the effects of all others seem to be additive.

Critical to the use of all vasodilators is the optimisation of conventional management prior to that use. None is particularly effective in the presence of acidosis, poor perfusion or severe ventilatory failure. Indeed, optimisation of these variables will often reverse pulmonary hypertension without recourse to vasodilators. Prior management will thus include the following:

Perfusion
- Assess: capillary return, peripheral pulses, BP, pH and base deficit
- Management
  — optimise circulatory volume (use plasma 10–20 mL/kg and observe effect, repeat as necessary)
  — consider using CVP measure (if BP remains low)
  — use dopamine 5–10 micrograms/kg per minute; observe effect
  — consider adding dobutamine 5–10 micrograms/kg per minute.

Ventilation
- Optimise $P_a CO_2$ to 4.5–6.5 kPa (30–50 mmHg).
- Do not hyperventilate ($P_a CO_2$ <3.5 kPa [25 mmHg]) as this may impair cerebral circulation and worsen barotrauma.
- If pH and perfusion are satisfactory then higher $P_a CO_2$ values may be tolerated.
- Use HFOV as indicated (there is evidence that HFOV and INO may have additive effects in term infants; in preterm infants HFOV may be better at improving V:P matching than INO).
- Use muscle relaxants as indicated, particularly in term infants.

- Consider the use of surfactant up to 6-hourly in term infants and extra doses in the very preterm.

General supportive care
- Optimise opiate dosage.
- Ensure adequate thermal control.
- Minimal handling (this will often improve baby's condition on its own).
- Appropriate use of antibiotics.

Monitoring
- Continuous transcutaneous or IA monitoring should be established out of choice.
- It may be useful to use saturation monitors in tandem to record pre-and post-ductal saturation if an UAC is not used.
- Transcutaneous P_aCO_2 monitoring is also invaluable in this situation.

INHALED NITRIC OXIDE

Investigations prior to INO therapy
- CXR — to exclude air leak, etc.
- Coagulation screen — INO may exacerbate bleeding tendencies; repeat each day during therapy.
- Cerebral ultrasound (intracranial haemorrhage has been a contraindication to INO use in many studies – the use of INO in the presence of significant haemorrhage must be considered carefully; repeat scan daily).
- Baseline methaemoglobin (metHb) estimation — aim to keep below 5%, monitor 12-hourly; no need to delay while this becomes available.

Suggested protocol for administration of INO
1. Monitor inspired NO and NO_2 continuously during use.
2. Commence NO at 5 ppm, increasing at 30 min intervals in 5 ppm steps to 20 ppm depending upon response (defined as increase in P_aO_2 greater than 3–4 kPa).
3. If no response to 20 ppm, a trial of 80 ppm for 60 min is indicated.
4. Failure at this level requires rapid weaning in 10 ppm steps back to 20 ppm (each step being held for 10–15 min).
5. Watch carefully for a fall in P_aO_2 during rapid weaning as this sometimes occurs and would indicate that the process should be done more slowly.
6. In the face of a good response to INO therapy, the dose should be weaned to the minimum consistent with this response. Generally this will be around 5 ppm. However, following a response at a particular dose level, weaning should be done slowly (8–12 hourly steps of 3–5 ppm down to a minimum of 2 ppm from whence INO may be stopped).

7. Sometimes weaning from INO can be very prolonged and the child may seem very sensitive to small drops and brief periods of disconnection. Care must therefore be taken even when the child appears better and stable.

8. Care must be taken when the child is disconnected from the ventilator for periods of time greater than a few seconds (e.g. during suction). If bag and mask ventilation is required, a T-piece should be used to provide flow at the same rate with the same concentration of INO as used on the ventilator.

9. Stop (or reduce) INO if airway NO_2 >5 ppm, metHb >5% or active bleeding is present.

USE OF OTHER VASODILATORS

Epoprostenol (Flolan (PGI_2; prostacycline)). This was the most widely used vasodilator prior to INO therapy becoming available. Start infusion (no bolus) at 5 nanograms/kg per min and increase in steps of 5–10 nanograms/kg per min to a maximum of 40 nanograms/kg per min. Higher infusion rates may sometimes be effective but use is limited by hypotension. Short half-life (3 min); rapid reversal of systemic hypotension over 15–30 min; may produce cutaneous flushing or geographic erythema.

Tolazoline. Give as an initial bolus of 1 mg/kg over 5 min to assess response; stop injection if effect is obtained or if BP falls. If effective without hypotension establish an infusion of 0.1 mg/kg per h. Side-effects include hypotension, prerenal failure, severe gastric and mucosal bleeding (gastric histamine effects) and rarely thrombocytopenia. Hypotension may take some time to resolve and requires urgent action. Rashes as for Epoprostenol.

Magnesium sulphate. This blocks calcium entry into cells and causes vasodilatation. Infuse 200 mg/kg of hydrated $MgSO_4$ ($MgSO_4 \cdot 7H_2O$) over 20–30 min. Larger doses may cause collapse and the sedative and hypotensive effects of this drug may limit its usefulness, as they may be slow to resolve. If effective, try 20–60 mg/kg per h by infusion, aiming to keep serum magnesium over 3.5 mmol/L. This intervention is the least well supported by published evidence.

Apnoea

Apnoea is a final common symptom for a range of diagnoses in neonatal medicine. Often associated with bradycardia and hypoxia, apnoea is a particular problem in the very preterm infant, until around 33–34 weeks gestation equivalent age and, as such, may simply represent immaturity of the cardiorespiratory control centre and periodic breathing. A diagnosis of 'apnoea of prematurity' is, however, one of exclusion having satisfied yourself that an underlying pathology is unlikely.

Apnoea may occur at the following times:

During ventilation

- Normal during high rate IPPV, HFOV or if overventilated, i.e. in association with an abnormally low $P_a\text{co}_2$:<3.5 kPa (25 mmHg)
- Arising de novo suggests that the ETT is displaced or blocked, or that new pathology has occurred (e.g. pneumothorax, septicaemia or IVH).

During the first day. This is associated with early-onset neonatal sepsis, undertreated respiratory disease or seizures. It is always likely to be significant and demands attention.

Subsequently

- Usually manifest as recovering from respiratory illness or later.
- It is important to rule out infection as a cause, especially when a series of apnoeas commence after a period during which the child has been stable (carry out an infection screen, including an LP, and commence antibiotics unless you are sure you know the cause of the problem).
- Consider:
  — infection: septicaemia, focal infection, catheter-related infection
  — respiratory: atelectasis, pneumonia
  — cardiovascular: congestive failure due to PDA/other cause
  — abdomen: NEC, GOR, other surgical cause
  — GU system: UTI
  — CNS: meningitis, seizures, haemorrhage
  — other: anaemia.

Investigations

Carry out investigations as appropriate following your clinical assessment.

Treatment

- Antibiotics, transfusion (if indicated).
- Commence methyl-xanthine treatment — we use oral/i.v. caffeine; alternatives are theophylline or aminophylline. If apnoeas persist, increase dose and consider measuring blood levels.
- If apnoeas persist, try nasal CPAP (4–5 cmH$_2$O) (see above).
- Consider prone lying and stopping feeds (occasionally reflux may cause apnoea).
- If apnoeas still persist, or if increasing frequency/associated with persisting cyanosis or poor circulation, intubate and commence IPPV, with circulatory support as necessary.

- On occasions it may be helpful to provide low-rate (S)IMV via a nasal prong to avoid reintubation; rates of 5–10 are usually sufficient; if more seem necessary it may be better to intubate and use slow-rate (S)IMV.

Drug therapy may be stopped after symptoms have settled for a few days, but many clinicians continue treatment until a gestational age equivalent of 33–34 weeks has been reached; others continue until out of oxygen if CLD present.

Chronic Lung Disease (CLD)

Defined as above (p. 78). In children who are developing or who have established CLD, there are several common management issues to consider.

Oxygenation

Although oxygen is carefully controlled to avoid hyperoxia in very preterm babies during their initial illness, at the end of the first month it is generally considered that the risk of initiating ROP is low and that it is more important to ensure adequate oxygenation to encourage tissue healing and growth. P_aO_2 should be maintained at around 9–10 kPa (65–80 mmHg) or, if using a saturation monitor, an S_aO_2 >94%. As soon as inspired oxygen falls below 30%, the use of low-flow oxygen via nasal prongs should be considered. This facilitates maternal involvement in care and cot nursing if appropriate. Using low-flow oxygen, the delivery rate is slowly reduced until satisfactory oxygenation is achieved in air. This process may take many months and children who are feeding well may be discharged home on nasal oxygen therapy to be weaned off at home.

Adequate oxygenation is mandatory to achieve good somatic growth.

Nutrition

Tissue healing and, by implication, resolution of CLD will be enhanced by optimal nutrition. Caloric requirements are increased to around 130–150 kcal/kg per day or more in the presence of CLD, secondary to the increased work of breathing. Minimum growth targets of 15 g/day should be carefully monitored. Dietetic help is invaluable. Long term growth may be enhanced by:

- optimising intake to 180–200 mL/kg
- using breast milk fortifiers or preterm formulae (see Ch. 15)
- monitoring alkaline phosphate levels and giving extra phosphate supplements if elevated — children with CLD are at greatest risk of metabolic bone disease

- current research is assessing whether vitamin A supplementation from birth may be effective in minimising CLD.

Use of steroids

Systemic steroids are invaluable in hastening weaning from ventilation in babies developing CLD. However, long periods of treatment with steroids carry significant risks, as in adults, and attempts must be made to use the minimum dose and course consistent with improvement. There is no evidence that steroids shorten oxygen dependency in a baby who is not ventilated. Although most trials have studied the effect of steroids at 3–4 weeks of age, most clinicians now commence treatment when weaning from the ventilator is delayed beyond 10–14 days. A multitude of doses and courses are in use; two suggested regimens are:

- Dexamethasone 0.5 mg/kg i.v. daily (usually given in the morning) for seven doses. If there is rapid weaning from the ventilator to room air, the course may be truncated.
- Dexamethasone 0.2 mg/kg i.v. 8-hourly for 3 days (may be prolonged to 7 days if effect delayed), followed by dexamethasone 0.1mg/kg 8-hourly for 3 days, then 0.1 mg/kg for 3 days and stop.

If markers (ventilator dependency, inspired oxygen concentration) deteriorate on lowest dose or immediately after course, move back one step and prolong the weaning phase, aiming to move to alternate morning doses of 0.1 mg/kg.

Dexamethasone may also be given orally if on full feeds.

Inhaled steroids are of unproven benefit in the management of CLD; nonetheless, many clinicians use metered-dose aerosols (budesonide or beclamethasone 200–400 mg 12-hourly via a suitable inhaler device, e.g. Aerochamber). Administration is difficult and the use of a self-inflating bag to encourage absorption may be necessary. Nebulised drugs have not been found to be effective. Disadvantages in the very preterm population are the encouragement of oral thrush and the possibility that the high doses necessary to achieve any effect may lead to systemic absorption and side-effects. Generally, inhaled steroids are introduced when weaning from dexamethasone has proved difficult.

Systemic, and to a lesser extent inhaled, therapy must be monitored carefully:

- BP twice weekly
- BG daily, urine glucose daily
- oral mucosa and perianal skin (risk of candidiasis)
- growth rate (especially linear growth) weekly.

Particular anxiety has been expressed over the development of steroid cardiomyopathy, which may complicate recovery from CLD when courses are prolonged, and the high rate of neurological sequelae in children with steroids. Most authorities recommend minimising the baby's exposure to steroids whenever possible.

Other medical interventions

Most children with CLD recover slowly and steadily. A few children with the worst symptoms may develop problems of CPAP, ventilator or steroid dependency. They may become very irritable (possibly secondary to hypoxia). A few will develop significant hypertrophy of the right ventricle and benefit from anti-failure treatment.

Several other interventions are occasionally used (much clinical variation in practice):

Diuretics may have significant effects in improving oxygenation even if right heart failure is not present. We use hydrochlorthiazide and spironolactone, monitoring electrolytes and alkaline phosphate as their use will increase urinary mineral loss, despite the use of spironolactone. If effective, continue until off nasal oxygen (usually 2–4 weeks).

Methyl-xanthines are used beyond the normal gestational age range because of theoretical advantage in enhancing diaphragmatic contractility, and continued until oxygen therapy is stopped.

Inhaled bronchodilators (ipatroprium bromide, salbutamol) may occasionally be of value but are not in widespread use.

Sedatives. In more irritable children, occasional doses of chloral hydrate may be helpful. Such treatment should not be commonly used and consideration as to why the irritability is present — hypoxia, cardiac failure, oral hypersensitivity — is mandatory.

Longer-term issues

Because of prolonged hospitalisation, there is a tendency to forget the needs of the family and the wider environment for the child. Appropriate and considered intervention by play therapists may be of value and the development of programmes of play and stimulation to encourage developmental progress, coupled with postural manipulation to discourage the development of deformity (scaphocephaly, extensor postures, hip adductor shortening), is encouraged.

The constant stimulation from interventions around the mouth (intubation, suctioning, gastric feeding, bottle feeding) may lead to difficulties in the establishment of feeding, which are very common in this group. Although there is little evidence for effective interventions, the early involvement of a speech therapist may head off some of these difficulties and a programme of oral desensitisation is only occasionally required.

Outcome

Children with CLD should be followed up in a suitable outpatient clinic with facilities for monitoring growth, respiratory function and neurodevelopment. Most will do well over time but there is a high rate of re-hospitalisation and admission to intensive care for respiratory illness and a significant post-discharge mortality, which recede in the second and third year. Long-term neuro-developmental problems may be more prevalent in this high-risk group. Respiratory function tends to improve, with minimal signs on CXR by 4–5 years and minor abnormalities on respiratory function testing at 9–10 years, although many will need therapy with bronchodilators and inhaled steroids in early childhood. The very long-term outcome for this particular at-risk group has not been documented.

SEVEN

Congenital heart disease*

Background

TRANSITION FOLLOWING BIRTH

Pulmonary artery pressure, which is higher than systemic pressure during fetal life, falls by half within the first 3 days after birth and to normal childhood levels by 6 weeks. The ductus arteriosus closes functionally (by vasoconstriction) by about 12 h of age and anatomically (by involution) over the next few weeks. We have used the terminology *persistent* ductus arteriosus (PDA), rather than patent ductus arteriosus, for a duct which remains open longer than this normal period of closure.

CONGENITAL HEART DISEASE (CHD)

Heart defects are the commonest congenital abnormalities (6/1000 live births):

- one-third will have mild heart abnormalities and never require any treatment
- one-quarter will present before the age of 1 month and these will include the infants with the most severe problems, of whom quarter will die
- 15% of infants with CHD have other extracardiac anomalies
- in the most severe group that present in the first month, a significant proportion have non-cardiac defects and these may contribute to the higher mortality rate.

In most cases, the cause of CHD is not known (Table 7.1).

ANTENATAL DIAGNOSIS OF CHD

A routine antenatal USS scan at 16–18 weeks gestation will detect less than 50% of all CHDs and under 50% of severe cases. AVSD,

---

* Note that the pulmonary circulation, persistent pulmonary hypertension of the newborn, persistent ductus arteriosus and the use of inotropic support are considered in Chapter 6.

single ventricle, hypoplastic left or right heart will be detected but not TGA and Fallot's, the commonest severe lesions. Scanning may miss isolated atrial or ventricular septal defects and CoA. A more detailed scan can detect a higher proportion.

Table 7.1 Associations with congenital heart disease

Chromosomal abnormalities	
Trisomy 21 (Down syndrome)	AVSD, VSD, TF
Trisomy 18 (Edwards syndrome)	VSD, PDA
Trisomy 13 (Patau syndrome)	VSD, PDA
XO (Turner syndrome)	CoA, AS
5p- (Cri-du-chat syndrome)	VSD
Catch 22	TF
Non-chromosomal syndromes	
Skeletal defects	
Ellis–van Creveld	Single atrium
Laurence–Moon–Biedl	TF, VSD
Holt–Oram	ASD, VSD
Fanconi	PDA, VSD
Thrombocytopenia with absent radius	ASD, TF
VACTER association	
Characteristic facies	
Noonan	PS, ASD, HOCM
Smith–Lemli–Opitz	VSD, PDA
De Lange	TF, VSD
Williams	Supravalvar AS, Peripheral PS
Skin lesion	
Leopard syndrome	PS
Neurofibromatosis	PS
Tuberose sclerosis	Fetal cardiac rhabdomyoma (resolves)
Situs inversus	
(Kartagener syndrome)	Dextrocardia
Ivemark syndrome	
(asplenia or polysplenia)	Complex heart disease
Intrauterine infection	
Rubella (especially in the first trimester)	PDA, peripheral PS
Parvovirus	Fetal cardiac failure leading to hydrops fetalis
Other maternal diseases	
Diabetes	HOCM, VSD
Systemic lupus erythematosus	Congenital heart block
Maternal drugs	
Thalidomide	TF, truncus arteriosus
Phenytoin	CoA
Fetal alcohol syndrome	VSD, ASD, TF
Lithium	Ebstein's anomaly

There are other syndromes associated with heart defects (e.g. Marfan syndrome and aortic aneurysm; Friedreich's ataxia and cardiomyopathy; Romano–Ward and arrhythmias) but these do not give rise to problems in the neonatal period and are not included in this table.

Suspected CHD in the newborn

Many cases are now anticipated because of fetal scanning. The place of delivery needs to be decided after consultation with a paediatric cardiologist and a plan of management agreed with the parents and written in the notes.

CHD presents in only three ways in the newborn period: (1) Central cyanosis, (2) Heart failure, and (3) Heart murmur.

CENTRAL CYANOSIS

- One-third of infants with CHD present with cyanosis, usually the more complex causes.
- It is important to differentiate heart disease from other causes of cyanosis (see Table 7.2). Non-cardiac causes should improve with 100% O_2.
- CHD may present as central cyanosis within 48 h of birth, or later depending on the underlying cause (Table 7.3).
- Central cyanosis is best observed in the tongue or mucous membranes, which are always well perfused.
- Cyanosis is clinically detectable if the arterial oxygen saturation is less than 75%, and sometimes at higher saturations because of the high neonatal haemoglobin. If in doubt, use a pulse oximeter (normal > 97%).
- Central cyanosis is more difficult to detect in dark-skinned babies and may be seen in infants with a normal P_aO_2 if there is polycythaemia.
- Peripheral cyanosis is common in the first few days in term infants and of no consequence.

Table 7.2 Causes of cyanosis

True central cyanosis with low oxygen saturation
Respiratory disease (e.g. RDS, MAS, choanal atresia)
Depressed respiration (CNS)
PPHN/PFC
CHD

True central cyanosis with increased deoxyhaemoglobin but normal saturation
Polycythaemia

Apparent cyanosis
Traumatic cyanosis
Sepsis
Shock
Methaemoglobinaemia

Table 7.3   Cardiovascular causes of cyanosis presenting at different ages

Detected within 48 hours
PPHN — Associations are:
- without associated lung disorder
  - idiopathic
  - associated with structural CHD
  - birth asphyxia
  - severe polycythaemia
  - hypoglycaemia
- associated with lung disorder
  - MAS
  - pneumonia
  - RDS
  - congenital diaphragmatic hernia

Transposition of the great arteries
Tricuspid atresia
Total pulmonary atresia or severe PS (with or without an intact ventricular septum)
TAPVD with obstruction

Detected within the first week
Ebstein's anomaly (with right-to-left shunt at atrial level)
AVSD

Detected after the first week of life
Tetralogy of Fallot
TAPVD (obstructed TAPVD may present earlier)

- Healthy term infants may also become centrally cyanosed when crying which causes a right-to-left shunt across the foramen ovale and ductus arteriosus which have not yet closed anatomically.
- Traumatic 'cyanosis' due to bruising may follow a face presentation, but the tongue should be pink in contrast to the lips and face.

Acyanotic CHD accounts for the other two-thirds of cases and is usually less complex than cyanotic heart disease. The presentation may be with heart failure or as a murmur.

HEART FAILURE

- Usually the result of a large left-to-right shunt or to obstruction of blood flow (Table 7.4).
- Clinical features:
  - increased heart rate and respiratory rate
  - hepatomegaly
  - cardiomegaly on CXR, often with pulmonary plethora
  - oedema is uncommon

— auscultation often unhelpful
— sweating often absent
— excessive weight gain not seen if feeding is poor.
● Differential diagnoses:
— other causes of respiratory distress (see Ch. 6)
— fluid overload
— PDA
— structural CHD
— arrhythmias
— myocardial disease
— systemic hypertension.

Table 7.4 Heart failure due to CHD presenting at different ages

Presenting within the first week
Aortic atresia/hypoplastic left heart
Endocardial fibroelastosis
Critical AS
Severe CoA
Systemic hypertension (due either to CoA or renal AS or certain types of CAH) may lead to cardiac failure in the newborn
Larger arteriovenous communications in the skin, brain, lung or liver

Presenting after the first week
VSD
PDA
More complex lesions such as TAPVD, AVSD, truncus arteriosus

HEART MURMUR

There are many more infants heard to have a heart murmur at their routine neonatal check than have CHD. Sorting this out is very important as, otherwise, unnecessary anxiety may be generated and inappropriate referrals made. The typical features of an innocent murmur are listed in Table 7.5.

Table 7.5 Typical features of an innocent heart murmur

● Symptom-free
● Systolic
● Short
● Soft
● Confined to a relatively small area of the chest
● The second heart sound is normally split
● Varies with phase of respiration
● There are no other abnormal cardiovascular signs

- The newborn infant, and particularly the preterm infant, is very small and therefore, not surprisingly, even innocent murmurs can be heard quite widely over the chest.
- Splitting of the second heart sound is almost impossible to distinguish, except by the cardiological cognoscenti.
- Haemodynamically benign heart murmurs may be heard in up to two thirds of otherwise normal healthy term infants (most commonly over the lower left sternal edge or the pulmonary area in the second left intercostal space).
- Transient murmurs of a PDA are heard in 15% of healthy term infants and in the newborn period are usually systolic rather than the continuous murmur typical of the older child.
- Murmurs consistent with a small muscular VSD (high-pitched, blowing and mid-systolic, well localised to the lower LSE) may disappear spontaneously.
- Transient high-pitched pansystolic murmurs of mild mitral or tricuspid regurgitation may be heard following perinatal asphyxia or with pulmonary hypertension, respectively.
- If a soft systolic murmur is found in an acyanotic infant who is otherwise well, referral to a paediatric cardiologist and immediate investigation are both unnecessary; the child should be seen at 4 weeks in a follow-up clinic. At 4 weeks, if the infant is still asymptomatic, thriving and there is an isolated innocent sounding murmur, the child should be seen again at 6 months. If the murmur persists then, ECG and CXR should be performed and either the parents should be told this is an innocent murmur or the child should be referred to a paediatric cardiologist for an opinion.
- Repeated and frequent follow-up is a waste of time and causes much anxiety .

Significant CHD may also present with a murmur in an acyanotic infant and the commonest lesions are as follows:

Persistent ductus arteriosis. This is one of the commonest lesions in the newborn period, particularly in the preterm infant (see below). The murmur may be either systolic or continuous. In the presence of central cyanosis (provided this is not due to RDS), such a murmur is suggestive of associated pulmonary atresia, severe PS or tricuspid atresia with blood flow to the lungs via a wide open ductus. PDA is also associated with CoA and VSD.

Ventricular septal defect. This is the commonest lesion in CHD, but only 10% of all VSDs ever become haemodynamically significant. Left-to-right shunt murmurs, such as those of a VSD or PDA, may not be heard until the second to fourth week of life when the pulmonary artery pressure falls below systemic arterial pressure.

Pulmonary stenosis. This is a common cause of systolic murmur, loudest over the upper LSE in the newborn period. If the PS is severe, the infant will be cyanosed because of right-to-left shunting through the foramen ovale.

Coarctation of the aorta. This accounts for 10% of neonates with severe CHD, is usually preductal and over three-quarters will have another associated cardiac malformation. Systemic blood flow to the lower body will be duct dependent and once the ductus arteriosus closes, clinical deterioration may occur as lower body perfusion is compromised. The commonest association is with a VSD. A rarer lesion is complete interruption of the aortic arch (associated with DiGeorge's syndrome); presentation is similar to that of CoA.

Aortic stenosis or other rarer causes of left ventricular outflow obstruction. An extremely important point is that many newborn infants with major structural cardiac defects do not have a loud heart murmur. CoA may present with severe heart failure but without an impressive murmur, and hypoplastic left heart syndrome and transposition of the great arteries usually present with cardiac failure and cyanosis, respectively, but with no murmur audible.

Essentially, an asymptomatic but significant murmur usually means AS, PS, acyanotic Fallot's or a VSD. After these come more complex lesions. A heart murmur explanation sheet with advice on what to look for (poor weight gain, slow to feed, breathless, sweaty, blue around the mouth) is useful for parents.

Isolated atrial septal defects never present in the newborn period.

Apart from these three classic presentations of cyanosis, heart failure or a murmur, a term newborn may present on the postnatal ward with a 'funny turn'. This may be a feature either of a cyanotic spell, an apnoea or cardiogenic shock (hypoplastic LV, coarctation). Classic symptoms of cardiac failure such as poor feeding or sweating on feeding are rarely seen in the newborn period.

CLINICAL DIAGNOSIS

Definitive clinical diagnosis is often very difficult in the newborn period because the physical signs are less easily elicited.

History
Important points are gestation, maternal drugs, problems in labour and early asphyxia, length of time for which membranes were ruptured and the presence of meconium, the type of delivery, and any CTG abnormalities (particularly bradycardia or tachycardia noted before the second stage of delivery).

Examination

Cyanosis

Is the infant centrally cyanosed, and if so, is there a non-cardiac explanation for this? (see Table 7.2).

Pulses

- Pulses are often difficult to feel and require experience to assess.
- If infant is distressed, try examination during a feed.
- Palpate both brachials and femorals.
- The assessment of bounding pulses is often best done on foot pulses.
- The arm should be gently extended to feel the brachial pulse.
- Unequal brachial pulses may be the result of an anomolous subclavian artery or CoA.
- Femoral pulses may be very difficult to feel, but anyone performing a neonatal check should always persist until they are certain the femoral pulses are present or return on another occasion to examine the infant sleeping.
- Radiofemoral delay is impossible to detect in such small infants but absence of femoral pulses means there is CoA until proven otherwise.
- If the examiner is unable to feel femoral pulses but can easily feel the dorsalis pedis or posterior tibial pulses (the dorsalis pedis is over the dorsum of the foot and the posterior tibial is behind the medial maleolus), then CoA is excluded.
- An infant with CoA may have femoral pulses present at the first neonatal check because the duct remains open.

Small pulse volume: ● cardiac failure ● hypoplastic left heart syndrome ● critical AS ● interruption of the aortic arch.

In CoA there are usually very full brachial pulses and upper limb BP is higher than lower limb BP. The full brachials and high arm BP with CoA only applies to babies with minimal symptoms. With failure, the brachials become weak or absent and BP falls.

Bounding pulses (any cause of a rapid run-off from the systemic circulation): ● PDA ● truncus arteriosis ● aorto-pulmonary window ● large systemic arterial-venous fistula.

Heart rate. Tachycardia is a non-specific sign in the newborn as it may be a feature of: ● crying ● pain ● respiratory distress. Nevertheless, persistent tachycardia, especially in an infant who is not crying, may suggest a compensatory response to small stroke volume: ● hypovolaemia ● obstruction to outflow ● poor myocardial contractility.

Tachycardia above 220/min suggests SVT (see below), whereas persistent bradycardia (less than 100 bpm) may be seen in complete heart block and magnesium toxicity (magnesium sulphate infusion is used to treat PPHN).

If a baby is in heart failure with a rate above 220 or below 100, it is likely that the rate is the cause and not the effect of failure.

Apex beat

It should be confirmed that the apex beat lies on the left side of the chest rather than the right. The heart may be pushed to the right by left pneumothorax or left diaphragmatic hernia, pulled to the right by collapse of the right lung, or there may be true dextrocardia. If this is associated with visceral situs inversus, it is of less concern. However, if true dextrocardia is associated with a right-sided liver and left-sided stomach, the incidence of CHD is very high. The other abnormality commonly found on palpation of the precordium in the neonate is a hyperdynamic apex beat associated with a PDA.

Cardiac murmurs

Innocent murmurs have already been discussed (see p. 113).

Systolic murmur, particularly if loud or harsh, is most likely in the first few days of life to be due to a PDA or an obstructive defect such as PS TF or AS. VSD, AVSD, ASD and CoA may be significant but not give rise to murmurs in the newborn period.

Diastolic murmurs are very rare in the newborn period and would suggest PDA, truncus arteriosus, or absent pulmonary valve.

Heart sounds

In the normal infant, the first heart sound is usually relatively loud and the second heart sound is usually single in the first 48 h of life. Even after this age, the fast heart rate and quiet heart sounds make the detection of splitting extremely difficult. Likewise, ejection clicks associated with valve stenosis may not be audible in the newborn period. The ejection click, together with full pulses and mild desaturation on oximetry, indicates a truncus arteriosus.

Blood pressure

If BP is elevated, it is the cause and not the result of failure.

Other

The infant should also be examined for dysmorphic features, other congenital abnormalities, evidence of any respiratory disease and hepatomegaly, which is an early and reliable sign of the failure of either ventricle in infancy.

Investigation of the centrally cynanosed infant

The major differential is between respiratory problems, CHD and PPHN. Careful clinical assessment is required. For example, babies with choanal atresia are not just blue — they have obstructed breathing.

Obtain arterial access. Catheterise the umbilical artery or the right radial artery (preductal) to obtain ABGs and direct BP measurements.

Interpreting an ABG:

- Ideally from right radial artery (avoids confusion from ductal shunting).
- Preferably from an indwelling arterial catheter (avoids P_aO_2 fall during handling).
- A raised P_aCO_2 suggests a respiratory or neurological disorder rather than a cardiac one.
- The pH may be low in CHD if complicated by cardiac failure, prolonged or profound hypotension, or persistent hypoxia.
- Capillary blood gases provide helpful information about pH and P_aCO_2 but are of little value in the assessment of the cyanosed infant.
- In the absence of respiratory disease, a low P_aO_2 suggests cyanotic CHD.
- A normal P_aO_2 in the presence of cyanosis suggests methaemaglobinaemia, (congenital enzyme defect or secondary to nitric oxide therapy). Treatment is with methylene blue (1 mg/kg as a 1% solution in normal saline).

Measure the haematocrit. If this is less than 70%, polycythaemia is unlikely to be the explanation for the cyanosed appearance.

Measure the blood sugar. Hypoglycemia may coexist with CHD.

Ask for an X-ray. Check that the umbilical arterial catheter is in the descending aorta. Look for the size and shape of the heart (the diameter of the heart should be < 60% of the diameter of the thorax). Enlargement of the heart may suggest:

- obstruction to outflow from the heart (e.g. in CoA or endocardial fibroelastosis)
- volume overload of the heart (as in VSD, PDA, AVSD, truncus arteriosus, TAPVD, arteriovenous fistula)
- a poorly functioning heart (cardiomyopathy or ischaemic myocardium)
- collection of fluid in the pericardial sack (hydrops fetalis or following cardiac puncture at resuscitation).

Beware the thymus, which may be very large in the newborn period and often 'sail-shaped' with a scalloped edge.

The boot-shaped heart of TF or PA, the egg on side with a narrow mediastinum of transposition of the great vessels, and the cottage loaf shape of supracardiac TAPVD are often diagnosed on the CXR after the diagnosis has been made by other means!

Assess the lung fields for:

- plethora
  — transposition of the great vessels
  — obstructed total anomalous pulmonary venous drainage
  — whenever there is a large left to right shunt (VSD, AVSD, PDA)
- oligaemia — right ventricular outflow obstruction (often accompanied by cyanosis as there is usually a right to left shunt at atrial or ventricular level).

This is notoriously difficult on a newborn CXR and both conditions tend to be overdiagnosed.

Also look for ground glass changes consistent with RDS, patchy opacification consistent with pneumonia or aspiration, and loops of bowel suggestive of congenital diaphragmatic hernia.

A normal chest X-ray does not exclude significant congenital heart disease.

Perform a full 12-lead ECG. Tables 7.6–7.8 give the normal ranges in the newborn period, the features of ventricular hypertrophy and abnormal morphology.

The ECG in premature infants. Calculate axis from the amplitude of R minus S waves in leads I and AVF. The ECG of the preterm infant differs from that of the term infant:

- The QRS axis is directed more leftward than in term infants
- The QT interval is 0.24–0.3 s in preterm infants
- The corrected QT (QT interval divided by the square root of the RR interval) is about 0.44 s, which is longer than for term infants.

Abnormal patterns in the neonatal ECG

- Incorrect placement of the limb leads? If in doubt, repeat the ECG.
- Right axis deviation may suggest hypoplastic left heart syndrome.
- A superior axis (between −30 and +210°) is always abnormal (e.g. tricuspid atresia, AVSD).
- In dextrocardia, an inverted P wave is seen in lead I.
- Many structural heart defects give rise to little or no cardiac hypertrophy in utero and therefore conditions normally associated with right or left ventricular hypertrophy may not show these signs on ECG during the newborn period.

Perform hyperoxia test ('nitrogen washout test'). An arterial blood sample is taken when the infant is breathing air and this will

Table 7.6 Normal ranges for cardiac parameters in the first week of life in a term infant

	Second centile	50th Centile (median)	98th centile
HR (bpm)	90	125	160
QRS axis	+ 60°	+ 135°	+ 195°
PR duration in lead II (ms)	80	105	160
QRS duration in lead V5 (ms)	20	50	75
QT duration in lead V5 (ms)	210	280	370[a]

[a]QT duration increases as HR slows (at a HR of 90bpm, the second centile is 280 ms, the mean 330 ms and the 98th centile 380 ms).

Standard ECG calibration: 10 mm amplitude is equivalent to 1 mV.
Q waves greater than 5 mm are rarely seen in any lead in the first week of life. Q waves greater than 3 mm in V5 or V6 suggest LVH, septal hypertrophy (as in the infant of a diabetic mother) or myocardial ischaemia (as in anomalous coronary artery).
The ECG is 'right dominant' at birth, i.e. voltages are larger in the right side of the chest leads and T waves are upright in V1 initially. T waves invert in the right side chest leads during the first week of neonatal life.

confirm a clinical diagnosis of central cyanosis. It is often more convenient to use pulse oximetry for the hyperoxia test. If the P_aO_2 is low, a second arterial blood sample should be obtained after the infant has been breathing 100% oxygen for 10 min. An oxygen analyser should be used to demonstrate that the F_iO_2 is continuously above 90% for this period. Possible results are as follows:

- In a normal child breathing 100% oxygen, the P_aO_2 rises above 50 kPa.
- In methaemaglobinaemia, the P_aO_2 rises above 50 kPa but the child remains cyanosed.
- In primary lung disease, the P_aO_2 may rise significantly or very little depending on severity of the lung disease but this should be obvious clinically.
- In cyanotic CHD, P_aO_2 rises modestly, if at all, and never rises above 15 kPa. The rise is particularly small in transposition of the great vessels and in conditions with low pulmonary blood flow.

The hyperoxia test is only valid if ventilation is adequate, and even if the infant is intubated and receiving positive pressure ventilation, severe lung disease or PPHN may result in a negative hyperoxia test very similar to that seen in cyanotic CHD.

Table 7.7 Electrocardiogram — features of hypertrophy

Voltage criteria

RVH
- R in V1
  ≥ 20 mm at any age
- S in V6
  ≥ 14 mm first week
  ≥ 10 mm 1 week–1 month
  ≥ 7 mm 1–3 months
  ≥ 5 mm > 3 months
- R/S ratio in V1
  ≥ 7 0–3 months
  ≥ 4 3–6 months
  ≥ 3 6 months–3 years
- Persistence of upright T wave in V1 after first week of life

LVH
- S in V1 ≥ 20 mm at any age
- R in V6 > 20 mm at any age
- Inverted T waves in V5 or V6 at any age
- Q wave > 4 mm in V5 or V6 at any age

Table 7.8 Electrocardiogram — morphology

Tall T waves
(>30% of the R wave in a left-sided chest lead) — hyperkalaemia
Flat T waves — myocarditis, hypothyroidism
Inverted T waves — normal in III (horizontal heart); may also indicate myocardial ischaemia or pericarditis or endocardial fibroelastosis. See RVH and LVH (Table 7.7)
Depressed ST segment — hypokalaemia
Elevated ST segment — myocardial ischaemia
Wide QRS complex (> 0.12 s) — conduction defect or artificial pacing
Delta wave (slow upstroke of R wave) and wide QRS — WPWS

Comparison of right radial and umbilical ABGs (or transcutaneous electrodes on the right upper chest and left lower abdomen or pulse oximeters on the right hand and either foot) allow comparison of pre- and post-ductal blood gases. If the pre-ductal P_aO_2 is more than 2 kPa higher than the post-ductal P_aO_2, this suggests that the duct remains patent with right-to-left shunting (either duct-dependent systemic circulation, e.g. CoA, or PPHN).

If the duct is patent and there is duct-dependent pulmonary blood flow, the direction of shunting will be from left to right and there should be no significant difference between pre- and post-ductal oxygen tension.

Echocardiogram and Doppler studies. Cardiac catheterisation remains the gold standard for cardiac investigations but has been superseded largely by echocardiography. In experienced hands, almost all cardiac conditions causing cyanosis or heart failure in the newborn can be diagnosed. In addition to two-dimensional views of the heart chambers and valves, Doppler measurements and colour flow Doppler allow the detection of shunts, small septal defects which are hard to visualise on two-dimensional views, and turbulent flow as a result of valve stenosis or persistent ductus. Assessment of the pressure gradient across a valve may also be made. Perhaps the most important contribution of echocardiography on neonatal intensive care units has been in the diagnosis of PPHN and PDA (see Ch. 6).

Management of CHD

GENERAL PRINCIPLES FOR THE NEONATE WITH SEVERE CHD

Do not defer supportive treatment while awaiting diagnosis. Stabilise the infant before transfer.

It is pointless to give O_2 unless a documented rise in P_aO_2 is shown.

Correct hypoglycaemia, acidosis and hypothermia, all of which cause pulmonary vasoconstriction, impair myocardial contractility and exacerbate PPHN.

Maintain plasma K^+ and Ca^{2+} concentrations in the normal range.

Consider PGE_2 infusion to produce relaxation of the smooth muscle in the wall of the ductus arteriosus regardless of the arterial P_aO_2.

Two groups of infants are duct-dependent and may benefit from a PGE_2 infusion:

Cyanosed infants with duct-dependent pulmonary blood flow. Eighty per cent of babies with cyanotic CHD show clinical improvement. Improvement is usually seen within 15 min of starting the infusion but the infusion should be continued even if there is no rapid response.

The best response is seen in infants:

- less than 4 days old
- with very low P_aO_2 with normal pH
- with tricuspid atresia
- with pulmonary atresia or critical PS
- with severe TF.

Those infants who show little response are those with:

- TGA

- PPHN
- TAPVD (these infants may become worse with PGE_2 infusion).

Even if a definitive diagnosis has not been made, PGE_2 is unlikely to cause harm (see 'side-effects' below) and therefore an infusion should always be started in babies with a $P_aO_2 < 5$ kPa who fail a hyperoxic test and have an oligaemic chest X-ray.

Infants with heart failure who have duct-dependent systemic blood flow

- Critical AS
- CoA
- Aortic atresia/hypoplastic left heart.

Heart failure is because of obstruction to flow of blood out of the left side of the heart. It may take up to 12 h for benefit to be seen and this manifests as improved systemic BP, improved urine output and resolving acidosis. Eighty per cent of infants with heart failure show clinical improvement.

If in doubt about the diagnosis, give PGE_2 infusion.

Prostaglandin E_2

Administration. PGE_2 is given by IV infusion (see Appendix 4). The dose is titrated against clinical response or side effects. Once P_aO_2 has risen (or heart failure lessened), the dose should be reduced in steps to 10 nanograms/kg per minute.

Side-effects of PGE_2. These occur in 20% of infants with CHD but are usually not severe and should not preclude the use of this valuable drug in an infant even if the exact cause of the CHD is uncertain. In order of frequency they are:

Cardiovascular effects: ● vasodilation ● oedema ● hypotension. These are most frequently seen with IA administration which, though effective, should be avoided except in an emergency as side-effects are more common.

CNS effects: ● jitteriness ● myoclonic jerks ● irritability ● fever ● apnoea occurs in < 10% of infants and is more common in babies less than 2 kg, those with cyanotic congenital heart disease, and if the dose is above 0.01 microgram/kg/min.

Respiratory effects: respiratory depression and apnoea.

Gastro-intestinal effects: diarrhoea.

Other considerations: IPPV should be available, the infant should be observed for 1 h prior to transport to a cardiac centre and both dopamine and plasma should be available in cases of hypotension. If jitteriness or fever occurs, the infusion rate should be halved. Arterial BP should always be monitored, ideally directly, during the infusion.

CARDIAC FAILURE

If medical treatment is required for cardiac failure in the newborn period, it is likely that this will be a prelude to corrective or palliative surgery as it suggests the lesion is at least moderately severe.

1. Restrict fluids by 30% until failure is controlled. Infants in cardiac failure have a higher metabolic rate and often increased work of breathing. The infants may need > 150 kcal/kg per day (180 mL/kg per 24 h of milk). If bottle-fed, this may be supplemented with Duocal which is a 50% fat: 50% carbohydrate source of extra calories. The feeds may need to be given by NG tube feeds if the baby is too breathless to suck.

2. Furosemide (frusemide) 1mg/kg 12-hourly and spironolactone 1 mg/kg 12-hourly initially; avoids the need for unpalatable K^+ supplements. Both can be increased to 2 mg/kg 12-hourly.

3. If diuretics are insufficient, digoxin 5 microgram/kg 12-hourly p.o. (check K^+ concentration) may help if there is low output but not if failure is associated with large shunt and dynamic heart. Rapid oral digitalisation is rarely essential, but if the child is acutely ill, IM. digoxin can be given 5 microgram/kg 6-hourly for 24 h and then 5 microgram/kg 12-hourly IV or IM. Therapeutic level = 1.5–3.0 nmol/L.

4. Give oxygen if saturation monitoring shows hypoxia.

5. Consider dopamine if there is clinically significant hypotension (acidosis, urine output < 0.5 mL/kg per h). Infuse IV at 5–10 µg/kg per min.

6. IPPV, with 6 cmH_2O PEEP, or CPAP may be used as a treatment for severe heart failure.

The best guides to effective therapy are liver size and tenderness, respiratory and heart rates, and daily weight gain (too much is as undesirable as too little).

ARRHYTHMIAS

Complete heart block

- Ventricular rate usually less than 60/min.
- Often systolic flow murmur because of increased stroke volume.
- P waves are dissociated from QRS waves and the the P wave rate is always faster than the QRS rate.

Associations are as follows:

- maternal SLE
- rarely familial
- following atrial septostomy
- following cardiac surgery.

Extrasystole

Ventricular extrasystoles are common and bigeminy, trigeminy and quadrigeminy (an extrasystole occurring with every second, third or fourth beat) are relatively common but benign arrhythmias which disappear spontaneously. Electrolytes should be checked, but if the infant is clinically well without other signs of CHD there is no requirement for continuous cardiac monitoring.

Supraventricular tachycardia

Background. The heart is usually structurally normal although 10% of infants will have WPWS. Other associated cardiac abnormalities include: ● Ebstein's anomaly ● cardiac tumour ● myocarditis ● post-cardiac surgery especially involving the atria.

Presentation

Fetal SVT may be detected as:
- fetal tachycardia on CTG, auscultation or USS.
- hydrops fetalis often with polyhydramnios. Antenatal USS shows oedema of the scalp, acites, pleural effusions, pericardial effusion and a rapid FHR with a dilated but structurally normal heart. Fetal SVT may be epidosic and if a hydropic infant is seen with a normal HR, CTG or USS should be repeated at intervals to look for episodes of fetal tachycardia.

SVT in the newborn. The younger the infant the less well the SVT is tolerated. Cardiac failure therefore rapidly develops at these high HR. This may result in poor feeding, pallor, cold peripheries, tachypnoea and grunting or vomiting. SVT may be associated with placement central venous lines in the right atrium.

Physical findings

These are pallor, tachypnoea and recession, poor perfusion with a weak rapid pulse which is too fast to count, systemic hypotension, gallop rhythm on auscultation of the heart, enlarged liver.

Investigations

ECG. Always obtain a full 12-lead ECG rather than relying on a heart monitor. The features of SVT are:
- HR 220–340/min. The maximum sinus rhythm in a baby who is crying is not above 220/min

- absolute regularity — there is no beat-to-beat variation
- QRS complexes are normal shape and width
- if P waves are seen, the axis is often abnormal.

CXR may show cardiomegaly and pulmonary congestion.

Electrolytes should be checked to ensure there is no hyperkalaemia.

Drug levels should be estimated if the infant is being treated with digoxin (for some other cardiac condition) or theophylline (for apnoea).

Management
Monitor the ECG throughout.

Vagal stimulation. The diving reflex stimulates the vagal reflex which may cause conversion to sinus rhythm.
1. Initially try facial cooling:
   - Fill a polythene bag with cold water and ice cubes.
   - Place this over the baby's forehead, eyes, nose, mouth and cheeks for 15 s.
2. If this fails, try immersion:
   - Wrap the baby in a towel and immerse the head and face completely in a basin full of water and ice for 5 s.
   - Ensure the nose and mouth are immersed and do not worry about aspiration as the baby will be rendered temporarily apnoeic as a reflex reaction to the cold water.
   - There may be a short period of nodal bradycardia before a return to sinus rhythm.
3. If vagal stimulation fails, try adenosine.

Adenosine
- Impairs conduction of electrical impulses through the atrio-ventricular node and is very effective in the treatment of SVT.
- Short half-life (15 s), so there is no cumulative effect and there is no depressant action on the myocardium.
- Give adenosine by a rapid bolus IV.
- Flush the line with saline immediately afterwards.
- Start with 0.05 micrograms/kg. IV.
- Increase in increments of 0.05 micrograms/kg. IV at 2-min intervals until sinus rhythm is restored.
- The maximum dose is 0.3 micrograms/kg.
- Adenosine is antagonised by theophylline.
- Adenosine has such a short half-life that SVT may recur unless a further regular antiarrhythmic agent is started.

Possible side-effects are sinus bradycardia, AV block and flushing, but these are rare and resolve within 40 s.

Flecainide
- A class 1 C antiarrhythmic drug.
- Use only after discussion with cardiologist.
- Give IV 2 mg/kg over 15 min.
- Return to sinus rhythm usually occurs within 10 min of the injection.

Hypotension and vomiting are uncommon, mild and transient.

Synchronised DC cardioversion
- Always successful in converting SVT to sinus rhythm.
- Repeated use causes myocardial damage.
- SVT may recur unless regular antiarrhythmic therapy is started.
- Establish IV access and have facilities available for intubation and positive pressure ventilation.
- Sedate with IV midazolam.
- Give oxygen by face mask.
- Use neonatal defibrillator paddles.
- Disconnect the ECG monitor from the infant.
- Apply one paddle to the apex of the heart and the other to the right sternal border and ensure there is no electrode gel bridging the gap between the 2 two paddles.
- Give an initial shock of 0.5–1 J/kg ensuring that the shock is synchronised.
- Because it is almost always successful, DC cardioversion should be first line treatment in the very ill infant.

Following a return to sinus rhythm:
- ECG for evidence of WPWS (slow upstroke of delta wave preceding QRS).
- Echocardiogram.
- There may be non-specific ischaemic changes on the ECG for 24 h afterwards and it may take 24 h for the CXR to return to normal.
- Colour and peripheral circulation should improve more dramatically followed by diuresis, with hepatomegaly and the gallop rhythm regressing over 24 h.
- Seek specialist advice.
- Regular antiarrhythmic: digoxin 5 μg/kg twice a day orally. In the presence of WPWS or pre-existing heart disease, digoxin alone may be unsuccessful but other drugs such as propranolol, flecainide or amiodarone require specialist advice. Fetal SVT can be treated by giving the mother digoxin or flecainide but again this requires specialist advice.

TRANSPORT OF THE BABY WITH CONGENITAL HEART DISEASE

- Discuss the case with the cardiac centre before arranging transport. Whilst it may seem urgent to transfer the child to the cardiac centre, the infant should always be stabilised first.
- Acidosis, hypoglycaemia and hypothermia should all be corrected initially and secure IV access established.
- PGE_2 infusion should only be used prior to or during transfer if facilities are available to intubate and ventilate the infant, but elective intubation for transport is unnecessary. A separate IV line is then necessary for volume administration since 5% of infants develop hypotension with PGE_2 administration. If the child deteriorates during transfer and after starting PGE_2, and there is uncertainty over the diagnosis, the infusion should be stopped since the child may have obstructed TAPVD.

EIGHT

Fluid and electrolyte therapy

The newborn baby is capable of adjusting to a wide range of fluid intakes. Breast milk production is low at first and the slow build-up of water intake over the first few days as milk production increases has traditionally been copied in the design of fluid regimes for well newborn infants. For orally fed and well children on IV fluids, this poses little problem as the baby copes well with low and high intakes (usually due to overprescription). For the sick or tiny infant, there is less margin for error, and careful attention to fluid and electrolyte management is essential.

Throughout fetal life, water comprises a decreasing proportion of body composition, from 90% body weight at 30 weeks, 60% of which is extracellular, to 80% and 45% by 40 weeks respectively. In the first few days, there is an increase in renal perfusion and GFR, which result in a diuresis. Body water decreases rapidly: initially, water is lost from the extracellular compartment and then from the intracellular water pool, producing a weight loss over the first few days of about 5%.

After preterm delivery, the reduction in body water brings body composition closer to that of the term infant. This normal diuresis may be delayed in sick infants and may be a factor in delayed recovery from RDS. Preterm infants have immature renal function and mechanisms for sodium homeostasis are less efficient than in the term baby; in the very preterm infant this may lead to high baseline losses.

Water balance

Water balance is controlled by renal perfusion and antidiuretic hormone (ADH).

Systemic perfusion is critical in maintaining renal plasma flow — BP and peripheral perfusion should be assessed in clinical context, not by the striving for fixed levels, and is probably adequate if renal function and urine output are normal.

ADH is secreted by the posterior pituitary and acts on the collecting duct. It is secreted in response to:

- a small rise in plasma osmolality (hypothalamic receptors)
- a fall in intravascular volume (left atrial stretch receptors)
- a fall in BP (carotid sinus receptors).

In the very preterm infant, the renal collecting duct is partially insensitive to ADH. However, in the sick infant, ADH continues to be secreted as a normal response to stress (e.g. pain, hypoxia, raised intrathoracic pressure, intracranial haemorrhage, hypoxic-ischaemic encephalopathy) and this may result in rapid swings in water excretion, even with a normal GFR.

SOURCES OF NON-RENAL WATER LOSS

The respiratory tract. Negligible if the infant is ventilated with humidified gas (usually >90% relative humidity).

Transepidermal evaporative loss. The very preterm infant loses water through the immature skin, and may lose up to 200 mL/kg if nursed exposed under radiant heaters. For tiny babies, humidification of the environment or the use of barriers, such as plastic wrappings or Vaseline, may reduce this to tolerable levels. These methods also reduce concomitant heat loss and energy expenditure. Humidification of close to 100% can be achieved in modern incubators with reduction of transepidermal water loss by about 50% in babies of 24–27 weeks gestation.

Gastrointestinal fluids. Babies with gut problems may have significant fluid losses which may be overt in the case of increased aspirates with obstruction (e.g. duodenal atresia, volvulus) or occult, such as with necrotising enterocolitis.

CLINICAL AND LABORATORY OBSERVATIONS TO ASSESS WATER BALANCE

Daily weights are possible in all but the sickest infants and provide an excellent guide to the adequacy of fluid replacement. A weight is critical in situations where there is ongoing diuresis or excessive losses (e.g. in a very preterm baby under a radiant heater). Charts should be available for the weights of items that cannot be removed during weighing of a sick child (e.g. ETT, splints) and the recorded weight should state any adjustment that is made.

Plasma sodium is the most reliable way of assessing water balance over the first few days, especially in the very preterm child who is experiencing large transcutaneous water losses. Water intake is adjusted to maintain plasma sodium in the normal range. Sodium may need to be measured 8–12 hourly in the first few days.

Other electrolytes. Creatinine is the most useful indicator of renal function in the newborn and should be measured each day in sick children. On the first day, the serum creatinine will reflect the mother's renal function, not the child's. Older laboratory methods showed interference by high bilirubin levels, but newer methods avoid this. In contrast, urea generation rates may be very variable, and high in preterm infants as a result of catabolism. A high blood urea in a sick infant does not therefore necessarily indicate dehydration or renal failure. Rely primarily on the creatinine concentration.

Urine output. The measurement of urine output by collection is often very difficult and inaccurate but can be estimated by weighing the nappy shortly after voiding. In boys, the use of a cut finger of a plastic glove, placed over the penis, may avoid evaporative losses. In the polyuric phase of renal failure or where water balance is critical, catheterisation may be necessary. During periods of intensive care aim for a urine output >1 mL/kg per h.

Urine specific gravity (SG, or osmolality) may give an indication of excessive urinary concentration if >1015, but should be interpreted with caution if there is blood, protein or glucose present in appreciable quantities on stick testing, all of which cause the SG to rise. It is easily performed at the bedside.

Urinary electrolytes. Urinary sodium, potassium, urea and creatinine may all be used to provide information about fluid balance. Sodium and potassium wasting may be common in the very preterm infant (high urinary concentration is found in the presence of low serum levels) and intake must be adjusted accordingly. Interpret high levels with caution if you have already increased intake. Urinary creatinine may be used to estimate urine volume as creatinine excretion is relatively constant, but this is rarely used in practice.[1] Similarly pre-renal failure may be distinguished from renal failure by consideration of the urine:plasma urea or osmolarity ratios, or fractional excretion of sodium (Ch. 10), if there is serious doubt.

Clinical assessment of hydration is the least useful method to assess the state of hydration during IV therapy as marginal over- or under-hydration will not be obvious. The classical signs of dehydration, such as dry mucous membranes, reduced tissue turgor and depression of the fontanelle, are all very late signs and their appearance implies poor fluid management or rapid changes in clinical condition. Although acute weight gain is the most sensitive sign of over-hydration, enlargement of the liver may be the most sensitive early sign of cardiac failure.

---

[1]Urine flow (L/day) = [90 × baby's weight (kg)]/urine creatinine (mmol/L).

NORMAL WATER INTAKE

In healthy breast-fed infants, water intake rises progressively to
about 150 mL/kg by the fifth postnatal day, forming the basis for
the conventional rising steps for IV fluids, and only applies to
relatively mature infants. There is much debate as to how much
fluid is enough. Generally babies cope with reasonable
maintenance volumes in the range 120–180 mL/kg after the fourth
day. We recommend the following daily intake volumes for well
babies >36 weeks:

- day 1 — 40 mL/kg
- day 2 — 60 mL/kg
- day 3 — 80 mL/kg
- day 4 — 110 mL/kg
- day 5 et seq. — 150 mL/kg

Volumes may be varied if increased energy intake is
required – (Ch. 15).

For babies requiring IV fluids, a suggested scheme for water,
sodium and potassium intake is shown in Table 8.1.

Adjust water intake after close assessment of the state of
hydration, urine output, insensible and observed losses, and
plasma electrolytes. Remember that water should be an
independent variable in your calculations and the concentration of
all solutes (e.g. sodium, potassium) must be adjusted if the rate of
water infusion is altered.

Always use birthweight in calculations until current weight
exceeds birthweight. It is difficult to assess normal weight in the
presence of hydrops or severe water overload. Usually a best
guess is used and then modified as oedema fluid settles.

Remember to include arterial flush solutions and infused
drugs (which also contain extra sodium) in your calculations.

Table 8.1 Guidelines for IV fluid and electrolyte administration (daily figures)

Age	Water[a]		Sodium[a]		Potassium[a]
	Preterm (mL/kg)	Term (mL/kg)	Preterm (mmol/kg)	Term (mmol/kg)	All babies (mmol/kg)
Day 1	60[b]	40	0	0	0
Day 2	90[b]	60	0	0	0
Day 3	120[b]	80	3–5[c]	1–2	2–3
Day 4	120–150	110	3–5[c]	1–2	2–3
Day 5 et seq.	120–150	120–150	3–5[c]	1–2	2–3

[a] Use birthweight or most recent weight, whichever is greater.
[b] Extremely preterm babies may have much greater requirements; monitor plasma Na+ (see text).
[c] Sometimes higher requirements — check plasma sodium daily.

Colloid infusions (HAS, fresh frozen plasma and blood) also contain a considerable amount of sodium, but are usually counted separately from crystalloid.

VARIATIONS FROM BASELINE RECOMMENDATIONS

There is much personal variation in the management of fluids in the sick infant, mainly relating to the maximum fluid volumes allowed. There is no convincing evidence that lesser maximum volumes prevent the development of a symptomatic persistent arterial duct or of CLD.

Reduce fluid intake in the following situations:

Anticipated neonatal encephalopathy. Where a child has been in poor condition at birth and is likely to develop symptoms of significant post-hypoxic encephalopathy, over-hydration may exacerbate cerebral oedema and renal impairment is common. Commence fluids at a maximum of 40 mL/kg and monitor urine output closely. Maintain fluid restriction until oliguria has resolved, which may take several days but maintain BP and perfusion. Beware the scenario where perfusion is poor and inadequate intake may cause persisting oliguria.

Severe RDS. Initially children with severe RDS may be relatively oliguric; a diuresis then precedes improvement in clinical condition. It is sensible to restrict fluids by one incremental step until a good urine output is achieved.

Symptomatic persistent arterial duct. The appearance of signs of a PDA (bounding pulses, hyperdynamic cardiac impulse, hepatic enlargement, ± systolic or continuous murmur) should prompt a mild restriction in fluid volumes — usually by one or two steps. Consider using a diuretic.

Fluid retention associated with raised intrathoracic pressure (e.g. pulmonary interstitial emphysema, hyperinflation) or intracranial pathology (usually secondary to ADH secretion).

Renal failure. Where there is prolonged oliguria, unresponsive to a fluid and diuretic challenge (e.g. 20 mL/kg 0.9% saline bolus and furosemide [frusemide]), reduce fluid intake to insensible losses (e.g. 20–30 mL/kg per day in a term baby) plus output calculated on a 6 hourly retrospective basis. Check electrolytes regularly and maintain perfusion aggressively using inotrope and minimal amounts of colloid, until renal output returns.

Increase fluid intake in the following situations:

Phototherapy. Increase IV intake by 20 mL/kg per day (this may not be necessary if adequate humidification and plastic wraps are used and leads to variation in local practice).

Increased non-renal losses. Replace gastric aspirates and stoma losses with appropriate fluids (e.g. Hartmann's solution or 0.9% saline as per unit policy). Replace protein-rich losses (e.g. chyle, CSF, abdominal paracentesis) with appropriate colloid if fluid balance is critical, serum albumin is low or losses are >20 mL/kg.

Increased renal losses. During the diuretic phase following renal failure or relief of obstruction, calculate fluid volumes 6-hourly based upon insensible losses (20–30 mL/kg per day) plus output calculated on a 6 hourly retrospective basis. Check electrolytes and state of perfusion regularly and adjust intake accordingly. Regular weights (e.g. 12-hourly) are of great value.

Sodium

Sodium is normally excreted via the kidney, controlled by the renin–angiotensin–aldosterone system. This control mechanism is as active in the preterm as in the term infant, but tubular unresponsiveness leads to sodium wastage at low gestations and in sick infants, in whom it may take up to 3 weeks to improve. Sodium losses from sweat and bowel secretions are negligible unless there is bowel obstruction.

Term breast milk has relatively little sodium (<1 mmol sodium/kg per day), implying that the kidney can conserve sodium and achieve positive balance and growth. Normal sodium requirements are usually 1–2 mmol/kg per day in term babies, and 3–5 mmol/kg per day in well preterm babies, but in very preterm infants, needs may be much higher secondary to tubular loss.

When there is a disturbance in electrolyte balance, monitor both serum and urinary electrolytes. It may be useful to calculate urinary sodium loss as fractional sodium excretion (F_eNa).[2] Normal F_eNa is <1% in healthy term infants, but values of up to 16% in sick, very preterm infants may occur due to renal salt wasting, without implying renal failure.

HYPONATRAEMIA

Defined as plasma sodium <130 mmol/L (note that some laboratories quote higher levels at the bottom of their normative range).

$$^2 F_e\text{Na} = \frac{\text{urine Na}}{\text{urine creatinine}} \times \frac{\text{plasma creatinine}}{\text{plasma Na}} \times 100$$

Causes

Water overload. Commonest cause *during* the first week in very preterm infants:

- In first 24 h due to excess administration of IV fluids to mother
- Excess administration to infant (commonest cause in first week)
- Secondary to ADH secretion (see above)
- Acute renal failure in oliguric phase before fluid restriction.

Increased sodium loss. Commonest cause *after* the first week in very preterm infants

- Excessive renal loss in preterm infants (worse during illness and diuretic or methyl-xanthine therapy, usually aminophylline rather than caffeine)
- Excessive bowel sodium loss during obstruction or, rarely, infection
- Rarely inherited tubular disorders or adrenal insufficiency (with low potassium and water loss).

Inadequate sodium intake
- During IV fluid therapy/IV feeding
- During oral feeding with unsupplemented breast milk or term formula in very preterm babies.

Management

Prevention
- Anticipate situations when losses may be high, such as in very preterm infants or following bowel surgery. Measure volume of losses and replace as appropriate.
- Use breast milk fortifiers and/or preterm formulae for feeding small infants.

Treatment (plasma sodium <130 mmol/L)
- Calculate sodium deficit: deficit in mmol = [(135 – plasma sodium) × 0.6 × body weight (kg)].
- Replace slowly over 24 h, where sodium levels are low (<125 mmol/L) replace half of deficit over 8 h and half over remaining 16 h. Add sodium replacements as 30% NaCl (5 mmol/mL) to bag or burette.
- If plasma sodium is <120 mmol/L with symptoms (irritability, apnoea, convulsions), resuscitation should be started with a bolus of 15–20 mL/kg plasma or normal saline (contains 150 mmol/L sodium).
- Where excessive ADH secretion (low urine volumes, fluid retention, high urinary sodium) or acute renal failure is suspected, restrict fluids rather than give more sodium.

HYPERNATRAEMIA

Defined as plasma sodium >145 mmol/L.

Causes

Net loss of water
- Transepidermal water loss in very preterm infants or during phototherapy.
- High rates of fluid loss occur during episodes of vomiting, diarrhoea or bowel obstruction (although both water and sodium are usually lost).
- Glycosuria may cause an osmotic diuresis in the sick or very preterm.

Management
- In the absence of circulatory compromise, rehydrate *slowly* over 24–48 h.
- If dehydration is marked, start with isotonic solutions (plasma or 0.9% saline) to reduce the risk of cerebral oedema.

Excess sodium
- Incorrect fluid prescription.
- Excess administration of sodium bicarbonate.

Management. Restrict sodium intake.

Congenital hyperaldosteronism (very rare)
- Give diuretic (spironolactone).
- Refer to endocrinologist.

Potassium

Renal excretion and conservation are similarly well developed in the newborn. Remember that plasma concentrations are buffered because the majority of body potassium is intracellular and therefore low plasma concentration is a late sign of whole body depletion. Breast milk supplies about 1 mmol potassium/kg per day. In sick infants, with normal renal function, 2–3 mmol/kg per day IV will establish positive balance. Where there is acute renal failure, oliguria or high plasma levels, potassium replacements should be withheld.

HYPOKALAEMIA

Defined as plasma potassium <3.0 mmol/L

Causes
- Inadequate intake — remember to add potassium to IV fluids after the first 48 h unless urine output is poor
- Bowel losses (usually during vomiting or diarrhoea)
- Alkalosis (buffering of pH causes renal potassium wastage)
- Diuretics — all cause potassium wastage, particularly loop diuretics, e.g. furosemide (frusemide)
- Hyperaldosteronism.

Management
- Increase potassium intake in infusion fluids or by adding to milk. Baseline requirements vary between 1–3 mmol/kg per day.
- Be wary of adding strong potassium solutions (2 mmol/mL) to bag or burette — recheck calculations carefully.

HYPERKALAEMIA

Defined as plasma potassium >7 mmol/L.

- Note that sick newborn infants seem to tolerate high potassium concentrations well.
- Use ECG as a guide to the presence of toxicity (tall P waves, long PR interval, arrhythmias).
- High plasma potassium results are common and often due to haemolysis which occurs during sampling — always recheck the result using a free-flowing venous sample.

Causes
- Catabolism in sick infants
- Acidosis — potassium moves out of cells in exchange for hydrogen ions to buffer acidosis
- Acute renal failure
- CAH (Ch. 11).

Management
- Establish ECG monitoring.
- Acutely, calcium infusion will lower potassium levels for up to 1 h — give 10% calcium gluconate 0.5 mL/kg over 4 min.
- Similarly, the correction of acidosis will drive potassium back into cells and reduce plasma levels for up to 2 h — give sodium bicarbonate 2 mmol/kg over 4 min.
- Use bowel binders to provide longer term background removal of potassium — give calcium Resonium 1 g/kg per day orally or rectally.
- For medium term reduction in levels (days) give salbutamol 4 mg/kg by IV bolus injection as required.
- A glucose/insulin infusion is often recommended but is less safe than salbutamol — give insulin 0.1 unit/kg with 4 mL/kg of 25% dextrose and monitor blood sugar closely.
- Seek specialist help for dialysis.

Calcium and magnesium

Serum calcium levels appear low in the newborn because of low albumin levels. There is a normal physiological fall in calcium concentrations after birth which reaches a nadir on the second day before rising. The measurement of ionised calcium gives a better guide to the physiological status of the baby, but levels are laboratory method dependent.

HYPOCALCAEMIA

Defined as total serum calcium <1.5 mmol/L (symptoms are rare above this value). Causes are:

- encephalopathy
- renal failure
- DiGeorge syndrome (Ch. 4)
- disordered maternal calcium metabolism
- maternal diabetes mellitus.

Early hypocalcaemia is difficult to interpret and rapidly resolves on milk or parenteral feeding. Symptomatic hypocalcaemia (tetany/seizures) is very rare with modern milk feeding. If a trial of therapy is needed a slow IV infusion of 0.2 mmol/kg (1 mL/kg 10% calcium gluconate) is generally given, observing the infusion site carefully and with ECG monitoring. Extravasation of calcium-containing fluid may produce local necrosis; hence avoid adding calcium to IV infusions (it is rarely necessary). Do not add to parenteral nutrition fluid, bicarbonate or phosphate solutions, as precipitation will occur.

HYPOMAGNESAEMIA

A low serum magnesium may accompany hypocalcaemia and produce refractory symptoms. Measure serum magnesium during investigation of seizures or if a low serum calcium persists despite replacement therapy.

Treat with 0.1 mL/kg 50% magnesium sulphate IM where hypocalcaemia or hypocalcaemic seizures persist despite calcium therapy. Oral therapy is occasionally required in chronic malabsorptive states.

HYPERCALCAEMIA

A serum calcium >2.8 mmol/L may result from:

- phosphate deficiency in very preterm babies

- prolonged calcium infusions without additional phosphate
- overtreatment with vitamin D.

Cessation of causative therapy or addition of phosphate therapy will rapidly resolve the issue.

NINE

Jaundice, liver disease and gastrointestinal disease

Jaundice and liver disease

Jaundice is a common neonatal problem and rarely pathological. For most infants it reflects immaturity of the conjugating enzyme system which is induced as bilirubin levels rise after birth, and is an example of adaptation to extra-uterine life (Fig. 9.1). It is important to maintain a sense of proportion when approaching a jaundiced child and their parent, in order not to provoke unnecessary anxiety and disruption to their evolving relationship. However, the clinical importance of neonatal jaundice lies in the potential for harm from very high serum levels of bilirubin and the need to identify rarer causes of jaundice which require complex investigation and management.

BACKGROUND PHYSIOLOGY

Bilirubin is a product of the metabolism of haem and, as unconjugated bilirubin, circulates in the blood bound to albumin. In this form it is lipid soluble and will cross the blood brain barrier. In high concentrations, bilirubin is neurotoxic leading to the condition of bilirubin encephalopathy or kernicterus, fortunately rarely seen nowadays. Features of neurotoxicity in the newborn period are non-specific but include irritability, lethargy, poor suck, hypertonia, seizures, fever or apnoea. There is a high mortality. If the child survives, long-term handicaps include severe learning difficulties, choreoathetoid cerebral palsy (resulting from deposition of bilirubin in the basal ganglia), high frequency sensory-neural deafness, dental staining and failure of upward gaze.

The liver excretes bilirubin (Fig. 9.2) by:

1 Transporting the bilirubin from plasma into the hepatocyte (probably involving specific receptors in the hepatocyte membrane).
2 Intracellular transport of the bilirubin by specific cytoplasmic binding proteins (known as ligandin or Y and Z proteins).

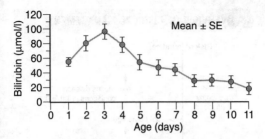

Fig. 9.1 Adaptation of bilirubin metabolism after birth in normal healthy term infants.

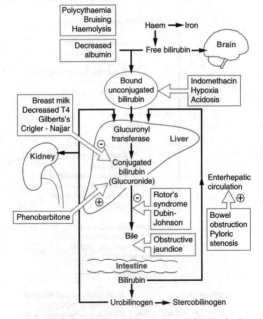

Fig. 9.2 Schematic of bilirubin metabolism — arrows indicate the site of interference for some causes of jaundice (- indicates inhibition and + enhancement of a particular step).

OVERVIEW OF CLINICAL MANAGEMENT

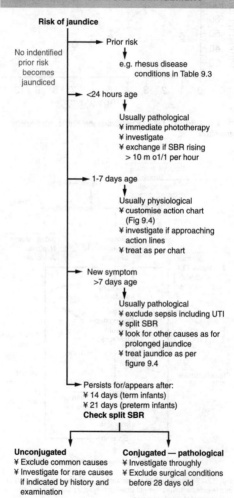

Risk of jaundice

No indentified
prior risk
becomes
jaundiced

→ Prior risk

e.g. rhesus disease
conditions in Table 9.3

→ <24 hours age

Usually pathological
¥ immediate phototherapy
¥ investigate
¥ exchange if SBR rising
> 10 m ol1 per hour

→ 1-7 days age

Usually physiological
¥ customise action chart
(Fig 9.4)
¥ investigate if approaching
action lines
¥ treat as per chart

→ New symptom
>7 days age

Usually pathological
¥ exclude sepsis including UTI
¥ split SBR
¥ look for other causes as for
prolonged jaundice
¥ treat jaundice as per
figure 9.4

→ Persists for/appears after:
¥ 14 days (term infants)
¥ 21 days (preterm infants)
Check split SBR

Unconjugated
¥ Exclude common causes
¥ Investigate for rare causes
if indicated by history and
examination

Conjugated — pathological
¥ Investigate throughly
¥ Exclude surgical conditions
before 28 days old

Fig. 9.3 Summary of clinical management of jaundice in the newborn.

3 Esterification with glucuronic acid (conjugation of bilirubin to glucuronic acid is catalysed by the microsomal enzyme uridyl diphosphate glucuronyl transferase, UDPTG, and both the monoglucuronide and diglucuronide are excretable in bile).
4 Excretion of the water-soluble conjugated bilirubin into bile.

Conjugated bilirubin excreted into the GI tract is converted to urobilinogen by bacteria. Most is excreted in the faeces, after conversion to stercobilinogen, and contributes to the normal yellow/brown colour of the stool. A small amount of urobilinogen is re-absorbed into the portal circulation and is excreted into the bile and urine. Urinary urobilinogen concentration is increased in both haemolytic jaundice (due to increased excretion of bilirubin into the bile and hence increased intestinal absorption of urobilinogen) and in hepatitis (due to impaired ability of the hepatocytes to re-excrete urobilinogen). If the biliary tree is obstructed, the stools are pale and the urine dark because bile cannot be excreted into the small bowel (no stercobilinogen to colour the stool) and the elevated plasma concentration of conjugated bilirubin spills over into the urine. Bilirubin is not normally detected in the urine of healthy infants as the plasma concentration of conjugated bilirubin (which is water soluble) is too low to exceed the renal threshold.

MEASURING BILIRUBIN LEVELS

Clinical assessment
- In a Caucasian infant, jaundice becomes visible in natural light when the plasma level exceeds 85–100 µmol/l. Jaundice may be made more apparent by blanching the skin of the nose with light pressure.
- In dark-skinned babies, colouring of the sclera is more reliable.
- In term babies, the appearance of jaundice progresses from the head caudally. Where the lower limbs are not jaundiced and the baby is >48 h old, the bilirubin level is rarely high enough to treat.
- Icterometers (devices to measure bilirubin colouring in the skin) are not reliable enough for clinical use at present.
- If the observer is inexperienced or unsure, or there are other risk factors for a pathological cause (see Table 9.1), blood should be taken for plasma bilirubin.

Blood sampling
- Capillary or venous blood may be used, though venous samples should be used to determine whether exchange criteria have been reached.
- After sampling protect from light (especially phototherapy units!) and, if sending to the laboratory, protect from light during transfer.

Table 9.1 Factors suggesting jaundice may have a pathological basis

Family history	1	History of jaundice or anaemia in a parent or sibling
	2	Ethnic group
Obstetric history	1	Infection
	2	Diabetes mellitus
	3	Drugs
	4	Rhesus -ve mother, or mother with rarer antibodies
Perinatal history	1	Delayed clamping of the cord
	2	Ill infants
	3	Vomiting, especially if bile-stained
	4	Pallor suggesting haemolytic anaemia
	5	Hepatosplenomegaly
	6	Petechiae suggesting congenital infection
	7	Cataracts

Measurement on the neonatal unit

- Spin blood in centrifuge to separate out plasma.
- Transfer plasma to cuvette to measure *total plasma bilirubin* using a photometric method.
- Results are less accurate at very high bilirubin levels and if there is a significant conjugated component.
- If the level is at odds with your clinical impression, repeat the sample using venous blood, repeat the measure and send a sample to the laboratory.

Measurement in the hospital chemical pathology department

This is required if:

- the levels are very high and an exchange blood transfusion is being considered
- it is necessary to know the contribution of conjugated and unconjugated bilirubin to the total level.

TREATMENT OF JAUNDICE

The aim of treatment is to prevent the unconjugated bilirubin in plasma from rising to neurotoxic concentrations, which may be lower in babies with the risk factors shown in Table 9.2. Treatment options are phototherapy and exchange transfusion.

Adequate fluid and calorie intake

Dehydration and hypoglycaemia exacerbate jaundice — ensure the baby has an adequate intake (Chs 5 & 6).

Table 9.2 Factors that increase the risk of developing kernicterus

- Prematurity
- Low plasma albumin concentrations
- The infant is ill (acidosis, hypoxia and hypoglycaemia all appear to increase the risk of kernicterus)
- Drug competition for bilirubin binding (theoretical): most of such drugs are not used (salicylates, rifampicin, sulphonamides, radiographic contrast agents) or do not displace significant amounts of bilirubin in neonatal doses (indomethacin, furosemide).
- Intralipid (theoretical): no supporting data but probably wise to stop infusion if approaching exchange levels

Phenobarbitone

Glucuronyl transferase activity can be induced by phenobarbitone over about 5 days, so routine use is of no value. Give phenobarbitone for 3 days before a HIDA scan. Prenatal treatment of the mother with phenobarbitone to decrease the severity of the jaundice from Rhesus haemolytic disease is now rarely undertaken. Phenobarbitone may help in total parenteral nutrition induced hepatitis and following the Kasai procedure for biliary atresia. The dose is initially 2mg/kg/day (i.e. considerably less than the maintenance dose for seizures which is 5mg/kg/day) but this dose can be increased to 8mg/kg/day if required.

SETTING BILIRUBIN LEVELS FOR PHOTOTHERAPY OR EXCHANGE TRANSFUSION

There are no firm guidelines for when to commence phototherapy or to perform an exchange transfusion. Most units have developed their own protocol. Ours is as follows:

- *In the first 24 hours.* **Phototherapy** should be started for all babies who are visibly jaundiced, until a diagnosis is reached and it is clear that the bilirubin level is not rising rapidly; **exchange transfusion** is generally indicated if the bilirubin level is rising at more than 10 μmol/l per hour.
- *After 48 hours.* Set levels for **exchange transfusion** which approximate to a bilirubin level in μmol/l of 10 times the gestational age in weeks. **Phototherapy** is commenced when the bilirubin level is rising rapidly beyond a figure 100 μmol/l below this.
- *For sick or acidotic infants.* Reduce both these levels by 50 μmol/l.
- *For well term babies on the postnatal wards.* Increase these levels by 50 μmol/l.
- *After 7 days.* Bilirubin levels should not rise rapidly unless there is some serious underlying condition. Where levels of jaundice simply persist at the same level but the child is well, we will often not use phototherapy.

These levels are plotted on a chart in the infants notes and updated with bilirubin levels as they are taken. An example is given in Figure 9.4 for a well baby of 30-weeks gestation. Note that it is only really necessary to commence phototherapy if you think you may have to perform an exchange transfusion. Bilirubin levels tend to peak at 3–5 days and using phototherapy to bring down levels that are not rising rapidly at this time is probably unnecessary. It is better to repeat the bilirubin level after 6 hours if you are unsure than to institute phototherapy, with its attendant disruption and maternal anxiety.

PHOTOTHERAPY

Phototherapy is used to reduce rising bilirubin levels to avoid an exchange transfusion. Non-ultraviolet light from the blue end of the physical spectrum converts unconjugated bilirubin into a more water-soluble isomer (sometimes known as photobilirubin or lumirubin), which can be excreted without conjugation and (because it is less lipophilic) is not neurotoxic. As blue light is unpleasant for staff and parents, white light is often used and the efficiency of phototherapy is improved by:

- increasing the area of exposed skin
- removing any covers over the infant
- decreasing the distance from the light to the baby.

A lamp with a minimum irradiance of $4\mu W/cm2$ per nm should be used. The light source should ideally be about 45 cm above the infant. If the infant is in an incubator there should be at least 5 cm space between this and the lamp to prevent overheating. The plastic used for the incubator walls will screen out infra-red energy and protect the infant from ultra-violet light but will not block the important energy in the 420-520 nm waveband. For infants nursed on radiant warmers rather than in an incubator, a spot phototherapy lamp with output in the blue spectrum may be used. The 'bili-blanket', a woven fibre optic blanket delivering light in the 425-475nm range for phototherapy, is now available but we have had disappointing results with this. The blanket remains cool avoiding burns, but it should not be used in extremely immature infants in whom skin lesions have been reported.

Indications for phototherapy (see above)

Standard phototherapy regime

- Investigations as indicated (see below).
- Explain your management to and reassure the child's parents before starting phototherapy — many parents find it upsetting but they should be reassured that they can handle the baby for feeding, changing and cuddling just as often as they wish with the baby out of the phototherapy unit and eyes uncovered. Intermittent phototherapy may be more effective than continuous.

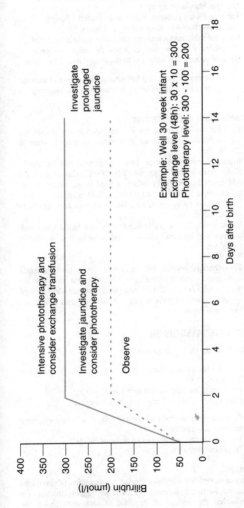

Fig. 9.4 Example of customised bilirubin levels for phototherapy and exchange transfusion for a well 30-week infant.

- The baby should be nursed naked lying on top of the nappy.
- The eyes should be covered.
- The infant's temperature should be measured 4-hourly.
- The infant should be turned every 2-4 hours.
- Serial bilirubin measurements should be made at least daily.
- Phototherapy can be stopped when the serum bilirubin has fallen to around 30μmol/l less than the appropriate threshold.

Phototherapy reduces skin bilirubin so that colour of exposed skin is a poor guide to the level of jaundice once phototherapy has started.

Complications of phototherapy

- Unstable body temperature. If a radiant warmer is used the servo-control should be set to maintain skin temperature at 36.5°C.
- Increased insensible water loss via the skin and the stools. Fluid intake should be increased by 20ml/kg/day to allow for this (see Chapter 5) for infants nursed in an incubator. For infants nursed under radiant warmers, fluid intake may need to be increased by as much as 200ml/kg/day in very low birth weight infants.
- Loose stools. This is partly due to increased faecal water loss, and partly to increased bile salts and unconjugated bilirubin in the bowel.
- Skin rashes.
- Phototherapy should not be given for a predominantly conjugated jaundice as conjugated bilirubin does not cross the blood brain barrier and is not neurotoxic but phototherapy used in such infants may cause skin pigmentation and a 'bronzed baby' will result.

EXCHANGE TRANSFUSION

Indications for exchange transfusion:

- Bilirubin in the appropriate zone corrected for gestation and illness (Fig 9.4)
- Early-onset haemolytic jaundice (see Fig. 9.5).

The objectives of an exchange transfusion are:

- To remove the antibody coated red cells in a Coombs positive haemolytic jaundice
- To raise the haemoglobin in an anaemic infant
- To remove bilirubin.

Consent

Practice varies but ideally informed written consent should be obtained from the parents. As with all urgent situations in paediatrics, the welfare of the child is paramount and if the parents are not available or withhold consent on any grounds, including religious grounds, this should be discussed with the child's consultant and the exchange transfusion should go ahead if this is thought to be in the child's best interests.

Technique
See Chapter 21.

Investigations before beginning exchange transfusion
See Chapter 21.

Complications
See Chapter 21.

Immediate after-care (see also Ch. 21)
● Continue phototherapy.
● Check serum bilirubin every 4 hours. After a 180ml/kg exchange, the serum bilirubin should be 45% of the pre-exchange level and only 13% of the infant's own red cells remain in the circulation. However within 30 minutes, serum bilirubin will have risen to 60% of the pre-exchange level. If you think you need to perform a second exchange (unusual) discuss with your consultant and re-evaluate the cause of the jaundice.
● Haemoglobin should be repeated weekly whilst an in-patient and a top-up transfusion considered if the infant requires oxygen or if the haemoglobin falls below 7g/dl.

Outcome
The mortality of exchange transfusion, excluding infants with hydrops, is 1% within 6 hours of completion of the exchange transfusion. Following exchange transfusion infants need careful developmental follow-up, a newborn hearing screen, and the neonatal screening test should be deferred for at least 4 days after the last exchange transfusion.

JAUNDICE IN THE FIRST 24 HOURS

This is a haemolytic process and *always* needs investigating. The most common causes are:

1 Rhesus haemolytic disease (mother Rh-, baby Rh+, DCT +ve) — see below.
2 ABO incompatibility (usually the mother is O+ve and the baby A+ve; blood film may show microspherocytes; DCT- or weakly +; exchange rarely required).
3 Other rarer blood group incompatibilities.
4 G-6-PD deficiency (usually affects boys only but rarely female carriers due to lyonisation, usually non-Caucasians). Rarer enzymopathies are deficiency of pyruvate kinase, pyrimidine-5-nucleotidase, glucose phosphate isomerase, triose phosphate isomerase, phosphoglycerate kinase.

5 Congenital spherocytosis (only 50% present with neonatal jaundice and a quarter of these will have a negative family history).

6 Congenital infection (toxoplasmosis is rare in the UK but cytomegalovirus and herpes virus occur and rubella is not excluded by an immunisation history). Congenital infection can cause unconjugated jaundice with a haemolytic anaemia but often has a conjugated component due to hepatitis.

7 Haemoglobinopathy (request haemoglobin electrophoresis if there is unexplained anaemia in the offspring of a family from the Mediterranean, Africa or the Far East).

If jaundice in the first 24 hours is not due to Rhesus haemolytic disease which has been anticipated antenatally (see p. 155), the following investigations are suggested:

- bilirubin level
- haemoglobin concentration
- blood film and reticulocyte count (automated measurement of reticulocytes may be unreliable due the large number of normoblasts in neonatal blood)
- baby's blood group
- direct Coombs' test (DCT) on baby's blood (but beware — ABO incompatibility or severe RHD may occur with a negative DCT)
- mothers blood group and haemolysins (these are IgG or IgM antibodies against red cell antigens); this specimen can also be used for a cross-match; 7 G-6-PD screen if the baby is not Caucasian
- congenital infection screen.

JAUNDICE BEGINNING ON DAY 2-5

This is likely to be physiological but always consider other causes:

- infection
- other causes of early jaundice (see above)
- true polycythaemia (see Ch 14).
- galactosaemia and other rare metabolic diseases
- familial non-haemolytic jaundice (Crigler–Najjar syndrome, Dubin–Johnson syndrome, Rotor syndrome and Gilbert's disease).

Consider further investigation only if the infant appears significantly jaundiced (approaching exchange levels) or if the baby is unwell:

- conjugated and unconjugated bilirubin
- infection screen including blood for malarial parasites if mother recently resident in an endemic region (note urinary

tract infection is rare before 7 days, after this suprapubic aspiration of urine must be included in any screen)
- tests for haemolytic disease (see jaundice beginning in the first 24 hours)
- urine for reducing substances in the absence of glycosuria (usually galactose, definitive diagnosis of galactosaemia requires assay of galactose-1-phosphate uridyl transferase activity in red blood cells)
- congenital infection screen including a urine sample for CMV culture
- blood and urine for amino acid and metabolic screen if the infant is ill or acidotic.

Dehydration and hypoglycaemia aggravate jaundice. In preterm babies, idiopathic jaundice may reach higher levels and last longer than in full term infants and is sometimes called 'jaundice of prematurity'.

JAUNDICE COMMENCING AFTER 5-7 DAYS

This is pathological and should be investigated. Rapidly rising bilirubin levels usually indicate infection (do not forget UTI) or haemolysis. Treat with phototherapy and exchange transfusion if rate of rise rapid (> 10 (mol/h). This is a different situation from the jaundice which commenced early and is slow to resolve.

PROLONGED JAUNDICE (JAUNDICE PERSISTING BEYOND 14 DAYS IN A TERM INFANT OR 21 DAYS IN A PRETERM INFANT)

The commonest cause for this is benign breast milk jaundice. This should only be accepted as a diagnosis, after investigation, if the baby is perfectly well and thriving. It is never a reason to stop breast feeding as these infants never require exchange transfusions. If there is concern that the bilirubin levels are very high, and beyond two weeks of age this is extremely unlikely, the baby may be given phototherapy but breast feeding should not be stopped.

The primary investigation must be a split bilirubin to differentiate between conjugated and unconjugated jaundice.

CAUSES OF PROLONGED JAUNDICE

1. *Persistence of any of the causes of neonatal jaundice beginning in the first 24 hours or between the 2-5 days, including:*

- breast milk jaundice
- delayed onset feeding (post surgery or a very preterm infant with increased enterohepatic circulation).

2. *Causes of unconjugated hyperbilirubinaemia (unconjugated fraction >85%):*

- urinary tract infection (presents with poor feeding/weight gain and jaundice)
- hypothyroidism
- drugs leading to haemolysis
- familial non-haemolytic jaundice (e.g. Lucey–Driscoll syndrome (a serum conjugation inhibitor), Crigler–Najjar syndrome, Gilbert's syndrome)
- pyloric stenosis (often after the neonatal period)
- trisomy 21.

3. *Conditions giving rise to conjugated hyperbilirubinaemia (conjugated fraction > 25µmol/l or >15% total)*

Conjugated hyperbilirubinaemia can arise from any pathology which prevents excretion of conjugated bilirubin from the hepatocyte into the duodenum. There is often a mixed conjugated/unconjugated picture, hence the definition of >15% conjugated. Clinically, the diagnosis will be suggested by hepatomegaly, splenomegaly, pale stools and dark urine. It may be preferable to describe this phenomenon as cholestasis emphasising that not only is there a retention of conjugated bilirubin but also bile acids and other components of bile leading to fat malabsorption and steatorrhoea. Infants with conjugated hyperbilirubinaemia account for a large proportion of the infants who develop haemorrhagic disease of the newborn (due to Vitamin K deficiency, see Ch. 14) as their abnormal liver function reduces their ability to synthesise clotting factors II, VII, IX and X even in the presence of adequate amounts of Vitamin K.

In the neonatal intensive care unit in the UK today, the most common causes of an elevated conjugated bilirubin, in decreasing order of frequency, are

1. total parenteral nutrition
2. idiopathic or cryptogenic hepatitis (no causes found but serious chronic liver disease is rare)
3. biliary atresia
4. alpha-1-antitrypsin deficiency
5. congenital infection
6. choledochal cysts
7. galactosaemia

The differential diagnosis of conjugated hyperbilirubinaemia is best considered as follows:

1. Liver cell injury with normal bile duct

- TPN-associated cholestasis — more likely the longer the duration of TPN, the lower the gestation of the infant, if there has been absolute absence of enteral feeding or sepsis. This is a powerful argument for early introduction of minimal non-caloric enteral feeding in the low birth weight infant.
- Infection
  - viral (hepatitis (A, B, non-A/non-B), rubella, cytomegalovirus, herpes, Epstein Barr virus, Coxsackie, adenovirus may all give rise to a giant cell hepatitis on liver biopsy)
  - bacterial (syphilis, *E coli*, group B Streptococcus, listeria, Staph spp.)
  - parasitic (toxoplasmosis)
- Metabolic with normal bile ducts
— more common: alpha-1antitrypsin deficiency; cystic fibrosis; galactosaemia
— less common: tyrosinaemia; fructosaemia; storage diseases (such as Gaucher's, Niemann–Pick); Rotor syndrome; Dubin–Johnson syndrome; Zellweger syndrome; Aagenaes syndrome (hereditary cholestasis with lymphoedema)

2. Excessive bilirubin load with normal bile ducts (also known as inspissated bile syndrome). This is seen in infants with hydrops fetalis or infants treated with intrauterine blood transfusions and is a result of severe red cell haemolytic disease leading to the sludging of bile pigments within the bile ducts.

3. Bile flow obstruction
- Extrahepatic biliary atresia. A disorder unique to infancy and characterised by obliteration of part of the extrahepatic biliary tree. This may be associated with abnormalities of the vasculature below the diaphragm, polysplenia, asplenia and chromosomal anomalies. The intrahepatic bile ducts remain patent in early infancy but may become affected and obliterated later. Without surgery, cirrhosis is inevitable and death usual by 2 years of age. Surgery is best performed before 4 weeks, and certainly before 6-8 weeks.
- Anatomical causes of bile flow obstruction
— Commonest: choledochal cyst.
— Others: spontaneous perforation of the bile duct; duodenal or low bile duct atresia; haemangioma; extrinsic compression by a tumour or fibrous band; bile plugs in the extrahepatic bile duct.
- Intrahepatic biliary atresia or hypoplasia. This may be associated with Alagille's syndrome (dysmorphic facies, peripheral pulmonary artery stenosis and intrahepatic biliary hypoplasia) or intrahepatic bile flow obstruction may occur secondary to anatomical causes of obstruction.

Management of cholestasis
The priorities are to prevent any further complications and to identify those conditions causing conjugated jaundice which can

be diagnosed and treated without proceeding to invasive biopsy or laparotomy.

1. The major life threatening complication is spontaneous intracranial haemorrhage due to coagulopathy from liver disease. Check prothrombin time, give Vitamin K parenterally (1mg if over 1.5kg and 0.5mg if less than 1.5kg). If the prothrombin ratio (infant's prothrombin time divided by control time) is more than 2 or there is active bleeding, give fresh frozen plasma 10ml/kg intravenously over 30 minutes.

2. Exclude hypothyroidism, septicaemia, urinary tract infection and congenital infections. Consider starting broad-spectrum antibiotics but remember that even if septicaemia is confirmed there may still be serious underlying disease (galactosaemia may present with E.coli septicaemia). The newborn screening test at 5-7 days should detect congenital hypothyroidism associated with high TSH levels but will miss hypothyroidism secondary to hypopituitarism.

3. Take blood samples for galactosaemia and fructosaemia and exclude galactose and fructose from the diet if the baby is ill until these results are available. The finding of non-glucose reducing substances in the urine does not necessarily prove galactosaemia since this may occur in normal infants in the first 2 weeks of life, particularly if there is liver damage, and definitive diagnosis requires measurement of galactose-1-phosphate uridyl transferase activity in red cells.

4. Exclude alpha-1-antitrypsin deficiency by determining whether the infant has the Pi zz phenotype.

5. Exclude cystic fibrosis by measuring blood immunoreactive trypsin level or looking for the commonest genetic abnormality (Δ-F508 mutation in 85% of CF) as a sweat test is not reliable below 6 weeks of age.

If the above have been excluded, look for causes of bile flow obstruction, most importantly biliary atresia (and other rare biliary tract problems, see Table 9.2). Remember to consider:

- Investigations as for jaundice beginning on 2–5 day.
- Investigate neonatal 'hepatitis' (HBsAg, Hepatitis C, congenital infection screen, alpha-1-antitrypsin phenotype, liver function tests).
- A fasting abdominal ultrasound scan should be done in all infants with prolonged conjugated hyperbilirubinaemia to exclude an extra-hepatic cause of biliary tree obstruction. (Right upper quadrant mass suggests a choledochal cyst.)
- Look at the colour of the stools. If the stools are white or grey, cholestasis is complete and biliary atresia must be suspected.
- Hepatic iminodiacetic acid tagged with technetium-99 (HIDA) excretion scan to demonstrate continuity of bile duct and duodenum, to exclude biliary atresia. Give phenobarbitone for 3 days prior to the HIDA scan to enhance excretion.

- Liver biopsy allows assessment for features consistent with biliary atresia, alpha-1-antitrypsin deficiency, cystic fibrosis and if some of the biopsy is stored snap frozen at -70°C this can be analysed subsequently for inborn metabolic errors. Diagnoses 75% cases of biliary atresia but must be done in an expert centre.

The primary aim is to distinguish biliary obstruction from neonatal hepatitis. In both conditions there may be hepatomegaly, coagulopathy and elevated transaminase levels. Of infants with biliary atresia, 90% have extra-hepatic atresia with absence or hypoplasia of the hepatic duct, cystic duct, common bile duct or any combination of these. The importance of distinguishing these two pathologies is that surgery for biliary atresia (Kasai procedure — a loop of jejunum sutured on to the porta-hepatis to achieve some biliary drainage) is much more likely to be successful if carried out within the first 6–8 weeks. If these investigations are equivocal then a laparotomy with operative cholangiogram should be undertaken.

Haemolytic disease of the newborn - Rhesus disease

Haemolytic disease of the newborn may be caused by a variety of blood group incompatibilities, the most important of which is the Rhesus D antigen. Individual genotypes may have any combination of C/c, D/-, E/e ('d' does not exist) as three antigens and in the presence of an antigen negative mother, an antigen positive fetus may elicit an antibody response. This is rarely of clinical significance in a first pregnancy, unless prior sensitisation has been caused by mismatched blood transfusion.

Many infants with early onset jaundice will have Rhesus disease but nowadays this is usually anticipated by investigation of maternal antibodies during pregnancy.

Antenatal management

Maternal blood group and antibody status is checked at booking and monitored during pregnancy. If elevated or rising titres of Rhesus (Rh) antibodies are detected, fetal investigation is indicated. Most severe Rh disease is now detected and treated before birth. Intrauterine transfusion appears relatively safe and well tolerated.

Management of possible Rhesus disease at birth

Babies of Rh-ve mothers may present with one of 4 scenarios:

1. **Rh-ve mother with no antenatally detected Rh antibodies**
- Cord blood should be taken for baby's blood group and DCT, irrespective of the partner's Rh status (may not be the biological father).

- A maternal Kleihauer test will indicate the likely size of any fetal-maternal transfusion during delivery and determine the dose of anti-D prophylaxis given.

Follow up
- Baby to postnatal ward with mother.
- Baby is Rh -ve or DCT -ve — no action is required.
- DCT +ve — monitor bilirubin levels until you are sure there is no ongoing haemolysis.

2. Rh-ve mother, low levels of antibody, no antenatal treatment ñ
- Cord bloods for group, Hb, DCT and bilirubin

Follow up
- Baby to postnatal ward with mother.
- **A named person** must be responsible for checking that these results are obtained and then arranging for therapy and subsequent bilirubin estimations if needed.

3. Rh-ve mother, antibody positive, fetal transfusions performed
- Cord bloods for group, Hb, DCT and bilirubin
- Bilirubin 4 hours later to estimate rate of rise (see 4 below).
- These babies may appear Rh-ve due to transfused blood and marrow suppression.

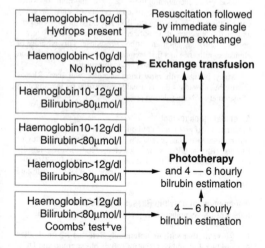

Fig. 9.5 Algorithm for the management of haemolytic disease of the newborn.

Follow up
- If rising bilirubin — manage as for neonatal jaundice.
- Often no early neonatal problems may follow (not even jaundice if there have been several fetal transfusions). These babies must be followed up with serial haemoglobin measurements every 1–2 weeks as frequent top up transfusions may be required due to up to 3 months of marrow suppression.

4. Rh-ve mother, antibody positive with rising or high titre, single or no IUT
- A moderately affected baby is anticipated.
- Ensure 1 unit of Rh-ve blood ready at delivery for exchange (sending maternal blood for cross matching, so that Rhesus negative blood is available is usually the responsibility of the obstetric team — but check!)
- Neonatal team present at birth, clinical assessment.
- Cord bloods for group, Hb, DCT and bilirubin.

Follow up
- If not jaundiced or pale and no hepatosplenomegaly — baby to postnatal ward with mother but ensure bilirubin is checked 4-hourly until it is clearly not rising.
- Not jaundiced/pale but hepatosplenomegaly present — consider admitting to NNU, repeat bilirubin within 4 hours (implies active disease).
- Jaundiced &/or pale — admit to NNU, and commence on phototherapy. Subsequent management depends on the cord haemoglobin results (see Fig. 9.3):
— Hb <10g/dl, baby ill — single volume (85 ml/kg) exchange transfusion immediately.
— Hb <10g/dl, baby well — double volume (170 ml/kg) exchange transfusion.
— Bilirubin rising >10 μmol/h — double volume exchange transfusion (it is thought that the earlier in the postnatal course this is done the less likely further transfusions may be required?).
- Hydropic baby at birth — resuscitate as outlined in Chapter 14 and transfer the baby as soon as possible to the neonatal intensive care unit for an urgent partial 'modified' (single volume) exchange transfusion.

Follow on care for babies with Rhesus disease
- Phototherapy should continue until the unconjugated bilirubin is down to satisfactory levels (see 'Setting Bilirubin Levels' and Fig. 9.4). In severe cases with liver disease or with the 'inspissated bile syndrome', the conjugated bilirubin may rise markedly at this stage. It is important to base your management on the unconjugated fraction unless the total bilirubin is rising very fast (> 10 μmol/L).

- In all DCT +ve babies who do not become jaundiced, check the haemoglobin weekly until the baby goes home, and than every 1–2 weeks until 12 weeks. Top-up transfusion may be required if the haemoglobin falls to less than 7g/dL, particularly if the reticulocyte count remains low. A DCT -ve baby (tested because mother Rh-) who never becomes jaundiced requires no follow-up.
- If treatment has been needed, give folic acid (250 micrograms/kg daily) until 6 months.
- Hearing assessment must be arranged on all infants who have required an exchange transfusion for hyperbilirubinaemia.
- All infants who receive an exchange transfusion should be seen in the neonatal follow-up clinic.
- Infants who have had repeated intrauterine transfusions tend to have bone marrow suppression at birth and may present at 4–6 weeks of age with failure to thrive or collapse with profound anaemia (as low as 2–4g/dl) if not monitored. These infants must be followed after discharge with 1–2 weekly haemoglobin estimations, top up transfusions as indicated (Ch. 14).

Complications of severe Rhesus Disease (now rare with good antenatal care)

- Thrombocytopaenia and leucopaenia due to marrow suppression (bleeding and infection risk).
- Coagulopathy due to liver dysfunction and thrombocytopaenia.
- Respiratory distress syndrome may complicate hydrops fetails.
- Inspissated bile syndrome — may be present at birth, due to biliary sludging, should resolve in time; avoid phototherapy (risk of bronzing).
- Late anaemia.

Summary

Jaundice is a very common condition in the newborn period. Because bilirubin encephalopathy and kernicterus are rarely seen now, it is tempting to become blase. Worryingly, several reports of clinical survivors of bilirubin encephalopathy have been reported recently, often in association with early discharge policies.

Do not forget that exchange transfusions carry a significant morbidity and mortality; by anticipation and attention to detail, these can usually be avoided by the early use of phototheraphy.

Although the commonest cause of conjugated jaundice is cholestasis related to TPN use, and usually resolves, careful evaluation is necessary to avoid missing a diagnosis of biliary atresia or choledochal cyst which will respond best to early surgery.

Gastrointestinal Disease

Gastro-oesophageal reflux (GOR)

GOR occurs when inappropriate relaxation of the lower oesophageal sphincter allows stomach contents to pass into the oesophagus. This may result in vomiting, aspiration of stomach contents into the lungs or oesophagitis. GOR is very common in infancy and is recognised more frequently in infants who are premature, on caffeine or following repair of oesophageal atresia.

- Mild symptoms in a thriving child require no treatment.
- GOR is almost universal in ELBW infants fed the large volumes of milk required for postnatal growth. It may present with apnoea and bradycardia, although most apnoea is due to immaturity or a sign of systemic illness.
- Simple measures such as elevation of the head end of the bed, prone nursing and alteration of feeding schedule from continuous to intermittent may suffice.

Follow-on treatments include:

- food thickeners made from carob seed or starch (Carobel or Thixo-D)
- Gaviscon which contains antacids and an alginate that forms a viscous layer on top of the stomach contents to prevent reflux (use with caution because of its high sodium content and tendency to constipate).

When the diagnosis is uncertain, there has been no response to simple measures, or there are complicating factors such as suspected oesophagitis, further investigation by pH monitoring, barium swallow to rule out hiatus hernia, or endoscopy may be helpful. The next lines of therapy are used where serious symptoms persist despite the above measures and the diagnosis has been confirmed:

- cisapride — a prokinetic agent, but not generally recommended for preterm infants and babies <3 months of age, because QT interval prolongation may occur
- ranitidine — reduces gastric acidity and helps resolution of oesophagitis

- omeprazole (proton pump inhibition) — reduces gastric acidity
- Further options include the use of a fundoplication with or without gastrostomy, which should not be contemplated without specialist advice.

Necrotising enterocolitis (NEC)

Necrosis of the bowel wall which may lead to perforation occurs most commonly in the terminal ileum and colon, but may be seen throughout the gut. NEC accounts for 10% of VLBW deaths and mortality is up to 30%. The exact cause is not certain and likely to be multifactorial. The immunological immaturity and poor gut defences may allow local infection by colonising bacteria, perhaps exacerbated by poor perfusion or gut hypoxia. Predisposing factors include prematurity, IUGR (especially where there is evidence of fetal hypoxia: absent or reversed end-diastolic flow velocity on umbilical artery Doppler), polycythaemia, septicaemia and early formula feeds. Possible preventive factors include feeding with expressed breast milk, early non-nutritive feeding, 12-hourly suppositories if bowels are not open, and the delaying of feeds if there is evidence of perinatal hypoxia. The relationship between umbilical catheterisation and NEC remains unclear. Milk feeds should probably be avoided when umbilical venous lines are used or in the first 48 hours where there have been abnormal Doppler velocities (see Ch. 2, p. 13).

DIAGNOSIS

This may be made by identifying pneumatosis intestinalis (intestinal submucosal air) on X-ray or at laparotomy. In the absence of pneumatosis, other symptoms lead to a 'high suspicion' of NEC and treatment is the same. Grading may be useful for prognosis:

Grade 1 (better prognosis). Cases have at least *two* of the following features:
- abdominal distension
- increasing or bilious aspirates
- blood in stool
- systemic illness — lethargy, hypotonia or apnoea
- X-ray — pneumatosis intestinalis, gaseous distension or frothy luminal contents.

Grade 2. In addition, cases have one or more of:
- abdominal tenderness or rigidity (guarding)
- tissue (mucosa) in stool

- abnormal or spontaneous bleeding (coagulopathy)
- total leucocyte count $<6 \times 10^9$/L at time of illness
- platelet count $<100 \times 10^9$/L at time of illness
- pneumoperitoneum or portal vein gas.

INVESTIGATIONS ON SUSPICION OF NEC

- Blood cultures
- Haemoglobin, white count, platelets
- Coagulation screen
- U & E, bilirubin, BG
- Albumin
- Plain radiographs — supine and right lateral decubitus
- Blood gas.

MANAGEMENT

- Stop feeds.
- Pass NG tube — put on free drainage and hourly aspirates.
- IV antibiotics — we use benzylpenicillin, gentamicin and metronidazole.
- Monitor circulation and perfusion (an IA line is useful) and use colloid and inotropes to correct shock (Ch. 6).
- Correct coagulation defect, thrombocytopenia (usually if $<30 \times 10^9$/L or bleeding) and anaemia if present (Ch. 14).
- Monitor girth (progressive increase may indicate perforation).
- Nutrition — put in long IV line after 24 h treatment and give TPN (Ch. 15).
- If NEC is confirmed, withhold feeds and give antibiotics for 7–10 days, depending on how quickly symptoms settle.
- If there is a high suspicion, but the diagnosis is not confirmed and the baby promptly recovers and appears hungry, feeds may be gradually reintroduced after 48 h.
- **Surgery**
  - a surgical opinion is useful early on in the illness unless symptoms are mild, as the decision to intervene with surgery requires repeated assessment in the absence of pneumoperitoneum.
  - indications for surgery include perforation or deterioration, e.g. worsening acidosis or thrombocytopenia, suggestive of the presence of necrotic bowel.
- Late complications include fibrosis resulting in stricture formation which may present as intestinal obstruction.
- Prognosis is excellent if there are no strictures or surgery is not required.

TEN

Renal disease

Background

The commonest renal problems in the newborn period are congenital abnormalities, transient renal failure due to perinatal asphyxia at term and UTIs. Those abnormalities of the GU tract requiring surgical management are dealt with in Chapter 16.

The liquor surrounding the fetus is largely the result of fetal urine production, the liquor then being swallowed and reabsorbed across the fetal GI tract. The fetus normally produces 300–800 mL/day of urine. Failure of production of fetal urine leads to oligohydramnios, whereas GI obstruction (e.g. oesophageal atresia) leads to polyhydramnios.

Diagnosis by antenatal fetal USS

Routine scanning at 16–20 weeks will identify most major abnormalities. Mild pelvicalyceal dilatation is the commonest abnormality requiring postnatal investigation (see below). More detailed USSs looking specifically for an abnormality of the GU tract are indicated as follows:

- *A positive family history* of congenital abnormalities of the GU tract.
- *Severe oligohydramnios* — may be associated with absent kidneys, dysplastic or hypoplastic kidneys or bilateral obstruction of the urinary tract (e.g. posterior urethral valves). If only one kidney is obstructed, urine will continue to be produced and excreted into the amniotic cavity. Oligohydramnios from any cause may result in pulmonary hypoplasia and postural deformities of the fetus (fetal akinesia syndrome).
- *A large placenta* — may be associated with the rare congenital nephrotic syndrome. Suspect if there is also oligohydramnios, IUGR and a raised maternal αFP level, particularly in amniotic fluid.

- *A single umbilical artery* — associated with an abnormality of the GU tract (most commonly renal aplasia or hypoplasia, hydronephrosis, obstructive uropathy) in less than 1 in 20 children. We do not routinely re-scan babies postnatally with a single umbilical artery if two normal kidneys were visualised on an antenatal scan.
- *Fetal abdominal mass* — **renal causes** (75%) include polycystic disease of the kidney, massive hydronephrosis, collections of urinary acites or renal tumours. **Other causes:** GI masses (15%); liver, biliary tree or spleen (5%); non-renal tumours (5%), e.g. neuroblastoma or teratoma.
- *Other fetal abnormalities.* A fetus who has one congenital abnormality is at greater risk of having another and in addition there are a number of syndromes in which renal abnormalities are a recognised feature (see Table 10.1).

Table 10.1 Dysmorphic syndromes with renal abnormalities

Syndrome	General features	Renal abnormalities
Skeletal malformations		
Spina bifida	Meningomyelocoele	Double ureter, horseshoe kidney, hydronephrosis
Hemihypertrophy	Hemihypertrophy	Wilms' tumour, hypospadias
Potter syndrome	Abnormal facies; lung and skeletal anomalies	Renal agenesis
Meckel syndrome	Encephalocele, polydactyly	Polycystic kidneys
Cerebrohepatorenal syndrome (Zellweger syndrome)	Hepatomegaly, glaucoma, brain anomalies, chondrodystrophy	Polycystic kidneys
Jeune syndrome	Thoracic asphyxiating dystrophy	Medullary necrosis, proteinuria, hydronephrosis, horseshoe kidneys
VATER syndrome	Vertebral abnormalities, anal atresia, TOF, radial dysplasia	Renal dysplasia
VACTERL syndrome	Same as VATER, plus additional cardiac and limb abnormalities	Renal dysplasia
Visceral abnormalities		
Prune belly	Hypoplasia of abdominal muscles, cryptorchidism	Urinary tract dysplasia
Tuberous sclerosis	Tuberous sclerosis, adenoma sebaceum	Cystic kidneys, kidney tumours

Table 10.1 *cont'd*

Beckwith–Wiedemann syndrome	Macroglossia, hypoglycaemia	Renal dysplasia, nephroblastoma
Facial or eye abnormalities		
Oculocerebrorenal syndrome (Lowe syndrome)	Cataracts, rickets, mental retardation	Proximal tubular defects
Aniridia–Wilms	Aniridia, cryptorchidism	Wilms' tumour
Meckel–Gruber syndrome (dysencephalia splanchnocystica)	Encephalocele, polydactyly, cryptorchidism, cardiac anomalies, liver disease	Polycystic kidneys
Melnick–Fraser syndrome (branchio-otorenal syndrome)	Preauricular pits, branchial clefts, deafness	Renal dysplasia
Oral-facial-digital syndrome, type I	Oral frenula and clefts, hypoplastic alae nasi, digital asymmetry	Renal microcysts
Chromosomal abnormalities		
Down syndrome (trisomy 21)	Abnormal facies, brachycephaly, CHD	Cystic kidneys and other renal abnormalities in 7%
Turner syndrome	Small stature, CHD, amenorrhoea, XO sex chromosones	Horseshoe kidney; duplications and malrotations of the urinary collecting system occur in 60%
Trisomy 13 (Patau syndrome)	Abnormal facies, cleft lip and palate, CHD	Cystic kidneys and other renal abnormalities in 60%
Trisomy 18 (Edwards syndrome)	Abnormal facies, abnormal ears, overlapping digits, CHD	Cystic kidneys, horseshoe kidney, or duplications occur in 70%
Metabolic abnormalities		
Galactosaemia	Cataracts, hepatic injury, brain damage	Renal tubular dysfunction
GSD (von Gierke's disease)	Hypoglycaemia, hepatomegaly	Renal tubular dysfunction
Hereditary tyrosinaemia	Failure to thrive, fever, hepatomegaly	Renal tubular dysfunction
Congenital infection		
Congenital rubella	Cataracts, cardiac anomalies, deafness, microcephaly	Various renal anomalies, renal artery stenosis with late hypertension
Miscellaneous syndromes		
Rubinstein–Taybi syndrome	Broad thumbs and toes, slanted palpebral fissures, hypoplastic maxilla	Renal anomalies

Presentation of renal disease in the newborn

The following suggest you consider further assessment of the GU tract:

- Dysmorphic syndromes (Table 10.1)
- External abnormality of the abdomen or genitalia (e.g. hypospadias, epispadias, ambiguous genitalia, bladder exstrophy)
- Fetal deformation (Potter sequence, arthrogryposis, pulmonary hypoplasia)
- A single umbilical artery (see fetal ultrasound diagnosis above)
- Any spinal abnormality
- Failure to pass urine within 48 h of birth
- Infection of the urinary tract
- Palpable renal mass
- Haematuria
- Glycosuria
- Proteinuria

Ninety per cent of healthy term infants pass urine within the first 24 h after birth and 99% by 48 h. Failure to pass urine by 48 h or observation of a poor stream, particularly in a male infant, should lead to a search for the causes in Table 10.2. Bladder catheterisation is essential to determine whether urine is present but either outflow is obstructed or urine has not been formed. Bladder drainage (urethral or suprapubic) should be discussed with a paediatric urological surgeon.

Table 10.2   Causes of failure to pass urine by 48 h

Inability to form urine
- Poor renal perfusion due to either hypovolaemia or hypotension
- Bilateral renal agenesis (Potter's syndrome)
- Acute tubular necrosis (due to perinatal asphyxia)
- Bilateral renal vein thrombosis
- Congenital nephrotic syndrome or congenital nephritis (most commonly due to congenital infection)

Obstruction to urinary flow
- Posterior urethral valves in a male infant
- Urethral stricture
- Urethral diverticulum
- Neurogenic bladder (in association with spina bifida)
- Drugs such as pancuronium which may lead to urinary retention

Infection of the urinary tract may lead to a non-specific presentation with poor feeding or weight loss, dehydration, temperature instability, vomiting, jaundice or lethargy.

Undescended testis (1% of term births, more common in preterms) is common and rarely associated with other GU tract anomalies. Follow up is required but further investigation in the newborn is not indicated.

A PALPABLE RENAL MASS IN THE NEWBORN PERIOD
(see Table 10.3)

- The lower poles of normal kidneys may be palpable:
  — on examination of normal neonates, particularly before the first feed if air has not been swallowed

Table 10.3 Causes of a palpable renal mass

Intrarenal
Solid
- Wilms' tumour
- Renal vein thrombosis (usually haematuria)
- Benign nephroma (rare neonatal problem)
- Horseshoe kidney
- Ectopic kidney (usually palpable in the pelvis)
- Bilateral enlargement following hypoxia or ischaemia

Cystic
- Hydronephrosis (due to reflux or anatomical or functional obstruction). May be accompanied by:
  — no megaloureter = PUJ obstruction
  — megaloureter = VUJ obstruction or VUR
  — large bladder = bladder outlet obstruction
  — prune belly syndrome
  A mass arising outside the urinary tract may also cause obstruction of the urinary tract
- Single cyst (benign renal cyst)
- Multicystic
  — dysplastic kidney
  — polycystic disease
    – infantile onset (autosomal recessive)
    – 'adult' onset (autosomal dominant)

Extrarenal
- An adrenal mass (e.g. neuroblastoma)
- Retroperitoneal haematoma (sometimes due to adrenal haemorrhage)
- The left 'renal' mass may be the spleen. The spleen tip is very commonly palpable in otherwise normal term infants
- A urinoma (there is perforation somewhere along the urinary tract but instead of free urinary acites forming, the collection of urine is walled off and forms a focal mass)
- An ovarian cyst

— if the infant has hypotonia involving the abdominal wall muscles
— if there is high GI atresia or a scaphoid abdomen associated with congenital diaphragmatic hernia.

- A postnatal USS is most useful in distinguishing the various causes of a palpable renal mass (see p. 174 for further investigation). Of normal neonates, 0.8% have a palpable abdominal mass (usually kidney or spleen).
- The commonest causes of a unilateral mass in the newborn are hydronephrosis, multicystic dysplastic kidney or renal vein thrombosis.
- The commonest causes of bilateral masses are bilateral hydronephrosis, polycystic kidney disease or renal vein thrombosis.
- The commonest cause of a midline mass is obstructive uropathy; rarer causes are a urachal cyst or hydrometrocolpos (the hymen bulges and accumulated secretions in the uterus may cause bowel obstruction, hydronephrosis or oedema and cyanosis of the legs; if not diagnosed at birth, the secretions decrease and the diagnosis will be missed until puberty when haemometrocolpos occurs).

HAEMATURIA

Frank haematuria is rare in the newborn but microscopic haematuria is common (Table 10.4). Test strips are extremely sensitive and detect red cells (5 red cells/mm^3 minimum) and free myoglobin or haemoglobin (0.02 mg/dL minimum). Intact red blood cells give a spotted reaction whereas free haemoglobin gives a uniform green on the test strip. However, the best discriminator is microscopy of fresh urine. Discoloration of the urine may arise due to other pigments (urate or phosphate crystals or bile pigments — see Ch. 9). Commonest causes of haematuria in the newborn are from perinatal asphyxia and DIC in a very sick low birthweight infant.

Table 10.4   Causes of haematuria

Non-glomerular
- Infection of any part of the urinary tract (urethritis, cystitis, pyelonephritis)
- Hydronephrosis without infection
- Coagulopathy (including haemorrhagic disease of the newborn)
- Vascular anomalies
- Wilms' tumour
- Vaginal blood ('withdrawal bleeding' in a female infant in the first few days after birth is not uncommon)
- Relief of obstructive uropathy
- Following SPA

Table 10.4 *cont'd*

Glomerular
Red cell casts, white cell casts or epithelial casts on microscopy suggest a glomerular cause but absence of casts does not exclude a glomerular problem
- Congenital nephritis (most commonly due to congenital infection including toxoplasmosis, CMV, syphilis)
- Alport's syndrome (hereditary deafness and nephritis)
- Trauma to the kidneys during delivery
- Arterial emboli — causes are:
  — from an UAC, especially if the tip is lying in the lumbar aorta. Such low-lying catheters should be sited with the tip below L2, but even this placement has been demonstrated to have a higher risk of renal and gut ischaemia than a high position with the tip of the catheter above the diaphragm between T4 and T8
  — from endocarditis associated with long-standing indwelling central venous lines for parenteral nutrition. Right atrial or tricuspid vegetations form and whilst most emboli are trapped in the pulmonary circulation, some may cross a patent foramen ovale
  — immune complex vasculitis due to low-grade ventriculoperitoneal shunt infection may also involve the kidneys
- Corticomedullary or tubular necrosis (usually secondary to perinatal asphyxia)
- Drugs (aminoglycosides or penicillins may rarely cause haematuria in the newborn)
- Renal vein thrombosis
- Polycystic or dysplastic kidneys

GLYCOSURIA

Glycosuria is extremely common in the newborn and is only very rarely a manifestation of renal disease (see Table 10.5).

PROTEINURIA

- Protein excretion in the urine falls with increasing gestational and increasing postnatal age.
- There is a wide range in the newborn and a normal term infant may excrete up to 1g albumin/L during the first 48 h of life.
- False-positive results are common as dipsticks will detect as little as 0.3 g/L urinary protein (see Table 10.6). Dipsticks also give false results if the urine specimen is old, if the dipstick is left in the urine too long or if the urine is alkaline.
- If significant proteinuria (Table 10.6) is found, a 12 or 24 h collection should be obtained, although this is technically difficult in the newborn (see below).
- Haematuria is inevitably accompanied by proteinuria.

Table 10.5   Causes of glycosuria

Hyperglycaemia

Transient hyperglycaemia
— Extremely common in very low birthweight infants receiving IV dextrose infusions or TPN
— Poor glucose homeostasis is a non-specific clue to infection in the newborn infant
— Due to 'stress' (e.g. following surgery or a prolonged convulsion)
— Due to drugs (e.g. steroids and theophylline)
— Iatrogenic (the infant is inadvertently receiving more than 6 mg/kg per min glucose and the metabolic threshold is exceeded)

Persistent hyperglycaemia
Neonatal diabetes mellitus due to delayed maturation of the insulin-releasing beta-cells in the pancreas. Insulin is present but in insufficient amounts. The condition usually resolves within 1–2 months of birth. Most infants do not develop insulin-dependent diabetes in later life

Normoglycaemia

Decreased renal threshold
— Isolated renal glycosuria (often due to prematurity; may be hereditary)
— Fanconi's syndrome

False positive dipstick test (i.e. presence in the urinary of reducing substances other than glucose)
— Galactose
— Fructose
— Alkaptonuria
Heavy proteinuria or heavy urate deposits may also give a false-positive Clinitest, but Clinistix reagent strips are specific for glucose

Table 10.6   Causes of significant proteinuria

Significant proteinuria = 0.1 g/m^2 per 24 h, but urinalysis sticks are very sensitive (1+ = 0.3 g/L, 4+ = 20 g/L)

Transient proteinuria
Common in the first 48 h of postnatal life

Persistent proteinuria
UTI
Congenital infections (syphilis, toxoplasmosis, CMV)
Renal vein thrombosis
Congenital nephrotic syndrome (sometimes familial)

Whilst the commonest causes of significant persistent proteinuria are given in the table, these are all relatively rare and much commoner is non-specific mild proteinuria which can be the result of almost any form of renal compromise (systemic infection, perinatal asphyxia, hypotension, DIC, cardiac failure). Haematuria is inevitably accompanied by mild proteinuria.

Investigation of the GU tract

Urinalysis is commonly carried out in newborn infants and is quick and cheap but false positives for haematuria, glycosuria and proteinuria are common, as indicated above.

COLLECTION OF URINE SAMPLES

Always send the sample fresh to the laboratory.

Bag urine specimen. Clean the genitalia with sterile water and allow to dry. Attach a Hollister urine bag which allows urine to be withdrawn from the bag as soon as voided without having to remove the bag. False positive rate is relatively high because of contamination of the urine specimen with skin commensals and faecal organisms in the nappy area. Care must be taken in very preterm infants as the adhesive used to affix urine bags may cause desquamation of the skin when the bag is removed.

Suprapubic aspiration (SPA). This is the 'gold standard' and the method of choice in the newborn (see Ch. 21). USS to detect a full bladder greatly increases the success rate of SPA but often stimulates micturition — be ready to collect a 'clean catch' specimen!

In-out catheterisation. This is a relatively simple procedure in the newborn, in both males and females, and can be done using a fine NG tube and sterile technique. It is essential if urine has not been passed since birth as a SPA is unlikely to be successful in the absence of a palpable bladder.

URINALYSIS

Colour
Normal urine is yellow — urobilinogen (see Ch. 9)
Dark urine
— normal but concentrated
— small amounts of blood cause smoky urine, larger amounts a
  frank red colour
— presence of clots suggests bleeding from lower tract
— free Hb or myoglobin causes dark red or black urine
— conjugated hyperbilirubinaemia: pale stools and dark urine of
  obstructive jaundice or hepatitis but not haemolytic jaundice.
Coloured urine — drugs (e.g. rifampicin — orange; methylene blue — green).
Cloudy urine — most commonly benign, due to phosphate or urate crystals; bacteriuria or pyuria are more significant.

Concentration (Table 10.7)
Specific gravity — easily measured at the bedside
Osmolality — (laboratory determination) better index of renal concentrating ability.

The relationship between these is not linear, e.g. glycosuria increases specific gravity by proportionally more than osmolality.

pH
Normal 4.6–8.0 depending on diet, but usually acidic (pH 5–6).
Alkaline urine (pH >8.0)
— urine infected with *Proteus* or *Pseudomonas*
— respiratory alkalosis
— metabolic alkalosis but not if hypokalaemic
— RTA (pH >6 is abnormal in the presence of metabolic acidosis in a term infant)
Acidic urine (pH < 4.6)
— starvation (ketonuria)
— urine infection
— respiratory acidosis
— metabolic acidosis (except RTA)
— hypokalaemic alkalosis.

MICROSCOPY

Red cells
Normally < 3 RBC/mm³ of uncentrifuged urine or < 2 RBC/high-power field of centrifuged urine (see Table 10.4).

White cells
Normally <3 WBC/mm³ of unspun urine or <5 WBC/high-power field of centrifuged urine. Infection can be present without white blood cells in the urine and pyuria can occur without a positive bacterial culture (e.g. TB, appendicitis, calculi).

Epithelial cells
Normal.

Table 10.7 Measurement of urine concentration

Specific gravity	Osmolality (mosmol/kg)
1.002	100
1.005	150
1.010	300
1.020	600
1.030	1200

Organism

Bacteria or yeast — always abnormal but may be a contaminant.

Casts

Hyaline casts — normal but often increased in febrile illness or cardiac failure

Red cell casts — suggest glomerular disease

Granular casts — occur in acute and chronic renal failure

White cell casts — occur in glomerulonephritis and infection of the upper tract

Epithelial casts — suggest tubular damage.

Crystals

Phosphate, urate and oxalate crystals are common and usually of no pathological significance. However, crystalluria may also indicate *Proteus* infection, hyperuricaemia or cystinuria.

ULTRASOUND SCAN

This is the best method for examining the *upper* renal tract. Ultrasonography can demonstrate the presence or absence of two kidneys, kidney size and position, echogenicity of the renal parenchyma (increased echogenicity is seen in hypoxic ischaemic damage), cystic abnormalities and any dilatation of the collecting system. Ultrasonography will detect gross hydroureter but may miss mildly dilated ureters and will also show dilatation and trabeculation of the bladder. Ultrasonography can distinguish between solid and cystic masses.

MICTURATING CYSTOURETHROGRAPHY (MCUG)

- Essential to examine the bladder for VUR and for abnormalities of the urethra, particularly for posterior urethral valves.
- The examination must be performed without anaesthesia or sedation as these drugs may alter bladder urodynamics.
- Should always be covered by additional antibiotic cover.

Give trimethoprim 4 mg/kg orally twice a day or, in a preterm infant, cephradine 25 mg/kg orally twice a day from 24 h before the MCUG until 48 h afterwards. The infant should then return to the regular nocturnal prophylactic antibiotic dose.

DMSA SCAN

- IV injection of DMSA labelled with the radioactive isotope technetium-$_{99}$.
- DMSA is used to assess structure and to look for scarring but is of less value in the newborn than in older children.

- DMSA scan may also give some guide to renal function as the percentage uptake of the isotope in each kidney may be calculated (a measure of GFR).
- DMSA may not be able to differentiate renal dysplasia from renal scarring.

DTPA SCAN

- IV injection of DTPA labelled with technetium-$_{99}$.
- To assess GFR.
- If excretion of the isotope increases following an injection of IV furosemide (frusemide), this suggests that any obstruction is functional rather than anatomical.

MAG-3 SCAN

- IV injection of MAG-3 labelled with technetium-$_{99}$.
- Often used in the investigation of obstructed uropathy and is now considered superior to DTPA scans.
- Again the function of each kidney can be assessed, and the response to diuretics such as furosemide (frusemide) observed.

INTRAVENOUS UROGRAPHY (IVU)

- Rarely carried out in the newborn.
- The dose of radiation is large for the amount of information obtained.
- Direct percutaneous puncture of a dilated collecting system is an alternative contrast technique to obtain detailed anatomical information about the structure and route of an abnormal collecting system.

INVESTIGATION OF ANTENATALLY DIAGNOSED URINARY TRACT PROBLEMS

The detection of a urinary tract abnormality on antenatal USS should have led to referral for antenatal counselling, ideally by a paediatric nephrologist, paediatric urological surgeon and obstetrician jointly. The parents will therefore be prepared for the fact that their child may be admitted to the neonatal unit and, in any case, is likely to have a number of postnatal investigations. The most common significant abnormalities detected antenatally are:

- *Unilateral hydronephrosis* — due to VUR; PUJ obstruction; multicystic dysplastic kidney (not to be confused with polycystic kidneys); VUJ obstruction; duplex systems; single kidney.

- *Bilateral hydronephrosis* — due to bilateral VUR, VUJ or PUJ obstruction; posterior urethral valves.

  Postnatally all children will require:

- Renal tract USS
- Even if there is no renal tract dilatation on the postnatal USS, MCUG is essential to exclude VUR
- If VUR is demonstrated, a DMSA scan will be necessary to look for cortical scarring
- If USS shows a multicystic dysplastic kidney, a DMSA scan will be necessary to confirm non-function of that kidney
- If obstruction is suspected, a DTPA or MAG-3 radionuclide scan will be necessary to look for evidence of obstruction.

Timing of investigation

If there are severe bilateral abnormalities or a palpable bladder, the paediatric nephrologist and paediatric urological surgeon should be involved early after birth. However, if the significant abnormality is unilateral only, US imaging can usually be delayed until after 48 h as some abnormalities can appear relatively minor soon after birth but become more prominent later. If the infant is well and feeding with no clinical signs or symptoms, USS can then be arranged on an outpatient basis if the mother wishes for an early discharge. All term infants with bilateral obstructive uropathy should receive trimethoprim prophylaxis (2 mg/kg each night) until all investigations have been carried out and the parents have met with the paediatrician to discuss these results. Babies with mild, unilateral dilatation of the renal pelvis only do not receive prophylaxis. Trimethoprim is not recommended for preterm infants because it acts as a folate antagonist; oral cephradine (25 mg/kg) at night is a suitable alternative.

INVESTIGATION OF A RENAL MASS (see Table 10.3)

In addition to abdominal USS, carry out:

- FBC
- Urea and creatinine
- Clotting studies
- Screen for increased urinary catecholamines
- BP
- SPA for urine electrolytes, microscopy and culture

  Depending on the cause, the following investigations may be indicated:

- MCUG
- DTPA or MAG-3 isotope scan
- IVU
- Aortogram

- Definitive histological diagnosis of a solid mass thought to be a tumour requires biopsy.

Management of specific problems

URINARY TRACT INFECTION

Background
Infection may cause symptoms (see below) or covert bacteriuria but we take a proven culture-positive diagnosis of UTI as:

- Any growth on culture of SPA. Every attempt should be made to confirm the diagnosis of UTI in the newborn by SPA. All too often a single positive bag culture is treated and the infant is then committed to invasive investigation.
- >100 000 organisms/mL in pure growth of a reliable (see p. 170) catheter or bag urine; ideally two consecutive growths of the same organism with identical sensitivities.

Accurate diagnosis and treatment are important to:

- alleviate symptoms
- prevent renal scarring
- detect underlying anomalies
- avoid unnecessary investigations.

Diagnosis
UTI is usually detected in the newborn period as a non-specifically ill or febrile infant, a baby who is not feeding well, or prolonged jaundice. Examination must include:

- blood pressure
- abdominal masses
- genitalia and spine for congenital anomalies
- observation of the urinary stream in boys.

Acute treatment
- IV treatment is preferred in the newborn infant because of the urgent need to avoid a localised UTI extending to a generalised septicaemia.
- Antibiotics should be started as soon as a urine sample has been obtained and IV ampicillin and gentamicin (as the usual organisms are *E. coli*, *Proteus*, *Pseudomonas* and *Streptococcus faecalis*) are a suitable combination in a term infant without congenital abnormalities (see appendix for drug doses).
- If the infant is known to have congenital abnormalities of the renal tract, urea and creatinine are a poor guide to renal function early in the newborn period (since they mirror the

maternal urea and creatinine until placental separation) and therefore IV cefotaxime is probably a safer choice.
- Sulphonamides should always be avoided, particularly in jaundiced babies, as they carry no advantage over trimethoprim but have additional side-effects.
- If the infant is well, he or she need not be admitted to the neonatal unit and can have the IV antibiotics via a heparinised cannula on the postnatal wards. If the infant is ill or not feeding well, he or she should be admitted to the neonatal unit for monitoring and IV fluids (see Ch. 8).

Investigation of a UTI

Every first proven UTI (see definition above) should be investigated irrespective of the child's age or sex. Do not defer antibiotic treatment whilst awaiting investigations. Discharge on regular chemoprophylaxis (see below) until investigations are complete. Controversy persists over the best combination of investigations (USS is especially operator-dependent) but one scheme is:

- USS as in-patient
- MCUG after 6 weeks

If these suggest VUR, consider DMSA for degree of renal scarring. If obstruction is suggested, consider DPTA or MAG-3 to assess function of each kidney.

The above investigations will show an anomaly in 30–50% (most commonly in boys), most commonly VUR. Many neonatal UTIs arise due to haematogenous spread and are themselves secondary to septicaemia.

Prevention

Follow-up 3-monthly with urine culture and BP check. The other important measures in the newborn period are:

- strict attention to hygiene with frequent nappy changes
- avoid constipation
- chemoprophylaxis pending investigation and for a minimum of 2 years if investigation shows an underlying abnormality (oral trimethoprim 2 mg/kg at night for a term infant or cephradine 25 mg/kg at night for a preterm infant).

Prognosis

VUR-related scarring accounts for 20% of adult dialysis. Most scarring is already present by 1 year of age — hence the need for prompt investigation in the neonatal period. 10% of children with renal scarring develop hypertension. VUR resolves spontaneously in 80% and chemoprophylaxis until resolution of VUR improves prognosis as much as surgical reimplantation.

NEPHROTIC SYNDROME

Background
This is extremely uncommon in the UK. Presentation may be with massive proteinuria, oedema, acites or hydrops fetalis. For the differential diagnosis of neonatal ascites and hydrops, see Table 14.2. Causes of nephrotic syndrome are:

- congenital nephrotic syndrome of the Finnish type — affects 1 in 2000 births in Finland. Autosomal recessive inheritance has also been described and the same pathology has been described in other countries
- congenital syphilis
- congenital CMV infection
- renal vein thrombosis
- nail–patellar syndrome.

Diagnosis
Massive proteinuria and low serum albumin.

Differential diagnosis
Oedema is an uncommon sign in the newborn and apart from the causes of hydrops fetalis (see Ch. 14), other causes include iatrogenic (excessive water and salt administration), acute renal failure and 'sick cell syndrome' (tissue injury due to hypoxia, ischaemia or hypothermia).

Outcome
Growth retardation, recurrent infection and progressive renal failure are all potential complications. Management consists of:

- detecting any treatable underlying cause (e.g. syphilis)
- symptomatic management of oedema and acites with spironolactone 1mg/kg twice a day and, if necessary, salt-poor 20% human albumin 1 g/kg IV over 3 h followed by furosemide (frusemide) 2 mg/kg IV.
- expert dietary advice to ensure optimal calorie intake
- renal transplantation has been carried out.

ACUTE RENAL FAILURE

Background
Transient acute renal failure (ARF) is relatively common in infants in the NICU care unit (Table 10.8), the commonest cause in term infants being perinatal asphyxia, and in preterm infants

association with severe disease affecting other systems (e.g. RDS, NEC, sepsis etc). ARF is defined as a sudden decrease in renal function resulting in retention of normal catabolic waste products (nitrogenous waste, phosphate, acid) and electrolyte imbalance. ARF is not synonymous with failure of urine production since biochemical renal failure may occur without oliguria in drug nephropathy and in polyuric ARF following relief of obstructive uropathy. Normal values for plasma creatinine in the newborn are given in Table 10.9 and for GFR in Table 10.10. Table 10.11 gives a number of biochemical indices which may help to distinguish pre-renal from intrinsic renal failure. In the newborn, GFR can be approximated from the plasma creatinine using the formula:

$$GFR = K \times l/\text{plasma creatinine}$$

where GFR is expressed in mL/min/1.73m^2, l is the body length in cm, plasma creatinine is in µmol/L, K is a constant (29 for infants <2.5 kg; 40 for infants > 2.5 kg).

Diagnosis

- A careful family and obstetric history is taken. The details of delivery, the CTG appearances and Apgar scores should be determined as these may suggest perinatal asphyxia. A history of oligohydramnios or IUGR may be significant.
- Careful physical examination is performed, looking for congenital abnormalities of the renal tract, and other systems and genitalia, and for abdominal masses and spinal disorders.
- Pre-renal renal failure is the commonest cause in the newborn and careful attention should be paid to signs of dehydration, evidence of vomiting, diarrhoea or other 'third space losses' (e.g. ascites in the peritoneal cavity, fluid in the lumen of an obstructed gut, hydothorax, etc.), history of blood loss etc.
- Take a careful history of any drugs that the baby and/or mother have been receiving. If the mother has been given a combination of diuretics and an angiotensin converting enzyme inhibitor for pregnancy-associated hypertension, this is strongly associated with neonatal ARF.

Investigations (see Tables 10.8–10.11)

1. Catheterise bladder using a sterile technique.
2. If there is urine in the bladder, send this for urinalysis, microscopy, culture, urine Na, creatinine and osmolality. If any urine is being produced, measure the hourly urine output and make a timed collection for protein excretion and an estimation of endogenous creatinine clearance, which is an approximation to GFR:

$$\frac{GFR}{(\text{mL/min})} = \frac{\text{urinary creatinine concentration (mmol/L)} \times 1000 \times \text{urine flow rate (mL/min)}}{\text{plasma creatinine concentration (µmol/L)}}$$

Table 10.8 Causes of acute renal failure in the neonate

Prerenal	Renal parenchymal (intrinsic renal failure)	Obstructive

Hypotension
  Septic shock
  Maternal antepartum
    haemorrhage
  Twin–twin transfusion
  Neonatal haemorrhage
  Major surgery
  Cardiac disease
    (typically CoA or
    hypoplastic left
    heart syndrome)
Congestive cardiac
  failure
Asphyxia
Dehydration
	Hypoperfusion related to:
	  Hypoxia
	  RDS
	  Sepsis
	  Diarrhoea
	  Dehydration
	  Haemorrhage
	  Shock
	  Surgical procedures
	Thromboembolic disease
	  Renal vein thrombosis
	  Arterial thrombosis or
	    emboli
	  Cortical necrosis
	  DIC
	Nephrotoxins
	Inflammatory
	  Neonatal nephritis
	  (usually congenital
	  infection)
	  Pyelonephritis
	Congenital abnormalities
	  Cystic dysplasia
	  Hypoplasia
	  Agenesis
	  Polycystic kidneys
		Urethral obstruction
		  Posterior urethral
		    valves
		  Stricture
		  Diverticulum
		Ureterocoele
		Ureteropelvic
		  obstruction
		Ureterovesical
		  obstruction
		Extrinsic tumours
		Neurogenic bladder
		Megacystis-
		  megaureter

Table 10.9 Plasma creatinine — 95% confidence limits of plasma creatinine (μmol/L) in neonates

Gestation (weeks)	Age (days)				
	2	7	14	21	28
28	40–220	23–145	18–118	16–104	15–95
30	30–192	20–132	17–107	15–95	13–87
32	27–175	19–119	15–97	14–86	12–78
34	24–158	17–109	14–88	12–78	11–71
36	23–143	16–98	12–80	11–71	10–64
38	20–130	15–89	12–72	10–64	9–59
40	18–118	13–81	10–66	9–57	9–53

3. Take blood simultaneously for plasma urea, creatinine, osmolality, Na, K, Ca, Mg and an ABG for acid–base status.
4. FBC and clotting studies to exclude DIC.
5. Plasma albumin.

Table 10.10 Glomerular filtration rate — 'normal' value in neonates and infants (mL/min/1.73 m²)

Gestational age (weeks)	Postnatal age (mean ± 1 SD)	
	First week	2–8 weeks
25–28	11.0 ± 5.4	15.5 ± 6.2
29–34	15.3 ± 5.6	28.7 ± 13.8
38–42	40.6 ± 14.8	65.0 ± 24.8

Table 10.11 Indices to differentiate between pre-renal and intrinsic renal failure

	Pre-renal	Renal
Ratio of urine/plasma concentrations		
Urea	>10	<10
Osmolality	> 2	< 1
F_eNa	< 1% term	>3%
	< 5% preterm	

$$F_eNa\% = \frac{100 \times U_{Na} \times P_{Cr}}{P_{Na} \times U_{Cr}}$$

Where F_eNa = fractional excretion of sodium; U = urinary; P = plasma; Cr = creatinine; Na = sodium. Values of F_eNa up to 16% may occur in the very sick preterm infant in the absence of renal failure.

NB. In both pre-renal and acute renal failure there is oliguria (less than 300 mL/m² per 24 h urine or less than 0.5 mL/kg per h). Total obstruction of the renal tract leads to anuria (apart from a small amount of bladder 'sweat'). The average 1 kg baby has a surface area of 0.1 m²; a term infant has a surface area of about 0.2 m².

6. Blood cultures.
7. Measure the BP to exclude hypotension or hypertension.
8. Urgent USS to check for the presence of kidneys, size of kidneys and to exclude obstruction.
9. ECG if hyperkalaemia is present.
10. CXR if there is evidence of fluid overload.

Immediate management

- If there is no evidence of obstruction or fluid overload, give 0.9% normal saline 20mL/kg over 1 h with furosemide (frusemide) 1 mg/kg IV.
- If the indices in Table 10.11 suggest pre-renal oliguria, repeat this fluid challenge after 1 h if there has been no response and increase furosemide (frusemide) to 3–5 mg/kg IV.

- If there is hypotension in the absence of fluid depletion start an infusion of dopamine at 5 µg/kg/min IV.
- If the infant responds to this approach, continue with standard maintenance fluid therapy (see Ch. 8).

Conservative management. If the indices in Table 10.11 suggest intrinsic renal failure, start conservative management for established renal failure:

- Keep a detailed fluid balance chart.
- Weigh the infant daily.
- Urine and electrolytes daily.
- Fluid restrict to insensible losses plus urine output:
  — Insensible losses are largely free water (through trans-epidermal and respiratory routes). Estimate insensible losses as 20–30 mL/kg per 24 h and replace with 10% dextrose to maintain blood sugar
  — Urine output is calculated on a 6-hourly retrospective basis and replaced as normal or half-normal saline depending on the Na excreted in the urine. Try to avoid giving additional Na in drug solutions or to keep IA and IV lines patent.

TPN provides an added load of Na, K, water and acids and should be avoided. If the caloric needs cannot be met by IV infusions of restricted amounts of 15% dextrose, this is an indication for dialysis. Complications of conservative management of ARF during treatment are shown in Table 10.12.

Table 10.12 Management of metabolic complications of renal failure

Complication	Treatment
Asymptomatic hyponatraemia	Fluid restriction
Symptomatic hyponatraemia	See p. 135
Hyperkalaemia	Ca resonium 1 g/kg per day oral or rectal
	Ca gluconate (10%) 0.5 mL/kg IV
	$NaHCO_3$ 2 mmol/kg IV
	Insulin 0.1 U/kg IV + 25% dextrose 4 mL/kg IV
Hypocalcaemia	Ca gluconate (10%) 1 ml/kg IV
Hyperphosphataemia	$Al(OH)_3$ 20 mg/kg three times a day orally, or $CaCO_3$ 20–50 mg/kg per day orally
Hypomagnesaemia	$MgSO_4$ (50%) 0.1 mL/kg IV
Acidosis (pH <7.2)	$NaHCO_3$ 1–3 mmol/kg IV/PO
Hypertension	Hydralazine 0.2 mg/kg IV every 4–8 h; fluid restriction, diuretics

Indications for dialysis

- Severe fluid overload or pulmonary oedema
- Severe persistent metabolic acidosis
- Severe hyperkalaemia (potassium > 7 mmol/L despite measures in Table 10.12)
- Plasma Na below 120 mmol/L.
- Plasma creatinine above 600 μmol/L.

Peritoneal dialysis is the method of choice for the dialysis of the newborn because access is relatively straightforward and intravascular anticoagulation is not necessary. Occasionally peritoneal dialysis may not be possible because of other considerations (e.g. peritonitis). Continuous arterio-venous haemofiltration is technically difficult but may be possible. Before embarking on peritoneal dialysis, expert nephrological advice should always be sought. Haemofiltration can also be used in the newborn.

Prognosis

Mortality rates in neonates requiring dialysis are high, usually due to the underlying problem rather than relating to the procedure itself. If the cause of ARF is acute tubular necrosis due to perinatal asphyxia or postnatal hypotension, renal function may recover after about 3 weeks and although dialysis is required continuously initially, once biochemical indices allow this may be reduced. However, ultimately more than half of the infants who survive neonatal ARF will develop chronic renal failure and be dialysis dependent.

SYSTEMIC HYPERTENSION IN THE NEWBORN

Background

- Systemic hypertension is rare in the newborn and for this reason is often missed. A term infant may present with cardiac failure or seizures.
- See Appendix 6 for systemic BP centiles by birthweight and postnatal age. BP increases with increasing gestation, increasing birthweight and increasing postnatal age. As a very rough guide, mean BP should be at least equal to the baby's, gestation in weeks. The lower limit of normal systolic BP in mmHg on the first day = (7.5 × birthweight in kg) + 30. The lower limit of normal diastolic BP in mmHg on the first day = (5 × birthweight in kg) + 10.
- Some infants will have a single BP measurement above the 97th centile (see Appendix 6), but many of these will be normal with subsequent measurement, especially if the infant is resting quietly.

Table 10.13   Causes of hypertension in the newborn period

Iatrogenic or accidental causes
Steroids*
UAC thrombosis
Excessive administration of
salt or water*
Inadvertent overdose of
dopamine or dobutamine

Vascular causes
CoA*
Renal artery stenosis*
Renal artery abnormalities
  Occlusion
  Aneurysm
Renal vein thrombosis
Segmental hypoplasia

Renal causes
Infantile-type polycystic kidney disease
Nephritis
Acute or chronic renal failure*
Cortical necrosis secondary to perinatal asphyxia*
Obstructive uropathy

Tumours
Neuroblastoma*
Wilms' tumour (nephroblastoma)
Ganglioneuroma
Leiomyoma
Phaeochromocytoma

Endocrine causes
CAH
Cushing's syndrome

Neurological causes
PVH
Cerebral angioma
Subdural haemorrhage
Cerebral oedema and raised ICP following perinatal asphyxia

Infections
Rubella (vascular problems)
Perinephric abscess

Pulmonary causes
CLD (independent of steroid use; onset at anytime; mechanism unclear;
frequently transient)

Increased catecholamines
Stress, hypoxia (although if sustained, hypotension results and PFC may
occur)

Miscellaneous
Closure of abdominal wall defects
Associated with ECMO

*Commonest causes.

- Less than 1% of infants will have systemic BP consistently above the 97th centile and this should be looked for specifically in the following groups:
  — any infant with congenital renal anomaly, renal disease or UTI
  — any infant suspected of having CoA
  — infants with perinatal asphyxia.

Other causes of systemic hypertension are given in Table 10.13.

Investigations

- Urine tests
  Always: urinalysis for blood, protein; microscopy for cells and casts; culture
  Then consider: VMA:creatinine and HVA:creatinine ratios (send spot sample followed by 6–24 h timed collection); save frozen urine for steroid profile
- Blood tests
  Always: FBC, U&E, creatinine, HCO_3^-, Ca^{2+}, PO_4^{3-}, albumin
  Then consider: 17-OH progesterone; aldosterone; plasma renin substrate and concentration; liaise with the laboratory first as these may require to be taken 'on ice' or into inhibitors and ideally 20 min after the infant has been lying supine quietly (with indwelling vascular catheter).
- CXR and ECG (always)
- Renal USS (always)
- Echocardiogram (always).

Further investigation depends upon the suspected cause:

- If there is a vascular cause, Doppler flow studies of aortic, renal artery and renal vein blood flow will also be required, as will a DMSA isotope scan to look for scarring of the kidney. Ultimately, arteriography may be required.
- If a renal cause is suspected, a DMSA isotope scan is necessary to look for renal cortical scars or infarcts. USS and MCUG can exclude VUR. A DPTA or MAG-3 scan are necessary if PUJ obstruction is suspected.
- If there is a palpable renal abdominal mass, this must be evaluated for the possibility of a tumour.

Treatment

1. Are you sure you have measured the BP correctly? Do not treat a single raised value, but if BP is persistently raised, treatment is indicated.
2. Treat any underlying cause if possible (e.g. CoA, see Ch. 7; cerebral oedema, see Ch. 12; endocrine disorders, see Ch. 11).
3. Significant (BP consistently >97th centile) symptomatic hypertension in the newborn may be treated initially with IV

agents and direct IA BP monitoring. These infants usually present with either cardiac failure or seizures. Asymptomatic hypertension can be treated orally.

4. Aim to reduce systolic and diastolic BP to less than the 95th centile for weight and postnatal age (see Appendix 6).

5. Aim for one third of the desired BP reduction in not less than the first 6 h; remaining two thirds over the next 24 h. All the drugs in Tables 10.14 and 10.15 may cause relative or absolute hypotension, which is as dangerous as hypertension.

6. a. Mild hypertension may respond to diuretics alone.
   b. Add a vasodilator (e.g. nifedipine or hydralazine).
   c. Add a beta-blocker if a vasodilator alone is ineffective, especially if there is reflex tachycardia — use with caution because of the risk of cardiac failure.
   d. Captopril should not be used in the newborn except with expert advice as there may be a rapid deterioration in renal function.

7. Once BP is consistently less than the 97th centile, convert to oral treatment.

BP measurement

This is difficult in the newborn and is only reliable if the infant is at rest.

Conventional mercury sphygmomanometer

- Systolic is more accurate and reproducible than diastolic.
- Use the widest cuff that can be applied to the right upper arm.
- Crudest method of measurement is to use the 'flush' method. The limb is gently squeezed to expel as much blood as possible and then the cuff inflated above systolic pressure (the radial pulse disappears). Cuff pressure is then lowered in 5 mm stages, pausing for 5 s at each stage. When the pressure in the cuff falls below systolic level, the limb will flush pink.
- Sphygmomanometry using a stethoscope over the brachial artery is technically impossible in the newborn.
- The alternative is to use a Doppler technique. An US probe is placed over the brachial artery prior to inflation of the cuff; pulsatile blood flow will be audible. When the cuff is inflated above systolic BP, the Doppler signal disappears but reappears when the cuff is deflated.

Automatic oscillometry (e.g. the Dinamap).

This method has become very popular because it is non-invasive, fairly quick, and requires relatively little training and expertise on the part of the observer. However, in the presence of oedema or hypotension the method can be unreliable. In particular, in the shocked, low birth weight infant, oscillometric devices over-estimate systolic blood pressure by as much as 10 mmHg.

Table 10.14 Intravenous antihypertensives (see text for choice of drug)

Drugs	Starting dose	Max. dose	Max. frequency	Onset	Duration	Possible disadvantages
Furosemide	1 mg/kg	5 mg/kg	Twice/day	30 min	12 h	Hypokalaemia, hypercalciuria
Hydralazine	0.2 mg/kg slowly	0.5 mg/kg slowly	Hourly	10–30 min	2–6 h	Tachycardia
Diazoxide	1 mg/kg slowly	3 mg/kg slowly	Hourly	1–5 min	4–24 h	Tachycardia, nausea, hyperglycaemia
Sodium nitroprusside	0.5 μg/kg per min	8 μg/kg per min	Onset immediate — needs IA monitor. Increase by 0.5 μg/kg per h every 5 min until BP starts to fall			Protect infusion from light, check infant's isothiocyanate levels

Table 10.15 Oral antihypertensives (see text for choice of drug)

Drugs	Starting dose	Max. dose	Max. frequency	Possible disadvantages
Vasodilators Nifedipine	0.125 mg/kg	0.5 mg/kg	12-hourly	Smallest tablet = 10 mg but the capsule can be opened to release the granules contained in it
Hydralazine	0.25 mg/kg	2.5 mg/kg	8-hourly	Tachycardia
Beta-blockers Propranolol	0.3 mg/kg	2.0 mg/kg	8-hourly	Bronchospasm
Diuretics Furosemide (frusemide)	0.5 mg/kg	2.5 mg/kg	12-hourly	Hypokalaemia
Spironolactone	0.5 mg/kg	2.0 mg/kg	12-hourly	Hyperkalaemia if renal impairment
Angiotensin-converting enzyme inhibitor Captopril	0.1 mg/kg	2.0 mg/kg	8-hourly	Caution with furosemide (frusemide) and in renal artery stenosis. Dose from 1 month; test dose required (see Appendix 4)

Using either of the above techniques, BP is usually recorded in the right arm. However, if any discrepancy exists between the arm pulses or between arm and leg pulses, BP should be recorded in all four limbs.

Direct arterial BP monitoring (see Ch. 21). This is the 'gold standard' but this invasive technique can only be justified in ill infants. It should be used in all children who have an indwelling arterial catheter already in situ for measurement of ABGs. It should be considered in the following categories:

- infants in the acute phase of RDS and requiring ventilation
- an infant in whom indirect methods of BP measurements suggest significant hypo- or hypertension
- any infant on inotropic drugs to support the circulation.

ELEVEN

Endocrine and metabolic disorders

Hypoglycaemia

This is defined as a whole blood glucose (BG) <2.6 mmol/L. The majority of babies with moderate hypoglycaemia will be asymptomatic. Symptoms which may be associated with hypoglycaemia include:

- convulsions
- abnormal neurological behaviour
- hypotonia
- lethargy
- apnoea.

Jitteriness is not a sign of symptomatic hypoglycaemia. For symptoms to be attributed to hypoglycaemia they should resolve with the maintenance of normoglycaemia.

GLUCOSE METABOLISM IN THE NEWBORN

The fetus receives a constant supply of glucose via the placenta. Insulin is an important fetal anabolic hormone and levels tend to be high. Glycogenolysis and gluconeogenesis are not active prior to delivery, but the newborn infant needs to switch to these pathways immediately after birth to maintain BG levels, especially if exogenous glucose supplies are delayed. There is commonly a transient fall in BG levels during the first 4 h after birth before the counter-regulatory hormones (glucagon, adrenaline, GH and cortisol) induce endogenous glucose production. When the BG concentration falls, healthy term infants utilise alternative cerebral fuels such as ketone bodies and lactate. The BG concentration in this group provides poor information on the adequacy of cerebral fuel.

Hypoglycaemia should not be screened for in healthy term newborn infants. There are, however, high-risk groups of babies (Table 11.1), who for various reasons do not adapt as quickly as normal and so are at risk of significant hypoglycaemia. There is little doubt that prolonged symptomatic hypoglycaemia has serious implications for neurodevelopmental outcome and that this is the high-risk groups of babies who are at particular risk of long-term adverse sequelae. However, there is no conclusive evidence that asymptomatic hypoglycaemia in healthy term babies carries an adverse neurodevelopmental prognosis.

In summary:
* At-risk infants — intervene if BG <2.6 mmol/L
* Other infants — only intervene if symptomatic.

CAUSES OF HYPOGLYCAEMIA (Table 11.2)

The most common causes of hypoglycaemia in the neonatal period are substrate deficiency secondary to immaturity of the enzyme pathways (preterm babies) or lack of adipose and glycogen stores (IUGR babies), poor activation of the enzyme pathways (perinatal asphyxia) or abnormal activation of the enzyme pathways antenatally (IUGR babies, mothers on various drugs). This results in reduced ability to respond to low blood sugars with glycogenolysis and gluconeogenesis. Some babies will have transient hyperinsulinism secondary to a mother with poorly controlled diabetes, maternal hyperglycaemia secondary to glucose infusion, or more rarely the infant has Beckwith–Weidemann syndrome.

GLUCOSE UTILISATION RATES (see Fig. 11.1 for glucose rate calculator)

Normal glucose utilisation rates are 4–6 mg/kg per min. Infants in the high-risk groups frequently require 6–10 mg/kg per min. Children requiring >10 mg/kg per min usually have a pathological basis for their hypoglycaemia, notably hyperinsulinaemia. *An insulin level >10 mU/L when the glucose concentration is <2.0 mmol/L is diagnostic of hyperinsulinism.*

Table 11.1 High risk groups for hypoglycaemia

* Babies < 37 weeks gestation — reduced ability to use alternative fuels
* Babies < 2.5 kg — reduced ability to use alternative fuels
* IUGR — reduced ability to use alternative fuels and paradoxically increased insulin levels
* Babies born to mothers with diabetes (including gestational diabetes) increased insulin levels
* Babies born to mothers on ß-blockers — side-effect
* Cold stress

Table 11. 2   Causes of hypoglycaemia

Increased glucose utilisation
Hyperinsulinism due to:
  Maternal diabetes
  Maternal dextrose infusions
  Maternal drug therapy
  Persistent hyperinsulinaemic hypoglycaemia of infancy[a]
  Beckwith–Weidemann syndrome
Hypothermia

Impaired glucose metabolism
Prematurity
IUGR
Perinatal asphyxia
Impaired glycogen synthesis — glycogen synthase deficiency
Impaired glycogenolysis — glycogen storage disease types I, III, IV, IX

Impaired ketogenesis and ketone body utilisation
IUGR
Prematurity
Perinatal asphyxia
Carnitine-mediated defects
Beta-oxidation defects
Ketone body formation defects
Ketone body utilisation defects
Mitochondrial respiratory chain disorders

Reduced gluconeogenesis
IUGR
Prematurity
Inherited metabolic defects
  Pyruvate carboxylase deficiency
  Phosphoenol-pyruvate carboxykinase deficiency
  Fructose1:6 diphosphatase deficiency
Endocrine causes:
  Panhypopituitarism
  Isolated ACTH, GH, cortisol or glucagon deficiency
  Adrenocorticol insufficiency (CAH)

Disturbance of glucose intermediary metabolism
Organic acidaemias
Disorders of amino acid metabolism
Carbohydrate disorders:
  Galactosaemia
  Fructose intolerance
  Glycerol intolerance

Miscellaneous
Liver disease
Haemolytic disease of the newborn
Polycythaemia
CHD
Septicaemia
Drug-related

---

[a] Previously known as nesidioblastosis. There has been a move away from a histological label to classification based on molecular studies, e.g. mutations in the ATP-sensitive channels of the beta-cells.

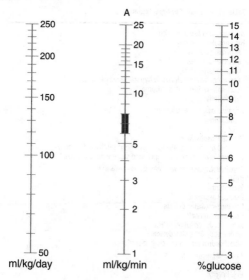

Fig. 11.1 Glucose rate calculator (reproduced with permission from Klaus M. H. and Fanaroff A.A. (1979). Care of the High Risk Neonate. London: W.B. Saunders).

MEASUREMENT OF GLUCOSE LEVELS

This should be done using one of the new generation blood sugar testing strips which are not affected by either the haematocrit or oxygen content of the blood. Values for BG using these methods correlate closely with laboratory whole BG measurements in contrast to the previously widely used BM stix.

PREVENTION OF HYPOGLYCAEMIA IN HIGH-RISK POPULATION

1. Take care to avoid hypothermia.
2. Commence feeds within 1 h of birth.
3. Feed regularly (3-hourly minimum) at breast or to at least 90 mL/kg per day with formula feed until 48 h old.
4. Measure BG before the second feed, i.e. at around 4 h:
   If >2.5 mmol/L:
   — observe feeding pattern
   — do not repeat BG unless feeding is poor or signs of neuroglycopenia are present

If <2.6 mmol/L:
— Give feed. If baby will not take offered feed consider NG or cup feed.
— Repeat BG 1 h after feed is finished:
— If normal: observe behaviour and feeding pattern over next two feeds. Do not repeat BG unless feeding is poor or there are signs of neuroglycopenia
— If <2.6 mmol/L: admit to NNU for IV glucose infusion whilst continuing enteral feeds if tolerated.

MANAGEMENT OF HIGH-RISK INFANTS WHERE ENTERAL FEEDS ARE CONTRAINDICATED

1. Commence IV 10% dextrose at 60 mL/kg per day within 1 h of birth.
2. Measure BG at 1 h, then 6-hourly for 24 h and subsequently once daily unless there are problems.
3. If BG <2.6 mmol/L and there are signs of neuroglycopenia, manage as described below (under neuroglycopenia).
4. If BG <2.6 mmol/L and asymptomatic:
   a. Increase IV 10% glucose infusion rate by 50% or increase glucose *concentration* to 15% and repeat BG after 1 h
   b. Try not to increase the volume of fluid other than as a short-term measure
   c. If glucose concentration >12.5% — central venous access is advisable
   d. Up to 20% glucose may be required
   e. Reduce glucose infusion slowly as indicated by BG measurements. It is usually possible to return to baseline requirements after 24 h unless pathology/IEM is present.

ENTERAL FEEDS IN THE HYPOGLYCAEMIC INFANT

- Try to continue enteral feeds if at all possible as milk contains nearly twice the energy of 10% glucose and promotes ketone body production and metabolic adaptation.
- Continuous NG feeds may be appropriate.
- If feeds are stopped during treatment, gradually reintroduce over 8–12 h whilst gradually reducing the IV glucose if the infant is well. Monitor BG every 4–6 h until the IV infusion is stopped.

MANAGEMENT OF NEUROGLYCOPENIA

This is suggested by drowsiness, coma or seizures in the presence of a BG <2.6 mmol/L (unusual until BG <1.0 mmol/L). If symptoms do not resolve when BG levels increase, a different diagnosis must be sought.

1. Establish IVI. Take blood (1–2 mL in a fluoride oxalate bottle and 1–2 mL into a lithium heparin bottle) for further investigation of cause (Table 11.3).
2. Give bolus of 5 mL/kg of 10% dextrose.
3. Infuse 10% glucose at 120 mL/kg per day (i.e. 8 mg/kg per min).
4. Attach urine bag to collect first urine sample passed following the hypoglycaemic episode (to investigate for an IEM — Table 11.3).
5. Check BG after 1 h:
   If >2.5 mmol/L — reduce infusion rate to 72 mL/kg per day (i.e. 5 mg/kg per min) and recheck BG after 1 h
   If <2.6 and symptoms resolved — repeat BG in 3 h
   If <2.6 mmol/L and symptoms persist:
   — increase 10% glucose infusion to 180 mL/kg per day (12 mg/kg per min). If fluid balance is critical, increase the glucose concentration rather than the volume but remember volume increments may be necessary as urgent treatment while more concentrated solutions are prepared
   — repeat BG in 1 h. If increased, reduce glucose infusion slowly over 4–6 h. If remains low, see below.

Table 11.3 Investigation of symptomatic or persistent hypoglycaemia

Mandatory
- Laboratory blood sugar*
- Plasma cortisol*
- Plasma insulin*

Consider
- Investigations for IEM:
  — plasma lactate, free fatty acids, hydroxybutarate (1.5 mL blood in fluoride oxalate bottle)*
  — urinary organic acids and amino acids*
  — urine-reducing sugars* or RBC galactose-1-phosphate uridyl transferase level
  — plasma triglyceride and urate*
- Infection screen including LP
- Investigations for hypopituitarism (especially if unstable temperature or small penis):
  — cerebral USS (+/− MRI or CT scan)
  — random GH, thyroid function tests
  — synacthen test
- Abdominal USS for hyperinsulinaemic hypoglycaemia

*These samples must be taken when the child is hypoglycaemic. Take: 1–2 mL in lithium heparin bottle; 1–2 mL in fluoride oxalate bottle; 6–10 mL of urine. Detailed investigation can subsequently be agreed with the metabolic laboratory.

6. If IV access is not possible use Hypostop massaged onto the buccal mucosa (0.5 mL/kg). Repeat at 10 min intervals if there is resistant hypoglycaemia; continue to seek IV access.

7. In the absence of risk factors (Table 11.1), investigation of the underlying cause is mandatory (Table 11.3) and should be done within 30 min of the hypoglycaemia.

MANAGEMENT OF PERSISTENT HYPOGLYCAEMIA DESPITE 12 MG/KG PER MIN OF IV GLUCOSE

1. Check infusion site.

2. Take blood for simultaneous insulin and glucose: in the absence of risk factors (Table 11.1) investigate for an underlying cause (Table 11.3) — take blood (1–2 mL in a fluoride oxalate bottle and 1–2 mL into a lithium heparin bottle at time of hypoglycaemia) and the first urine sample (6–10 mL) passed following the episode of hypoglycaemia.

3. Discuss with senior colleague.

4. Insert percutaneous silastic long line to secure an uninterrupted glucose infusion, particularly if the glucose concentration is ≥15%.

5. Commence hydrocortisone 2.5–5 mg/kg IV b.d. (**NB.** May be of little benefit in hyperinsulinism).

6. If no response and there is hyperinsulinism (i.e. insulin >10 mU/L when blood glucose <2 mmol/L or glucose:insulin ratio <0.3) use diazoxide 1.7–5mg/kg PO. 8-hourly (observe for hypotension) and chlorthiazide 10 mg/kg 12-hourly (watch for dehydration).

7. If hyperinsulinism does not respond to the above and glucose infusion rate >20 mg/kg per min, give somatostatin (as octreotide, 1 µg/kg subcutaneously every 4 h).

8. Glucagon 20 µg/kg stat IM (repeated 6–12 hourly if necessary) can be used but may result in increased insulin.

9. Suspect persistent hyperinsulinaemic hypoglycaemia of infancy if infant is macrosomic with very high glucose utilisation rates and high insulin. Seek senior specialist help urgently.

Hyperglycaemia

Defined as a BG >8 mmol/L. Glycosuria (≥+++) is usually present.

AETIOLOGY

● Frequent in extremely preterm infants treated with 10% dextrose or TPN

- Stress response to: sepsis, cold, pain, post-surgery
- Neonatal diabetes is extremely rare and usually transient but may last several months. Suspect if:
  — IUGR infant/wasted
  — hyperglycaemia on enteral feeds
  — no other potential aetiology
- Glycosuria in the absence of hyperglycaemia reflects a decreased renal threshold.

TREATMENT OF HYPERGLYCAEMIA

1. Identify underlying cause.
2. Reduce concentration of glucose infusion or glucose within TPN.
3. Occasionally, insulin 0.05–0.1 IU/kg per h as a sliding scale will be required. We commence insulin if the BG remains above 10 mmol/L with glycosuria despite a reduction in the administered glucose concentration or because we wish to maintain calorie intake with TPN.
4. Glycosuria may cause an osmotic diuresis and electrolyte disturbance. Monitor fluid balance and serum electrolytes carefully.

Neonatal hypothyroidism

This occurs in 1:3000 newborn infants. Untreated, it is a significant cause of learning difficulties: the later treatment is started, the greater the degree of irreversible brain injury. 90% of cases are sporadic and due to thyroid agenesis, hypoplasia or an ectopic thyroid; 10% are as a result of a defect in thyroxine synthesis and are autosomal recessive in inheritance.

CLINICAL SIGNS

Most babies do not have diagnostic features — hence the need for a universal screening programme. Suspect hypothyroidism where there is:

- prolonged jaundice
- hypotonia
- lethargy
- poor feeding
- poor weight gain
- umbilical hernia
- delayed passage of meconium
- large tongue.

INVESTIGATIONS AND DIAGNOSIS

- Routine neonatal screening on day 6 for raised TSH:
  - — 15–30 mU/L: repeat test age 1month
  - — 30–45 mU/L: repeat test at 2 weeks
  - — >45 mU/L: immediate referral for thyroid function tests and treatment.

  NB. This test will fail to detect those infants with secondary hypothyroidism due to:
  - — hypopituitarism: infants with panhypopituitarism present with poorly developed genitalia and low blood sugars
  - — isolated deficiencies of the TRH–TSH pathway
- T_4 and TSH — always do these tests if hypothyroidism is suspected even if screening test was normal. Transient hypothyroxinaemia may be seen in sick preterm infants.
- X-ray knee — may show delayed maturation of upper tibial and lower knee epiphyses.
- Isotope scan[123] I-sodium iodide scan for detection of thyroid tissue.
- If TSH low, consider TRH stimulation test, GH, cortisol etc.

TREATMENT

- L-thyroxine
  - — 8–10 µg/kg per day for preterm infants
  - — 5–8 µg/kg per day for term infants

  Give as crushed tablets. Adjust dose on basis of subsequent thyroid function test results.
- Refer to a paediatric endocrinologist.
- Consider a trial off treatment after 2 years of age, as it may be transient.

Congenital hyperthyroidism

This can be life-threatening and should be considered in:

- babies born to mothers with Graves' disease now or in the past, even if not on treatment and asymptomatic.
- infants born to mothers with autoimmune disease associated with thyroid-stimulating immunoglobulin.

PATHOLOGY

Maternal thyroid-stimulating IgG crosses the placenta and stimulates TSH receptors of the fetal/neonatal thyroid, resulting in transient neonatal thyrotoxicosis.

CLINICAL SIGNS AND SYMPTOMS

These are: preterm or SGA, palpable goitre with bruit, irritability, restlessness, jitteriness, staring eyes, eyelid retraction, exophthalmus, tachycardia, cardiac failure, arrhythmia, abnormally increased appetite, weight loss or poor weight gain, diarrhoea and vomiting.

- The diagnosis is unlikely without an enlarged thyroid and/or tachycardia.
- Onset may occur in utero, be immediately after birth or be delayed for up to 10 days due to the protective effect of maternal antithyroid drugs or blocking antibodies.
- May be fatal.
- Self-limiting illness — treatment rarely required after 2 months.

MANAGEMENT

- Observe on postnatal ward for 4 days.
- 8-hourly, temperature, HR and observation
- Warn parents of the signs of thyrotoxicosis and the need to seek medical help if symptoms develop following discharge from hospital.
- Perform thyroid function tests on day 4 if asymptomatic; earlier if there are symptoms. Thyroid function tests do not need repeating if child remains well.

TREATMENT

If there are any signs of thyrotoxicosis, commence treatment with:

- propranolol 250–750 micrograms/kg 8 hourly — to control stimulatory effects of thyroid hormones
- carbimazole 250 micrograms/kg 8 hourly — prevents synthesis of thyroid hormones
- ± digoxin — if there are signs of high output congestive cardiac failure. Care must be taken when giving associated propanolol
- ± diuretics.

Treatment should be continued for up to 2 months and then slowly withdrawn.

Congenital adrenal hyperplasia

CAH is an autosomal recessive deficiency of essential enzymes involved in the synthesis of cortisol and aldosterone (Table 11.4).

Table 11.4 Clinical presentation of adrenal enzyme deficiency

Enzyme deficiency	Male genitalia	Female genitalia	Salt loss	Salt retention	Cortisol	Aldosterone	Androgens	Plasma ACTH
20–22 desmolase	Ambiguous	Normal	+	–	↓	↓	↓	←
3β-hydroxysteroid dehydrogenase	Ambiguous	Ambiguous	+	–	↓	↓	→*	←
17α-hydroxylase	Ambiguous	Normal	–	+	↑	↑	↓	←
21-hydroxylase	Normal	Ambiguous	±	–	→	↓/→	←	←
11β-hydroxylase	Normal	Ambiguous	–	+	→*	→*	←	←

→*, replaced by biologically active precursors.

The incidence is 1 in 10 000; 90% of cases are due to 21-hydroxylase deficiency and 5% to 11ß-hydroxylase deficiency.

Suspect in the newborn period if there is:

- ambiguous genitalia
- salt losing crisis — infant presents after first week with vomiting and/or collapse, hyponatraemia (Na+ <130), hyperkalaemia (K+ >6.5 mmol/L) and often hypoglycaemia
- previous family history or unexplained neonatal death.

INVESTIGATION AND DIAGNOSIS

- Plasma 17-hydroxyprogesterone
  - normal values: <50 nmol/L in first 36 h of life
                    <18 nmol/L thereafter
  - 21-hydroxylase deficiency: often >1000 nmol/L
- Plasma 11-deoxycortisol — if 11ß-hydroxylase deficiency suspected
- Serum ACTH — normal range: 10–80 pg/mL
- Daily plasma electrolytes
- Monitor BP and weight
- Plasma renin and angiotensin
- Urine to specialist laboratory for identification of specific metabolites.

TREATMENT

Acute crisis

- Volume replacement with 10–20 mL/kg of 0.9% saline and 5% glucose over 30 minutes followed by maintenance fluids of 0.45 or 0.18% saline and 5% dextrose at 150 mL/kg per day
- Hydrocortisone 25 mg stat followed by 5 mg/kg per day then taper to 15–20 mg/m^2 per day.

Maintenance treatment

- Hydrocortisone 6.6 mg/m^2 8 hourly
- Fludrocortisone acetate 2–5 micrograms/kg daily
- Occasionally supplementary salt (2–4 g NaCl/day) may be necessary for the first few weeks
- Close monitoring of growth
- Refer to a paediatric endocrinologist.

Ambiguous genitalia

The diagnosis of ambiguous genitalia is usually made at birth although detailed fetal USS may raise suspicion in the antenatal period. A child's sexual identity is determined by five interrelated factors: chromosomes, gonads, internal genitalia, external genitalia and hormonal production from the adrenal glands and the gonads. Ultimately, however, the most important factor in assigning a child's gender is the long-term functional sexual potential of the child. Male development is a more complex process than female development and more prone to disruption. The commonest cause of a masculinised XX infant is CAH due to 21-hydroxylase deficiency.

DIFFERENTIAL DIAGNOSIS

Children with ambiguous genitalia can be divided into four subgroups:

Masculinised XX female — i.e. 46XX with normal ovaries and female internal genitalia but virilised external genitalia:

- Virilising CAH
  - 21-hydroxylase deficiency
  - 11β-hydroxylase deficiency
  - 3β-hydroxysteroid dehydrogenase deficiency.
- Iatrogenic — maternal progesterone or androgen ingestion.
- Maternal or fetal androgen-producing tumour.

Incompletely masculinised XY infant

Disorders of testicular differentiation:
- Mutations in genetic control of testis determination, e.g. SRY, SF-1, SOX9 and others.
- Mixed gonadal dysgenesis.
- Pure gonadal dysgenesis.
- Drash anomalad (associated glomerulonephritis and Wilms' tumour).

Disorders of testicular function:
- Enzyme defects in corticosteroid and testosterone synthesis
  - 20,22-desmolase (cholesterol side-chain cleavage)
  - 3β-hydroxysteroid dehydrogenase
  - 17α-hydroxylase.
- Enzyme defects in testosterone synthesis
  - 17,20-desmolase
  - 17β-hydroxysteroid dehydrogenase.
- Defects in MIF synthesis/action.

Disorders of androgen-dependent target tissues:
- Enzyme defects in testosterone metabolism — 5α-reductase deficiency.

- Androgen receptor defects
  — partial or incomplete testicular feminisation
  — complete testicular feminisation.

Malformation disorders involving genitalia.

True hermaphrodite — i.e. ovarian and testicular tissue either in separate gonads or in an ovotestes with variable karyotype, e.g. mosiac 46XX/46XY(13%) and 46XX(58%).

Mixed gonadal dysgenesis — i.e. a unilateral testis with Wolffian structures and a contralateral streak gonad with Müllerian structures and a 45XO/46XY or 46XY karyotype.

ASSESSMENT

History

- Maternal drug exposure
- Parental consanguinity
- Family history of ambiguous genitalia, neonatal death.

Examination (including medical photography)

- Presence/absence of palpable gonads (if palpable, likely to be testes)
- Length and girth of phallus (average length at 30 weeks gestation is 2.5 cm, rising to 3.5 cm at term with a girth of 1–1.5 cm)
- Position of urethral orifice
- Labial/scrotal fusion
- Pigmentation of external genitalia (suggests CAH)
- Asymmetry of external genitalia (suggests chromosomal mosaicism or gonadal intersex)
- Position of vaginal orifice if present
- Associated anomalies, i.e. imperforate anus.

Investigation

- Karyotype
- Hormonal assessment:
  — 17-hydroxyprogesterone and testosterone on days 1 and 3
  normal values of 17-hydroxyprogesterone:
  <50 nmol/L in first 36 h of life
  <18 nmol/L thereafter
  >1000 nmol/L in CAH
  normal values of testosterone:
  <0.05 nmol/L pre-puberty
  >2 nmol/L post-HCG stimulation test
  NB. Levels are difficult to define in infancy due to early neonatal and later infancy surges secondary to LH release; however, these surge levels can be valuable in assessing

Leydig cell capacity, avoiding the need for HCG stimulation test.

- Consider in incompletely masculinised XY infant:
  — basal LH, FSH and HCG stimulation test
  — plasma dihydrotestosterone
  — adrenal androgens
  — plasma MIF
  — urinary androgen and dihydrotestosterone:testosterone derivative ratios
  — assessment of androgen sensitivity of phallus to IM testosterone oenanthate
- Serial plasma sodium and potassium measurements
- Abdominal USS and retrograde genitogram
- Assessment of functional potential in liasion with paediatric urologist/plastic surgeon.

MANAGEMENT

The major aims of initial management are assignment of appropriate gender, parental support and prevention of life-threatening complications, especially salt losing crisis in some forms of CAH. *Do not attempt to assign a sex to the baby immediately following birth.* Explain to parents that a number of investigations will be required before this is possible. Discourage the use of neutral names and the early registration of the child's birth. Definitive medical and surgical management will depend on the underlying diagnosis. A paediatric endocrinologist should be involved in diagnosis, counselling and follow-up.

Inborn errors of metabolism (IEM)

It is important to consider an IEM as a potential cause of any severe neonatal illness and to have a systematic approach to diagnosis and management. IEMs may present acutely in the neonatal period (Table 11.5) or later in life when they are often precipitated by stress, change in diet or drugs. IEMs may also present as chronic degenerative disorders. This section focuses on IEMs presenting in the neonatal period.

CLINICAL PRESENTATION

The presenting features of an IEM are often non-specific with poor feeding, lethargy, hypotonia and vomiting. Presenting features in some IEMs are described in Table 11.5. The history (Table 11. 6) and examination (Table 11.7) may provide several diagnostic clues.

Table 11.5 Specific presentation of IEM

Metabolic acidosis
Organic acidaemias
Lactic acidosis
Maple syrup urine disease
Renal tubular acidosis
Exclude cardiac or respiratory disorder

Respiratory alkalosis
Hyperammonaemia, e.g. urea cycle defects, organic acidaemias

Vomiting
Galactosaemia
Hereditary fructose intolerance
PKU
Organic acidaemias[a]
Urea cycle defects[b]
CAH

Septicaemia
Galactosaemia
Tyrosinaemia
Organic acidaemias[a]

Convulsions
Disorders of aminoacid metabolism[c]
Organic acidaemias[a]
Urea cycle defects[b]

Coma
Disorders of amino acid metabolism[c]
Organic acidaemias[a]
Urea cycle defects[b]

Unexplained hypoglycaemia
Maple syrup urine disease
Methylmalonic acidaemia
Propionic acidaemia
Glycogen storage diseases, especially type I
Galactosaemia
Hereditary fructose intolerance
Fatty acid oxidation defects
Exclude endocrine disorder

Cardiomegaly
Glycogen storage disease type II
Fatty acid oxidation defect (not all!)
Mitochondrial myopathy

Jaundice and/or liver dysfunction
Galactosaemia
Hypothyroidism
Tyrosinaemia
α1-antitrypsin deficiency
Niemann–Pick C
Fatty acid oxidation defects

Table 11.5 *cont'd*

Hypotonia
Zellweger's
Glycogen storage disease, type II
Non-ketotic hyperglycinaemia

---

[a] Organic acidaemias, e.g. propionic acidaemia, methylmalonic acidaemia, isovaleric acidaemia.
[b] Urea cycle defects: carbamyl phosphate synthetase deficiency, ornithine carbamyl transferase deficiency, citrullinaemia, arginosuccinic aciduria, hyperargininaemia, N-acetyl glutamate synthetase deficiency.
[c] Disorders of amino acid metabolism, e.g. non-ketotic hyperglycinaemia, maple syrup urine disease.

Table 11.6   Factors in the history which increase the suspicion of an IEM

- Family history
- Unexplained sibling death, especially male
- Consanguinity of parents
- More than one feature of an IEM present
- Symptoms associated with feeding, fasting, infection, surgery
- Improvement when milk feeds are stopped with relapse on reintroduction
- Infant well in first few hours or days. Symptoms develop with the onset of intense catabolism and the introduction of feeds containing proteins

Table 11.7   Clinical clues in examination suggesting an IEM

- Examination is usually normal
- Odour, e.g. isovaleric acidaemia (body smells of smelly feet), maple syrup urine disease (urine smells sweet like maple syrup)
- Cataracts — infants with galactosaemia develop cataracts within the first week of life
- Dysmorphic features, e.g. Zellweger syndrome, pyruvate dehydrogenase deficiency
- Tachypnoea — organic acidaemias
- Extreme hypotonia from birth
  - non-ketotic hyperglycinaemia
  - Zellweger syndrome
  - Menke's syndrome
  - glycogen storage disease, type II
- Severe hepatomegaly — galactosaemia
- Abnormal hair
  - arginosuccinic aciduria (brittle)
  - Menke's syndrome (kinky)

INVESTIGATION OF AN IEM

Quantities of 1–2 mL of blood in a lithium heparin bottle, 1–2 mL of blood in a fluoride oxalate bottle and 6–10 mL of urine (in a sterile container without preservatives) should be collected when the child is unwell. Also consider collecting blood onto a Guthrie card and whole EDTA blood. These can be saved by the laboratory and may be important for confirmation of any diagnosis.

A metabolic screen performed when a child is well (e.g. once milk feeds have been excluded) may result in a missed diagnosis. If a result is required urgently or the child has specific signs discuss further investigations with the clinical chemistry laboratory. Ideally samples should be taken before any blood transfusion is performed.

General

Blood:
- pH, P_aCO_2, HCO_3^-, BE
- Na^+, K^+, Cl^-, measure anion gap = $(Na^+ + K^+) - (Cl^- + HCO_3^-)$ [normal <16]
- Ca^{2+}, PO_4^{2+}, Mg^{2+}
- LFTs including total/conjugated bilirubin
- Glucose
- Coagulation.

Primary investigations

Blood:
- Amino acids
- Ammonia
- Triglyceride, urate, erythrocyte galactose-1-phosphate uridyl transferase (if hypoglycaemic).

Urine:
- Simple screening tests, e.g. pH, glucose, reducing sugars, ketones, ketoacids, cystine/homocystine, sulphite stix.
  These spot tests can be misleading and should not be done in isolation. Always do urine amino and organic acids in addition.
- Sugar chromatography
- Amino acids
- Organic acids
- Mucopolysaccharides
- Oligosaccharides and sialic acid.

Secondary investigations (after discussion with biochemist and consideration of clinical presentation and initial results)
- Plasma lactate
- CSF — lactate and glycine

- WBC enzymes
- Biotinidase
- Blood spot acyl-glycines
- Very long-chain fatty acids.

Confirmatory investigations
- Enzyme analysis in blood, fibroblast culture, liver biopsy
- DNA analysis for specific mutation.

MANAGEMENT

Management whilst awaiting results when IEM felt likely
1. Stop all protein intake.
2. Rapidly induce an anabolic state using a high energy intake:
   — 15–20% glucose
   — lipid solution e.g. 20% intralipid
   — insulin 0.05 IU/kg per h
   These should be given via a Silastic long line or central line.
3. Correct any electrolyte imbalance.
4. Treat metabolic acidosis with sodium bicarbonate solution (0.5–2 mmol/h).
5. Treat with antibiotics — metabolic decompensation may be precipitated by infection.
6. Carnitine 100 mg/kg per day oral or IV should be started whilst a diagnosis is being made.
7. Removal of toxic intermediaries using arteriovenous haemoperfusion or peritoneal dialysis (e.g. ammonia in urea cycle defects or propionate in propionic acidaemia) may be required.
8. Vitamin cocktails should, in general, not be used without a specific diagnosis but can be given if infants continue to deteriorate (see Table 11.8) in the hope that a cofactor-responsive metabolic disease is present.
9. If there is hyperammonaemia (ammonia>180 μmol/L) commence sodium benzoate 250 mg/kg as a bolus followed by 250 mg/kg per day as an infusion (once urine has been obtained for organic acid analysis). If ammonia >400 μmol/L, dialysis will be required.
10. Specific treatment of individual IEMs should always be discussed with a consultant experienced in the care of metabolic illness.

Management of the child who dies unexpectedly when IEM is being considered
A postmortem examination should be carried out as soon as possible after death (and preferably within 4 h). Consideration should be given to discussing the importance of an early

postmortem with parents and the pathologist before the child's death. If the child dies prior to a metabolic investigation or before the availability of results, obtain:

- 20 mL of urine into a sterile container — store in 5 mL aliquots at –70°C. If not possible, store at –20°C
- 5-10 mL blood into a lithium heparin bottle — separate plasma as soon as possible and store in small-volume aliquots at –20°C. Packed RBC can be stored at 4°C for up to 48 h otherwise store at –20°C
- 5 mL blood into an EDTA bottle for later DNA analysis (store at –20°C)
- Skin biopsy — divide into three pieces. Place one piece in sterile saline, store at 4°C and send for fibroblast culture. This sample can later be used for enzyme assay or DNA analysis. Place another piece into formalin, stored at room temperature for histology, and the final piece into gluteraldehyde for EM stored at 4°C.
- CSF — obtain via a ventricular tap or LP, freeze immediately and store at –20°C. Use for organic and amino acid assay.

If full postmortem is refused or postmortem within 4 h is not possible, perform (following consent) biopsies of liver and muscle and consider biopsies of brain, kidney and heart if there is a strong clinical indication of a primary defect affecting one of these organs. Take three needle biopsy specimens of each organ. Snap-freeze one specimen in liquid nitrogen for biochemical analysis. Place one specimen into formalin, stored at room temperature for routine histology, and one piece into gluteraldehyde, stored at 4°C for EM

It is essential that close liaison occurs with the clinical chemistry laboratory, preferably before any samples are taken, so that they can be processed appropriately.

Table 11.8 Vitamin cocktail

Vitamin	Amount (mg/day)
B12	1
Biotin	100
Thiamine	50
Riboflavin	50
Nicotinamide	600
Pyridoxine	100
Folic acid	15
Ascorbic acid	3000
Pantothenic acid	50
Carnitine	300

Neonatal screening test

All babies born in the UK are screened for PKU and congenital hypothyroidism. Sophisticated analysis of dried blood spots is now possible and an increasing array of disorders may be detected on the neonatal screen, e.g. raised IRT and DNA analysis in CF and sickle cell disease.

- Screen is performed on day 6.
- Delay 48 h after transfusion.
- If protein intake is inadequate, phenylalanine may remain low even if the baby has PKU. Repeat test 48 h after commencing full enteral feeds or TPN.
- Test at latest by 14 days of age when phenylalanine will have increased in PKU regardless of protein intake.

FURTHER READING

Blau N, Duran M, Blasovics M E (eds) (1996) Physicians guide to the laboratory diagnosis of metabolic diseases. London: Chapman and Hall Medical.

Holton J (ed) (1994) The inherited metabolic diseases. Edinburgh: Churchill Livingstone.

Scriver C R, Beaudet A L, Sly W S, Valle D (eds) (1995) The metabolic and molecular basis of inherited disease. New York: McGraw-Hill.

TWELVE

Neurological problems

Examination of the nervous system

Neurological examination requires practice and patience. In addition to illness, factors which may influence the neurological status include drugs administered to baby or mother, gestational age, systemic illness and hunger. Standardised neurological examination is required for research purposes or for monitoring progress of an infant during treatment, e.g. in neonatal myasthenia. Suitable schemes are those of Dubowitz and Amiel-Tison (see bibliography). The neurological scale of the Dubowitz gestational assessment proforma (Fig. 12.1) is also a valuable scheme and provides a simple numerical score for sequential examinations; at the very least you should be familiar with this.

The examination should ideally take place when the infant is quiet, but alert. Examination of the head and neck, vision and hearing may be carried out with the baby clothed; the remainder should be carried out with the baby completely undressed. Assess the following:

- Measure maximal OFC and plot on centile chart.
- Note head shape, separation or fusion of cranial sutures, tension of anterior fontanelle.
- Look in the mouth — a high-arched palate may indicate abnormal motor function of the tongue in utero; tongue fasciculation is seen in spinal muscular atrophy.
- Observe the sucking response — is there a gag reflex, are secretions cleared from the pharynx?
- Watch the face during normal movements or crying (best) — is there facial asymmetry?
- Do the pupils react to light, is there a normal 'red' retinal reflex?
- Does the baby show visual fixation — a term infant should fix on a bright object or face at 30 cm.

- Is there an acoustic blink? Responses to auditory stimuli are present in early fetal life but formal assessment requires standardised procedures in a soundproofed room.
- Assess general posture and limb and truncal movements by observation.
- Assess passive limb tone during flexion of the elbows and knees — in standardised assessments, the flappability of feet and arms are examined and then the scarf sign, heel–ear, popliteal, adductor and ankle angles (Fig. 12.1); these should be performed gently and, with practice, rapidly become repeatable reliable signs.
- Demonstrate deep tendon jerks, e.g. biceps and knees — these may be absent in neuromuscular disorders — and evaluate ankle flexion for clonus.
- Is there any asymmetry in these assessments?
- Assess passive truncal tone and head lag on pulling to sit and in ventral suspension.
- Sensation to pinprick may be gently assessed in babies with myelomeningocele, including the anal reflex, but is usually omitted unless it is likely to be helpful (these children may also have poorly developed natal clefts and a patulous anus).
- Evaluate the neonatal reflexes, e.g. palmar and plantar grasp, traction response, rooting, sucking. Where the infant is neurologically depressed, check the Moro response:
  — allow the head to fall quickly back a few centimetres into your hand
  — the arms should abduct and then adduct and flex, leg movements are less consistent
  — the baby should cry during this procedure and therefore *it is avoided* unless there are concerns about the neurological status.
  Other neonatal reflexes are well described (stepping, Galant's) but of little additional help in localising a neurological lesion.
- During your examination, observe the posture of the thumbs and feet. Fixed adduction of the thumb across the palm (cortical thumb or 'fisting') or persisting flared extended toes are abnormal signs and should be noted.
- Examine the spine for pits, hairy patches or cystic swellings.
- The skin should be examined for rare evidence of neuro-cutaneous syndromes: pigmented (neurofibromatosis) or depigmented (tuberous sclerosis) lesions or the port wine stain in the trigeminal area of Sturge–Weber syndrome.

If you find an abnormality, make sure it is clearly documented and seek confirmation from a senior.

Neurological criteria

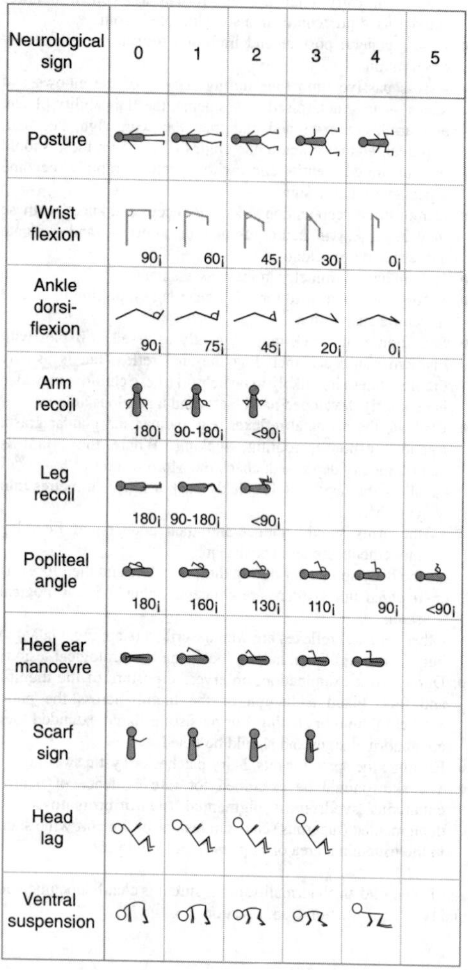

Neurological sign	0	1	2	3	4	5
Posture						
Wrist flexion	90¡	60¡	45¡	30¡	0¡	
Ankle dorsiflexion	90¡	75¡	45¡	20¡	0¡	
Arm recoil	180¡	90-180¡	<90¡			
Leg recoil	180¡	90-180¡	<90¡			
Popliteal angle	180¡	160¡	130¡	110¡	90¡	<90¡
Heel ear manoevre						
Scarf sign						
Head lag						
Ventral suspension						

Fig. 12.1 Dubowitz neurology chart.

Some notes on techniques of assessment of neurological criteria

Posture. Observed with infant quiet and in supine position. Score 0: Arms and legs extended; 1: beginning of flexion of hips and knees, arms extended; 2: stronger flexion of legs, arms extended; 3: arms slightly flexed, legs flexed and abducted; 4: full flexion of arms and legs.

Wrist flexion. The hand is flexed on the forearm between the thumb and index finger of the examiner. Enough pressure is applied to get as full a flexion as possible, and the angle between the hypothenar eminence and the ventral aspect of the forearm is measured and graded according to diagram. (Care is taken not to rotate the infant's wrist while doing this manoeuvre.)

Ankle dorsiflexion. The foot is dorsiflexed onto the anterior aspect of the leg, with the examiner's thumb on the sole of the foot and other fingers behind the leg. Enough pressure is applied to get as full flexion as possible, and the angle between the dorsum of the foot and the anterior aspect of the leg is measured.

Arm recoil. With the infant in the supine position the forearms are first flexed for 5 seconds, then fully extended by pulling on the hands, and then released. The sign is fully positive if the arms return briskly to full flexion (Score 2). If the arms return to incomplete flexion or the response is sluggish it is graded as Score 1. If they remain extended or are only followed by random movements the score is 0.

Leg recoil. With the infant supine, the hips and knees are fully flexed for 5 seconds, then extended by traction on the feet, and released. A maximal response is one of full flexion of the hips and knees (Score 2). A partial flexion scores 1, and miminal or no movement scores 0.

Popliteal angle. With the infant supine and his pelvis flat on the examining couch, the thigh is held in the knee-chest position by the examiner's left index finger and thumb supporting the knee. The leg is then extended by gentle pressure from the examiner's right index finger behind the ankle and the popliteal angle is measured.

Heel to ear manoeuvre. With the baby supine, draw the baby's foot as near to the head as it will go without forcing it. Observe the distance between the foot and the head as well as the degree of extension at the knee. Grade according to diagram. Note that the knee is left free and may draw down alongside the abdomen.

Scarf sign. With the baby supine, take the infant's hand and try to put it around the neck and as far posteriorly as possible around the opposite shoulder. Assist this manoeuvre by lifting the elbow across the body. See how far the elbow will go across and grade according to illustrations. Score 0: Elbow reaches opposite axillary line; 1: Elbow between midline and opposite axillary line; 2: Elbow reaches midline; 3: Elbow will not reach midline.

Head lag. With the baby lying supine, grasp the hands (or the arms if a very small infant) and pull him slowly towards the sitting position. Observe the position of the head in relation to the trunk and grade accordingly. In a small infant the head may initially be supported by one hand. Score 0: Complete lag; 1: Partial head control; 2: Able to maintain head in line with body; 3: Brings head anterior to body.

Ventral suspension. The infant is suspended in the prone position, with examiner's hand under the infant's chest (one hand in a small infant, two in a large infant). Observe the degree of extension of the back and the amount of flexion of the arms and legs. Also note the relation of the head to the trunk. Grade according to the diagrams.

If the score for an individual criterion differs on the two sides of the baby, take the mean. *For further details see Dubowitz et al., Pediat. 1970, 77, 1.*

Hypotonia — the 'floppy infant'

There are many causes of hypotonia in the neonatal period (see also Table 12.1):

- Acute causes, including hypoglycaemia and sepsis, are life-threatening and must be ruled out promptly. Suspect if a baby has poor respiratory effort or requires ventilation and has a normal CXR.
- Most commonly there is an associated acute encephalopathy (see below).
- Investigation of hypotonicity without other signs of systemic illness requires a systematic approach, which is dependent on the clinical signs. Generally, central causes may be differentiated from neuromuscular causes by the presence or absence of deep tendon reflexes, respectively.
- Investigations include EMG, nerve conduction studies, muscle biopsy, CPK, metabolic screen, karyotype and Tensilon test — assess neurology (use neurological score), give edrophonium chloride (1mg intramuscularly) and reassess: in neonatal

Table 12.1 Neonatal Hypotonia

Common causes:
Prematurity
Neonatal encephalopathy
 Hypoxia
 Hypoglycaemia
 Infection
Drugs administered to baby or mother

Rare causes:
Neuromuscular (anterior horn cell, peripheral nerves, muscles)
Spinal muscular atrophy
Congenital muscular dystrophy
Congenital myopathy
Congenital myotonic dystrophy
Neonatal myasthenia

Metabolic
IEM
Renal tubular acidosis
Hypothyroidism

Central CNS origin
Chromosomal disorders
Connective tissue disorders
Prader–Willi syndrome
CNS malformations
Benign congenital hypotonia

myasthenia there is a dramatic improvement in tone and activity.

- In the dysmorphic child, consider Prader–Willi syndrome or congenital myotonic dystrophy. If either is suspected, send an EDTA sample to cytogenetics.
  — deletion of the long arm of chromosome 15 at q11/q13 is observed in 70% of cases of Prader–Willi syndrome using the FISH technique
  — congenital myotonic dystrophy is most severe if the mother is affected; make sure you examine both parents for the typical facies and failure to relax their grip on grasping.

- If muscle biopsy is contemplated, refer to a paediatric neurologist. Muscle biopsy may be easier to interpret when the infant is a few months old, but if the infant is likely to die or if it will alter acute management, it can be done in the neonatal period. If the infant dies without a diagnosis, it is important to obtain fresh tissue for evaluation.

- Prognosis depends upon the underlying cause.

Neonatal encephalopathy

Encephalopathy may occur following a hypoxic or ischaemic insult before, during or after labour and delivery; it may also follow septicaemia, meningitis and metabolic disturbances and may be a clinical feature of structural brain anomalies, including those associated with karyotype abnormalities. Infants born prematurely, who are growth restricted or have a congenital anomaly, are at increased risk during the birth process. The most usual scenario is the infant whose perinatal period is complicated by fetal hypoxia. The establishment of causation to events occurring during the birth process is often a difficult task. Paediatric staff should refrain from written or verbal comment regarding the quality of management of midwifery or obstetric complications and refer such questions from relatives to the relevant professionals concerned.

Warning signs of fetal hypoxia (see Ch. 2)

Management at delivery (see Ch. 3)

POST-RESUSCITATION CARE OF THE INFANT WITH SUSPECTED PERINATAL HYPOXIA

Initial assessment

- Look for risk factors for infection and maternal disease/medication.

- Examine carefully, looking specifically for congenital malformations, dysmorphic features, skull or limb fracture, nerve palsy.
- Perform a neurological assessment. Encephalopathies are best graded by their severity using the scheme as described by Sarnat & Sarnat (1976) or that modified by, for example, Levene & Lilford (1995) (Table 12.2).

Basic management plan

Although no specific therapies are as yet available to treat post-hypoxic injuries, good supportive care maintaining perfusion, oxygenation and avoiding fluid overload, temperature disturbances or persistent seizures may avoid secondary hypoxic injury.

- Nurse in a thermoneutral environment (Ch. 3).
- Expose to allow observation of abnormal movements or seizures.
- Anticipate hypoxic injury in all organ systems and not just the CNS (commonly kidneys, heart, lungs, liver and coagulation).
- An indwelling arterial line is important to allow blood gas monitoring and accurate BP measurements.

Fluid management

Post-hypoxic oliguria is common and may persist for several days. It may be impossible to differentiate this from inappropriate ADH secretion secondary to CNS injury. If liberal fluids are allowed, there is a risk of hyponatraemia and of cerebral oedema, which could worsen the CNS injury. Fluids are therefore restricted and perfusion supported with inotropes if necessary until urine output is established (usually for 48 h). This restriction will cause a relatively low glucose supply and steps may need to be taken to ensure this is maintained without fluid overload (see below).

- Until urine flow is established:
  - glucose 10% at 40 mL/kg maintenance
  - 12-hourly serum electrolytes, creatinine, urea
  - daily urine electrolytes and specific gravity or osmolality
  - 6-hourly BG.
  - measure all urine output and all additional input from infusions, etc.
- Hypoglycaemia must be treated promptly and glucose infusion increased accordingly. It may be necessary to insert a central venous line to permit the use of concentrated glucose solutions (>10%), rather than increase the volume of water infused by increasing the volume of 10% dextrose solution with consequent hyponatraemia.
- We usually keep encephalopathic children (Grade 2 or 3) without enteral feeds for 48 h to minimise the risk of NEC (see Ch. 9).

Table 12.2 A clinical grading system for neonatal encephalopathy (Adapted from Sarnat & Sarnat (1976) Arch Neurol 33: 696–705 and Levene & Lilford (1995) Fetal and Neonatal Neurology & Neurosurgery 405–425, Ch. 24)

	Grade 1 — Mild	Grade 2 — Moderate	Grade 3 — Severe
Level of consciousness	Hyperalert	Lethargic	Stuporose
Neuromuscular control			
Muscle tone	Normal	Mild hypotonia	Flaccid
Posture	Mild distal flexion	Strong distal flexion	Intermittent decerebration
Tendon jerks	Overactive	Overactive	Decreased or absent
Clonus	Present	Present	Absent
Complex reflexes			
Suck	Weak	Weak/absent	Absent
Moro	Strong — low threshold	Weak, incomplete — high threshold	Absent
Autonomic function			
Overall	Generalised sympathetic	Generalised parasympathetic	Both systems depressed
Pupils	Dilated	Small pinpoint	Variable, often unequal, poor light reflex
HR	Tachycardia	Bradycardia	Can be either
Bronchial/salivary secretions	Sparse	Profuse	Variable
GI motility	Normal or decreased	Increased; diarrhoea	Variable
Seizures	None	Common; focal or multifocal	May be absent or difficult to control

Respiratory support

Ventilation is necessary for respiratory failure, or apnoea in grade 3 encephalopathy. Meconium aspiration and pulmonary hypertension may also be present (Ch. 6). Aim to keep $P_a o_2$ and $P_a co_2$ in the normal range. The $P_a co_2$ should not be allowed to fall to less than 3.5 kPa or cerebral vasoconstriction will lead to further risk of ischaemia. If muscle relaxants are used following a difficult resuscitation, neurological assessment becomes very difficult. Continuous EEG monitoring is then recommended.

Blood pressure and perfusion

Maintenance of normal systemic BP is the most effective way of ensuring adequate cerebral perfusion. Hypoxic injury to the myocardium may result in decreased contractility, bradycardia and ischaemic changes on the ECG, and may be manifest as hypotension. It is important to use inotropes early and to avoid overloading a failing myocardium. If hypotension is present (Appendix):

- seek and treat hypovolaemia with 10 mL/kg HAS or blood; repeat once if necessary
- start dopamine infusion at 3 microgram/kg per min and build up to 10 microgram/kg per min.
- start dobutamine infusion at 5 microgram/kg per min, increasing gradually to 15 microgram/kg per min.

Metabolic

- Monitor electrolytes, creatinine, glucose as above.
- Check Ca^{2+} daily (hypocalcaemia may occur).
- Acidosis — metabolic acidosis secondary to acute hypoxia will usually be corrected by adequate ventilation, correction of hypovolaemia with colloid and improvement in cardiac performance with inotropes. Ensure perfusion and BP are adequate before considering half correction with bicarbonate.

Haematology

- Monitor Hb at least daily. Anaemia may be secondary to concealed intracranial haemorrhage or external trauma, e.g. cephalhaematoma or subaponeurotic haematoma.
- Perform coagulation screen, give vitamin K routinely on admission (Ch. 15) and correct as necessary (Ch. 14).

Liver function

Check LFTs after 24 h — raised liver enzymes indicate hypoxic liver injury; repeat as indicated.

Neurological assessment

Record daily neurological assessment including agreed grade of encephalopathy (Table 12.2). The prognosis is related to the worst grade of encephalopathy, but accurate grading may be difficult if the infant is heavily sedated with anticonvulsants.

Cerebral oedema

If present on USS (slit-like lateral ventricles, parenchymal shadowing — 'bright brain'), maintenance of normal systemic BP and avoidance of water overload are the mainstays of treatment. Steroids have not been shown to be effective. Mannitol 20% 0.5 g/kg IV over 20 min may temporarily reduce ICP, but should not be used in the presence of cardiac or renal failure or intracranial haemorrhage.

Convulsions — see below

Neuroimaging

Perform daily cerebral USS, over the first few days, to assess focal brain injury (typically basal ganglia), size of lateral ventricles and echogenicity of cerebral parenchyma. Doppler assessment of flow velocity in the anterior or middle cerebral arteries provides an index of resistance to flow and is related to subsequent outcome, but should not be used in isolation to predict outcome. Where available, MRI and spectroscopy provide the most detailed, non-invasive assessment of the pattern and extent of brain injury. Correlation of long-term outcome with early MRI abnormalities is being studied; MR or CT images taken in the second week are better predictors to date.

EEG

Early seizures or a marked burst–supression pattern on EEG (in first 6 h) may be a good predictor of outcome if available. For later prognosis, it is useful to examine background electrical activity.

OUTCOME

Good prognostic features

- Grade I encephalopathy (as worst grade — no later disability is likely)
- Absence of fits in first 24 h
- Resolution of fits, off anticonvulsants by 7 days of age
- Ability to suck and feed by 7 days of age.

Poor prognostic features (i.e. risk of severe disability or death)

- Grade II encephalopathy (risk: 20–25%)
- Grade III encephalopathy (risk: 75–90%)
- Duration of encephalopathy grade II or III > 5 days

- EEG evidence of unreactive or discontinuous waveform
- Scan evidence of thalamic or extensive parenchymal haemorrhage or infarction.

Where encephalopathy has a non-hypoxic cause, the outcome relates to the underlying condition. Severe disability following perinatal hypoxia usually comprises dystonic quadriplegic cerebral palsy with severe learning difficulties, often with cortical visual loss and occasionally hearing impairment. Some of these children will go on to develop infantile spasms and a severe seizure disorder. Outcomes with less disability can occur. Careful long-term follow-up and early referral to community disability services are vital.

Neonatal convulsions

Seizures occur in approximately 0.5% of newborn infants (causes are given in Table 12.3). They are often subtle and may be manifest in a variety of different ways. If convulsions affect primarily motor tone, there may be clonic or tonic movements of one or all limbs, or alternating episodes of floppiness. Seizures may also present as episodes of apnoea, eye rolling, chewing, sucking or nystagmus. It is essential to have a high index of suspicion in this age group.

Examination
Careful examination should be carried out for signs of sepsis, congenital abnormalities and trauma.

INVESTIGATION

In all cases:
- Blood glucose (immediate bedside test)
- U&E
- Ca^{2+} and Mg^{2+}
- FBC and differential white count and platelets
- Blood culture
- LP — protein, glucose, Gram stain and culture
- pH and blood gas
- Cranial USS to exclude haemorrhage.

Additional investigations in selected cases:
- CT/MRI to exclude brain malformations and ischaemic injury
- Urine for drug toxicology screen
- Metabolic screen, including plasma ammonia, amino acids, lactate, urine amino acids and organic acids, CSF glucose

Table 12.3 Causes of neonatal convulsions

Birth trauma and hypoxia
Neonatal encephalopathy
Tentorial tear
Subarachnoid or subdural haemorrhage
PVH

Congenital malformations of the brain

Metabolic
Hypoglycaemia
Hypocalcaemia
Hypomagnasaemia
Hypo- or hypernatraemia
Hyperammonaemia
Hyperglycinaemia

Infections
Bacterial meningitis
Viral encephalitis

Drugs
Withdrawal from drugs of abuse
Inadvertent administration of ergometrine or local anaesthetic

Other rare causes
Kernicterus
Fifth day fits
Pyridoxine deficiency
Hypertension
Cerebral vein thrombosis
Benign familial neonatal seizures

- Screen for intrauterine infections (remember to ask for appropriate investigations, e.g. including herpes simplex virus titres in an acutely ill child)
- EEG may be useful if there is clinical uncertainty as to whether abnormal movements are seizures.

TREATMENT

Treat the underlying disorder, e.g. hypoglycaemia, sepsis, drug withdrawal.

Anticonvulsant drugs
- Not all seizures need treatment.
- If there are more than three fits per hour, a single seizure lasts more than 5 min, or seizures are associated with prolonged low oxygen saturations, they should be treated.
- Polypharmacy should be avoided if possible.

- No drug has been shown to be better than any other at controlling seizures, which tend to cease once the (usually) acute brain insult has resolved. Hence maintenance therapy is best left until an ongoing seizure disorder is identified several days into the course of the illness.
- Phenobarbitone is the usual first choice. Give 20 mg/kg IV and follow with 10 mg/kg 30 min later if seizures continue. This should give adequate blood levels for several days and maintenance is not required until levels fall. If seizures recur, consider a further dose of 10 mg/kg or add a second drug.
- Second-line drugs are:
  — clonazepam: may be given as bolus doses (preferred) or infusion (see drugs section); use with caution as it rapidly accumulates and causes deep sedation and increased secretions
  — paraldehyde: may be given rectally or preferably as a continuous IV infusion for frequent seizures
  — lignocaine: relatively underused, this is a good anti-convulsant and produces lasting improvement in the EEG in about 70% of cases; cannot be used if phenytoin has been given; use with ECG monitoring as there is slight risk of arrhythmias
  — midazolam: may be given by infusion to ventilated infant, additive effect with lignocaine.
- If seizures persist despite two drugs, an EEG is performed; consider pyridoxine IV if EEG demonstrates persisting spike and wave pattern.

Diazepam is generally avoided because of respiratory depression. Shorter acting benzodiazepines are being studied.

Once seizure control is achieved, aim to gradually reduce and withdraw anticonvulsants in the first week, if possible. Maintenance therapy, if required, may be with phenobarbitone, clonazepam or sodium valproate.

PROGNOSIS

Depends upon the underlying condition (q.v.).

Opiate withdrawal

Infants born to mothers who abuse opiates and other drugs in pregnancy are more likely to be premature or of low birthweight. Theoretically there is a reduced risk of RDS if the mother has used heroin.

- *Neurological symptoms* of withdrawal syndrome include sleeplessness, hyperreflexia, convulsions, restlessness/irritability and tremors. *Non-neurological symptoms* include sneezing, tachycardia, vomiting, fever, nasal stuffiness, sweating, yawning, fist sucking, diarrhoea and respiratory depression.
- Heroin withdrawal symptoms begin soon after birth, peak by 4 days and disappear by 2 weeks. Barbiturate and methadone withdrawal syndromes present later and symptoms may last many weeks.

MANAGEMENT

- Close observation of the infant for signs of withdrawal for a minimum of 4 days after birth.
- The mother should be aware of the signs of withdrawal so that she may seek help for the infant if there are problems after discharge. On the postnatal ward, it is helpful to teach mothers about the signs of withdrawal to facilitate this.
- Breast feeding is allowed if the mother has not been on large doses of methadone (>20 mg/day).
- Drug therapy is indicated if the infant develops six of the above symptoms or convulsions.
- For opiate-addicted mothers, the baby is commenced on oral morphine at a dose of 40 micrograms/kg 4-hourly and doses are titrated against symptoms. The dose is reduced gradually once symptom control is achieved. Many babies only need one or two doses and it is important not to over-treat and prolong admission.
- If morphine does not adequately treat the symptoms, chlorpromazine may be used. Convulsions may require treatment with phenobarbitone (see above).
- Since 1–2% of the maternal drug dose appears in breast milk mothers should be warned not to suddenly stop breast feeding, but gradually to tail off.
- Close liaison with the primary care team is required at discharge.

Nerve palsies

Brachial plexus injury in the neonatal period is usually due to birth trauma, e.g. traction injury occurring following shoulder dystocia (see Ch. 5). The injury involves some or all of the brachial plexus roots C5–T1, which may be stretched or avulsed from the spinal cord.

Central nervous system malformations

NEURAL TUBE DEFECTS

These conditions are seen rarely since the advent of preconception folate supplementation, antenatal screening and selective termination of pregnancy.

Anencephaly

There is failure of formation of structures above the brain stem. The condition is lethal.

Encephalocele

Herniation of brain tissue through a midline defect in the skull — 80% occur in the occipital region, the rest occur anteriorly. The lesion is covered by skin. Other congenital anomalies should be excluded. USS or MRI will identify underlying hydrocephalus or cerebral malformation which is associated with poor neurodevelopmental progress. If there is no brain tissue in the sac, most children develop normally. The encephalocele is usually removed surgically within the first few weeks of life.

Spina bifida

Failure of fusion of the vertebral bodies in the midline. Several distinct lesions are defined.

Spina bifida occulta. A defect in the vertebral arch, but with intact spinal cord and skin closure. A range of similar defects may be identified during routine newborn examination:

- *Dermal sinus* — a deep pit from the skin to the spinal canal may occur anywhere along the spine, but is commonest in lumbosacral area and not common with dimples occurring below the level of S2 (i.e. in the natal cleft). There may be a sentinel hairy patch (see below) or naevus. Detailed USS before 6 weeks of age should identify a sinus. Early referral is necessary to avoid the potential risk of ascending meningitis.
- *Lipoma* — a fatty swelling is present over the spine at birth and may extend into the spinal canal.
- *Diastometamyelia* — an overlying hairy patch may signal that a bony or fibrous spur divides the spinal cord (this is also commonly associated with myelomeningocele; see below)

Infants with spina bifida occulta have no neurological deficit at birth, but tethering of the spinal cord may progressively develop during childhood. All babies should be referred for detailed imaging of the spine by USS or MRI and the opinion of a neurosurgeon if a lesion is confirmed.

Meningocele

Herniation of meninges through bony defect with skin cover, usually lower lumber or sacral region. The prognosis is good; neurosurgical referral is necessary.

Myelomeningocele

The meningeal sac and spinal cord tissue herniate through a defect in the lumbar or thoracic spine; the open lesion oozes CSF and there is usually severe neurological abnormality. Careful assessment in liaison with a neurosurgeon is important.

General
- Exclude other congenital abnormalities.
- Ensure the baby is not sedated due to administration of maternal medication.

Neurological
- Assess motor and sensory level and size of lesion.
- Is there skin cover or is the spinal cord exposed?
- Examine for hydrocephalus and scoliosis.
- Determine degree of muscle wasting and deformity, e.g. talipes.
- Assess sensory level using gentle pinprick.
- Is the anus patulous with dribbling of meconium?
- Is the bladder palpable and does spontaneous micturition occur?

Ultrasound will identify hydrocephalus and MRI the presence of the Chiari malformation, i.e. herniation of the cerebellar vermis through the foramen magnum.

Further management. Having carefully assessed the baby at birth, a treatment plan is developed with the parents. If the diagnosis is made antenatally, the parents will already have been counselled and be familiar with many of the likely problems ahead. If active treatment is agreed, the lesion is usually closed on the first day in order to minimise the risk of infection and achieve good skin cover. If the baby is treated conservatively and survives, the lesion will epithelialise and hydrocephalus may develop. This will require shunt placement to ease dressing and for cosmetic appearance. A ventriculoperitoneal shunt may be necessary to treat hydrocephalus in approximately 50% of babies, either at the first operation or within 2 weeks of back closure.

Follow-up is by a multidisciplinary team including neurosurgeon, orthopaedic surgeon, urologist and developmental paediatrician and is lifelong. Parents may need to learn intermittent urinary catheterisation at an early stage.

OTHER CEREBRAL MALFORMATIONS

Holoprosencephaly

A severe developmental defect of the forebrain. It is frequently associated with chromosomal anomalies and facial abnormalities. The prognosis is poor.

Hydranencephaly

A bilateral vascular accident involving the territory of the internal carotid artery resulting in widespread loss of cerebral tissue. Small islands of cerebral tissue remain posteriorly. The prognosis is poor.

Microcephaly

Examine carefully for dysmorphic features. Check karyotype and screen for intrauterine infections. Enquire about maternal drugs or alcohol in pregnancy and consanguinity. Exclude underlying cerebral dysmorphism. Idiopathic microcephaly may be auto-somal recessive or X-linked.

Dandy–Walker malformation

A posterior fossa cyst continuous with the fourth ventricle with hypoplasia of the cerebellar vermis associated with several chromosome abnormalities, including triploidy and trisomies 13 and 18.

Acquired haemorrhagic and ischaemic brain injury

PREMATURE INFANTS

Periventricular haemorrhage (PVH)

The commonest site of intracranial haemorrhage in premature infants is PVH arising from the subependymal germinal matrix which is situated between the caudate nucleus and thalamus. During the mid-trimester of pregnancy the germinal matrix is the site of vigorous glioblastic activity and is richly supplied with blood via thin walled capillaries which may rupture initiating haemorrhage into the basal ganglia, lateral ventricles or brain parenchyma. Parenchymal haemorrhage occurs in 15% of infants with PVH. It is unlikely that haemorrhage extends directly from the ventricles into the cerebral cortex, rather that obstruction of blood flow in the terminal veins as a result of blood clot in the ventricles results in venous infarction of the periventricular white matter and secondary haemorrhage. Predisposing factors include variability in BP, oxygenation and CO_2 levels (especially hypercapnia) which leads to surges in blood flow in the fragile capillaries. The incidence of PVH increases with reducing gestational age below 32 weeks, but appears to have decreased in frequency over recent years. PVH is reported in approximately 10–15% of infants <32 weeks gestation. Scans may be normal at birth and haemorrhage develops during the first week, with maximal frequency between days 3 and 5.

Clinical signs. Most frequently, the haemorrhage is silent and diagnosed on routine USS (see below). Symptoms suggestive of PVH are: ● sudden collapse ● bulging fontanelle ● seizures ● anaemia ● hypoxia.

Classification. Haemorrhages are frequently graded according to various systems. It is better to report what is seen, most usefully described by the site and extent of lesion and its relationship to the ventricle. Haemorrhages may be subependymal (i.e. confined to the germinal matrix – SEH), intraventricular (IVH, where they may or may not distend the lateral ventricle) or parenchymal.

Prevention

General measures:
● Optimal use of antenatal steroids to minimise respiratory illness
● Maintain systemic perfusion
● Try to avoid rapid swings in BP and blood gases
● Intervene early in respiratory illness
● Use of surfactant
● Minimise infant–ventilator mismatch, using fast rate or synchronised ventilation.

Specific measures. There have been numerous studies of the protective effects of drugs such as pancuronium, ethamsylate, indomethacin, phenobarbitone and vitamin E. Of these, only indomethacin has been shown to have a protective effect after systematic review, but there are concerns about potential ischaemia as its use is associated with a reduction in CBF. None can be unreservedly recommended or universally adopted.

Management
● Treat anaemia with blood transfusion.
● Check coagulation screen during acute bleed.
● Anticonvulsants for seizure control.
● Repeat USS regularly to assess the extent of haemorrhage and monitor ventricular size (see p. 229).

Complications
● Post-haemorrhagic ventricular dilatation may occur due to failure of reabsorption of CSF owing to the presence of blood

in the ventricular system (tends to become a problem at 14–21 days) and may progress to hydrocephalus (see p. 235).
- Parenchymal haemorrhage may resolve or organise as cystic periventricular leucomalacia or a porencephalic cyst.

Prognosis
- Infants with SEH or uncomplicated IVH have a prognosis that is similar to infants of the same gestation without haemorrhage.
- Approximately 50% of infants who develop post-haemorrhagic ventricular dilatation requiring shunt placement will develop cerebral palsy.
- Parenchymal haemorrhage which evolves into PVL is associated with a high risk of cerebral palsy and associated disability. Depending upon definition and the study, up to 80% are reported to have cerebral palsy.

Periventricular leucomalacia (PVL)
PVL refers to necrosis of white matter in a characteristic distribution adjacent to the superolateral angles of the lateral ventricles. It is associated with 'watershed' or 'boundary zone' areas, with the least adequate cortical blood supply. As for haemorrhagic parenchymal lesions, cysts may develop. In the absence of a clear haemorrhage, it is thought that these reflect ischaemic injury. PVL may often coexist with PVH. Clinically, similar risk factors have been described to those in PVH, excepting that several studies have suggested that hypoperfusion secondary to low $P_a\text{co}_2$ levels may be important in its pathogenesis. Thus too high and too low $P_a\text{co}_2$ levels may be associated with different types of preterm brain injury.

Diagnosis. Early USS reveals typical 'flare' in the periventricular white matter, often difficult to distinguish from the normal peritrigonal blush. Many flares resolve without cyst formation. Over the course of 10–14 days, others may evolve into cysts, which in turn are reabsorbed later in the first year, leading to ventricular dilatation secondary to loss of brain tissue. The incidence of flares is approximately 12% and of cystic lesions 3% of infants <1500 g at birth.

Prognosis. This depends on the number and distribution of cysts. Anterior cysts alone, or cysts confined to the centrum semi ovale, are associated with a good prognosis. Cysts in the occipital region or widespread cysts are associated with cerebral palsy. It is important to differentiate pseudocysts (cysts lying immediately adjacent to the ventricular wall of no certain significance) and choroid plexus cysts (good prognosis in the absence of dysmorphic syndrome).

CEREBRAL USS IN THE PRETERM INFANT

Ultrasound scanners are widely available in neonatal units. Interpretation of the findings is a skilled job and should not be undertaken without training and supervision. In this section we describe the basic technique and suggest a scheme for reporting scans, but before embarking on cerebral USS, the reader is directed to a more detailed text. The aim of scanning is to identify major abnormalities which may influence care and prognosis. Major landmarks are shown in Figs 12.2 and 12.3.

Machines and recording your examination

- The best pictures are taken with a 7.5 or 10 mHz probe. A 5 mHz probe may miss parenchymal changes.

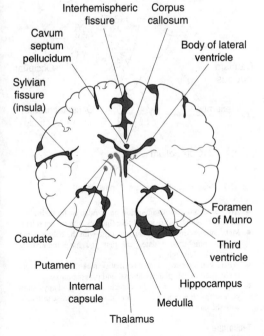

Fig. 12.2 Coronal section.

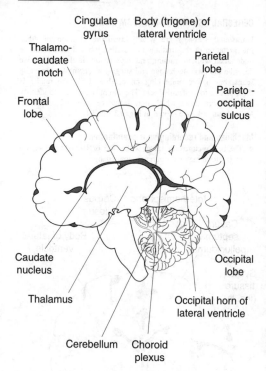

Cingulate gyrus

Body (trigone) of lateral ventricle

Thalamo-caudate notch

Parietal lobe

Parieto-occipital sulcus

Frontal lobe

Caudate nucleus

Thalamus

Occipital lobe

Occipital horn of lateral ventricle

Cerebellum

Choroid plexus

Fig. 12.3 Parasaggital view – long axis of lateral ventricle.

- Always record your examination on a video or by taking still pictures to allow discussion of your findings with the consultant.
- Make sure the record is clearly marked with the baby's name, hospital number and date, and that you have marked the orientation (left/right).
- Where you have found an abnormality, make sure its presence is recorded in two planes (coronal and parasagittal).
- Report your findings in the clinical notes and always show your scans to a consultant before discussing the scan results with the parents.

Technique

1. Clean ultrasound head with alcohol solution and allow to dry.

2. Cover transducer with ultrasound jelly.
3. Apply transducer to anterior fontanelle in coronal section (transducer axis in line with the ears). Scan from frontal fossa to posterior, keeping transducer in the coronal plane (make sure that you keep the transducer in plane). Record appearances in standard planes (Fig. 12.4) plus any abnormality you see. Display the images as if viewed from the front of the head, i.e. with the baby's right side on the left of the screen. *Remember to label the sides.*
4. Rotate transducer through 90° and scan in sagittal and parasagittal planes. Record appearances as above (Fig. 12.5).
5. Common errors are encountered by not turning down the gain (snowstorm effect) or by not varying the depth of scanning to maximise the picture on the screen with loss of definition.
6. Wipe jelly from fontanelle and clean transducer.

Reporting your findings

Describe what you see and try not to ascribe grading systems to the appearances as different units and individuals have different systems. The easiest way of reporting your scan is to identify three basic elements:

- Is there PVH present? Describe by extent (subependymal, intraventricular and parenchymal), size with reference to the ventricles (small, — usually with no ventriculomegaly or distension; large — enlarged ventricular systems or distension of ventricles) and position in the ventricle.

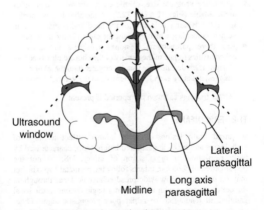

Fig. 12.4 Standard planes in coronal section.

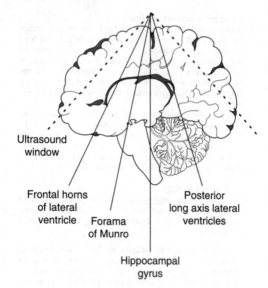

Ultrasound window

Frontal horns of lateral ventricle

Forama of Munro

Hippocampal gyrus

Posterior long axis lateral ventricles

Fig. 12.5 Standard planes in parasagittal and sagittal section.

- Assess the ventricle size; centile charts for ventricular index are available (Figs 12.6 and 12.7). Remember hydrocephalus implies a dynamic enlarging of the head and is distinct from ventriculomegaly, which may also be due to cortical atrophy.
- Are there parenchymal lesions? Describe in terms of echodensities (relate to the density of the choroid plexus echoes — significant densities are usually brighter than these) or cystic changes, again by extent, by reference to the ventricle and size.

Other findings can then be reported if present.

THE TERM INFANT

Acquired brain lesions in term infants reflect a range of pathologies and many are acquired before birth, characterised by early resolution or organisation of injury. USS is not the investigation of choice in infants following perinatal hypoxia, but may on occasions show widespread echogenic areas throughout the cortex, together with focal haemorrhagic lesions in the basal ganglia, all tending to be rather poor prognostic signs. Other lesions are described below.

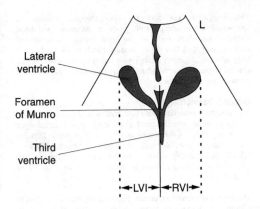

Coronal View

LVI = Left Ventricular Index
RVI = Right Ventricular Index

Fig. 12.6 Assessing ventricle size: standard measures.

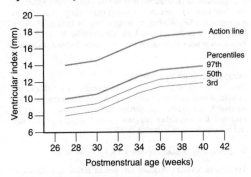

Fig. 12.7 Chart to assess ventricular growth.

Subcortical cystic leucomalacia

Ischaemic lesions extending into the deep white matter of the cortex may be seen in term and preterm infants with severe encephalopathy (see above). These changes organise as subcortical leucomalacia, with cysts in the more peripheral vascular 'boundary zone' in the term infant. Inexperienced scanners may find that the cysts are difficult to see as they are truly subcortical. Severe disability, including spastic quadriplegia, cortical blindness, microcephaly, severe cognitive impairment and seizures, are common sequelae.

Subdural haemorrhage

This is usually associated with birth trauma leading to a dural tear or rupture of the superior cerebral bridging veins. Clinical signs are usually those of the accompanying encephalopathy. Massive haemorrhage is associated with shock, coma and death. USS is not reliable in excluding subdural lesions although larger lesions causing displacement of midline structures may be seen; CT or MRI are of more value.

Treatment is usually expectant. Subdural tap may be helpful to decompress convexity haemorrhage causing midline shift. Neurosurgical advice should be sought. Approximately 50% of survivors are neurologically abnormal at follow-up.

Subarachnoid haemorrhage (SAH)

This may be primary haemorrhage due to rupture of capillaries or veins within the subarachnoid space or secondary to blood tracking into the ventricular system following PVH. SAH may be asymptomatic or presentation may be with convulsions, apnoea or the symptoms of coexistent post-hypoxic injury. Diagnosis is suspected by LP yielding uniformly bloodstained CSF or by bright echoes in the sulci on USS. Confirmation is by CT scan. Prognosis is usually good; post-haemorrhagic hydrocephalus is a rare sequel.

Intraparenchymal haemorrhage

Most cases of primary intraparenchymal haemorrhage are associated with fetal or neonatal coagulopathy. Thrombocytopenia, vitamin K deficiency and clotting factor deficiency should be excluded (Ch. 14). Other rare causes include protein C deficiency and heparinisation (e.g. during ECMO).

Diagnosis may be confirmed by USS, CT or MRI.

Treatment. Correct coagulation abnormalities and thrombo-cytopaenia if platelets <30 ×10^9 /L (Ch. 14). Surgical evacuation of haemorrhage is not necessary unless there is gross shift of the midline.

Prognosis. Roughly one-third of infants die, one-third are handicapped and one third are neurologically normal.

Hydrocephalus

Excessive accumulation of CSF resulting in excessive growth of the head. Obstruction to the normal pathway of CSF flow and absorption lead to ventricular dilatation. The cause may be congenital or acquired (Table 12.4).

ASSESSMENT

- Cerebral USS may demonstrate underlying congenital malformation.
- Investigations for intrauterine infections (typically *Toxoplasma*, occasionally CMV).
- Plot head circumference serially (e.g. weekly at first).
- US measurement of ventricular index (VI). This is a measure of the horizontal width of each ventricle, measured in the coronal plane at a level just posterior to the foramen of Munro. Ventricular growth charts are available (see Fig. 12.7).
- Examine for signs of raised ICP, i.e. apnoea, drowsiness, vomiting, increased limb tone, bulging fontanelle, separation of sutures.

MANAGEMENT

Intervention is generally required when the VI measures 4 mm over the 97th centile for gestation (see Figs 12.6 and 12.7).

- Drugs, such as acetazolamide, which are thought to reduce CSF production, have not been shown to avoid shunt placement and in one recent study were associated with increased morbidity and mortality.

Table 12.4 Causes of hydrocephalus

Congenital
Aqueduct stenosis
Arnold–Chiari malformation
Dandy–Walker malformation
Associated with cerebral malformation, e.g. encephalocele
Congenital infection, e.g. CMV, toxoplasmosis
Cerebral tumour

Acquired
Post-haemorrhagic
PVH
Subdural haemorrhage
Subarachnoid haemorrhage

Post infective
Neonatal meningitis or encephalitis

Table 12.5 Potential sequelae of very preterm birth

Major disabling conditions
Cerebral palsy (all types are found)
Sensorineural (high tone) hearing loss
Blindness (due to cicatricial ROP or cortical injury)
Developmental retardation

Other major conditions
Respiratory problems (sequelae of CLD)
Impairment of growth

Other problems
Feeding difficulties (oromotor dysfunction)
Specific language delays
Later educational problems
Attention deficit disorder
Clumsiness

Table 12.6 Follow-up checklist

- Record parental concerns and recent medical history, including immunisations
- Review diet and feeding
- Plot growth parameters on centile chart
- Review development — it may be useful to use a developmental screening tool (e.g. the Denver Chart or Schedule of Growing Skills)
- Review medication — including iron and vitamin supplements for very preterm babies (see Ch. 15)
- Physical examination — in particular:
  — cardiovascular: murmurs present?
  — Respiratory: signs of chronic respiratory problems?
  — Neurology: evolving signs of cerebral palsy?
  — Hips
  — Development: can you confirm your review findings?
- Record your findings and discuss the next appointment with the parents
- Complete any local audit forms (e.g. see Table 12.7)

- Removal of CSF by LP or ventricular tap may alleviate symptoms of raised ICP and temporarily control rapid head growth, but carries a risk of introducing infection into the CSF. In a randomised trial, this did not improve the rate of shunt placement or of long-term sequelae.
- Definitive treatment for hydrocephalus will usually require placement of a ventriculoperitoneal shunt.
- Recent alternative strategies include intraventricular fibrinolytic therapy, ventricular drainage/lavage and, in some centres, neuroendoscopic third ventriculostomy. These measures may delay the need for shunt placement as the child grows and recovers from other neonatal illnesses, but none

have been shown to improve long term outcome. The complications of shunt placement, e.g. blockage and infection, are considerable: 40% failure rate over 2 years, and 80% failure rate over 20 years. Thus any attempts to avoid insertion should be welcomed.

PROGNOSIS

This depends on the aetiology of the hydrocephalus. Children with aqueduct stenosis do very well. Extremely premature infants with post-haemorrhagic hydrocephalus and parenchymal lesions have a very high incidence of neurological abnormality. It is suggested that, in uncomplicated hydrocephalus, IQ will be normal if the cerebral mantle is 3 cm. or more by 5 months of age.

Withdrawal of treatment in an infant likely to be severely handicapped

Sadly there are some infants born with congenital abnormalities of the brain and nervous system in whom severe physical and/or mental disability may be predicted. A similar outcome may be anticipated in normally formed infants who suffer brain injury, e.g. grade III encephalopathy, severe parenchymal haemorrhage or PVL.

The assessment of severe brain damage is not easy. The diagnosis of brain death (BPA 1991) may be established in term infants from the age of 2 months. These criteria cannot be safely applied to less mature babies, owing to the rapid developmental changes seen in late gestation and the early weeks of life, which result in the presence or absence of brain stem reflexes being an unreliable test. An assessment of likely outcome is therefore made on the basis of a combination of repeated clinical examination, diagnostic brain imaging and assessment of function, e.g. evoked cortical potentials and EEG activity.

A decision may be reached by the parents and neonatologist, in discussion with all members of the team of specialist doctors, nurses and therapists caring for the baby, that it is inappropriate to continue extraordinary means to keep the baby alive or that such measures should not be initiated should the baby deteriorate. If the parents are kept fully informed of the results of all scans, laboratory investigations and clinical progress of their baby that contribute to the difficult decision-making process, it is unlikely that there will be surprise or conflict between the views of the professionals and family. The culture and religious beliefs of the family must be respected. It is important that the views of the parents are sought and incorporated into the plan of continuing care for the baby. It must be emphasised that the parents should not feel they are being asked to decide alone whether their baby should live or die, but rather to participate in planning appropriate continuing care, i.e. warmth, nutrition and contact. Such a care plan will no longer include intensive care. Thus, although *intensive* care may be withdrawn, *care* is always continued.

Neurodevelopmental follow-up

Babies who are admitted to NICUs are at increased risk of subsequent impairment of motor and/or cognitive function. The two greatest risk groups are those with grade II or III encephalopathy (see above) and those of very preterm gestation (see Fig. 1.5). These groups should be closely followed up after discharge. They may need the help of a team of professionals, including a paediatrician, physiotherapist, occupational therapist, speech therapist, dietician, health visitor, audiologist and ophthalmologist. Early identification of any of the listed impairments (Table 12.5) will permit a multidisciplinary approach to the planning of health, social and educational services for each child. Other children who have been admitted for intensive care also require follow up for varying lengths of time depending upon the underlying condition. Follow-up arrangements will be made according to local policy, but high risk groups will usually be followed up until 2 years of age. The age corrected for gestation (chronological age minus weeks of prematurity) is used for all assessments up to 2 years.

The neonatal follow-up clinic serves a number of functions:

- to provide continuity of care for parents who have often got to know medical staff well during their child's stay in the NICU
- to detect both emerging medical and developmental problems, and to provide counselling and intervention as required
- to provide data for service monitoring.

Where problems are identified, the appropriate local service should be involved and it is often more appropriate for children with disabilities to receive their ongoing care from these services rather than the neonatal follow-up clinic. A brief checklist of items to address during the clinic visit is given in Table 12.6.

Nationally, criteria for severe disability have been defined at 2 years, to help parents and professionals in discussions and service provision (Table 12.7 and Fig. 1.5). It should be remembered that comparisons of the incidence of adverse outcomes between different NICUs may largely reflect the severity of illness of the babies admitted rather than the technical abilities of the unit staff. Intra-unit differences may be compensated for to some extent by correcting for disease severity over the first 12 h using the Clinical Risk Index for Babies (CRIB) score, which is based upon:

- birthweight
- gestation
- presence of malformation
- minimum and maximum F_iO_2 with normal P_aO_2 values in first 12 h
- Worst base excess in first 12 h.

Although follow-up information is used to calculate disability rates at 2 years, further problems may become apparent over the early school years (e.g. attention deficit, poor fine motor skills, cognitive and academic problems). Before discharging the child from follow-up, the paediatrician should ensure that, in particular, very immature children (<27 weeks gestation) are identified to the community child health service as children at particular risk of these later problems.

Table 12.7 Standard minimum dataset for classification of health status at 2 years of age. (Adapted from Disability and Perinatal Care. National Perinatal Epidemiology Unit/ Oxford Health Authority 1994)

Domain (Key questions)	Criteria for disability (criteria for severe disability underlined)
Malformation Does the child have a malformation?	Any anomaly detected at birth or apparent within the first 2 postnatal years, which is likely to result in death, disfigurement or disability, and which is likely to require medical or surgical treatment (other than a simple cosmetic procedure) <u>Any malformation which, despite physical assistance, impairs the performance of daily activities</u>
Neuromotor function Does the child have any difficulty walking?	Non-fluent gait Abnormal gait reducing mobility <u>Unable to walk without assistance</u>
Does the child have any difficulty sitting?	Sits unsupported but unstable Sits supported <u>Unable to sit</u>
Does the child have any difficulty with hand use?	Some difficulty feeding with one hand Some difficulty feeding with both hands <u>Unable to use hands to feed self</u>
Does the child have any difficulty with head control?	Unstable but no support required <u>Unable to control head movement without support</u> <u>No head control</u>

Table 12.7 *cont'd*

Seizures

Does the child have seizures?	No treatment required
	No seizures on treatment
	Seizures despite treatment <1/month
	Seizures despite treatment >1/month

Auditory function

Does the child have any difficulty hearing?	Hearing impaired, not aided
	Hearing impaired, corrects with aids
	Hearing impaired, uncorrected even with aids

Communication

Is there any difficulty with communication?	Unable to comprehend word/sign out of familiar context
	Unable to comprehend word/sign in cued situation
	Uses single-words-only vocabulary >10 words
	Vocabulary <10 words
	Unable to produce >5 recognisable sounds
	No vocalisation

Visual function

Does the child have any difficulty with vision?	Normal vision with correction
	Not fully correctable
	Blind or sees light only

Cognitive function

Does the child have any learning difficulty (function assessed on standardised test)?	<2 standard deviations below mean (approximately >6 months behind at 2 years)

Other physical disability

Does the child have any other disability (Any restriction in performing an activity in the manner considered normal for a human being)?	*Respiratory*
	Limited exercise tolerance, no drug treatment
	Limited exercise tolerance, on drug treatment
	Requires continual oxygen therapy
	Requires mechanical ventilation
	GI
	Requires special diet
	Has stoma
	Requires tube feeding
	Requires parenteral nutrition
	Renal function
	Renal impairment known, no treatment
	Renal impairment drug or dietary treatment only
	Requires dialysis
	Growth
	Height or weight below 3 percentile for age
	Height or weight velocity <3 percentile for age
	Other function
	Describe (A description of the disability is necessary to allow later allocation of severity grading)

THIRTEEN

Fetal and neonatal infection

The sterile environment of the amniotic fluid and uterus protects the fetus from infection. Transplacental infection may be acquired during maternal bacteraemia (including syphillis, Group B Streptococcal (GBS) and listeria infections) or viraemia (e.g. rubella, varicella zoster virus and CMV) or occassional during infections with other organisms such as toxoplasma or malaria.

The fetus is also at risk from ascending infection from the vagina (particularly if the membranes are ruptured). During vaginal delivery the infant may be exposed to a number of potential pathogens in the birth canal: GBS, *E. coli*, *N. gonorrhoeae* and herpes simplex virus). 1 in 50 preterm infants and 1 in 1000 term infants will develop systemic infection in the neonatal period. This increased risk occurs because of both physical and immunological differences:

- Impaired physical defences
  - Thin, fragile skin
  - Skin sterile at birth; no competition from normal flora
  - Invasive procedures, e.g. IV access, intubation.
- Decreased humoral immunity
  - IgG crosses placenta in small amounts from 12 weeks. Passage in substantial amounts occurs after 34 weeks. At term, levels are higher in fetal than in maternal blood. Majority are IgG_1 or IgG_3 subclass. Relative lack of IgG_2 inhibits rapid responses to capsular polysaccharides of some organisms, e.g. GBS. Half-life of passively acquired IgG in neonatal plasma is 3–6 weeks. Nadir in IgG levels is reached at 3 months, after which endogenous production of IgG takes over
  - IgM does not cross placenta, and therefore there is no passive immunity to Gram-negative organisms
  - IgA does not cross placenta. Found in breast milk.
- Decreased cellular immunity — B and T cells immature but normal adult numbers.
- Decreased white cell function
  - normal numbers of neutrophils
  - decreased chemotaxis, phagocytosis and opsonization

- Deficient complement system — mediators of the complement pathway, especially the alternative pathway, are low.

Postnatal infection may be acquired from the environment, staff and parents or may occur by direct invasion. Table 13.1 describes measures to reduce cross-infection.

Table 13.1 Prevention of cross-infection

- Adequate spacing of infants
- Strict handwashing policy
  - remove jewellery, watches etc.
  - wash hands using antiseptic solution
  - after handling re-clean hands — alcohol solution can be used and is well tolerated
  - re-wash hands if soiled
- Gloves
  - initial handling of infant
  - if in contact with blood
- Gowns/masks — ineffective; use to protect own clothes only
- Minimal handling
- Strict readmission policy — do not readmit infants to neonatal unit from home if any risk of infection. Admit to paediatric ward instead
- Equipment
  - sole use preferable
  - clean other equipment, e.g. cold light source with alcohol swab between babies
- Staff/parental infections
  - immunise all staff against measles, rubella, tuberculosis and hepatitis B
  - treat paronychia, local skin infections
  - cover cuts when on duty
  - proven group A streptococcal throat infection: treat with penicillin and exclude from work until symptoms are clear
  - herpes simplex virus
  - cold sores: do not kiss baby; if recurrent, start acyclovir with prodrome
  - herpetic whitlow: no direct patient care
  - varicella zoster virus (VZV): if non-immune and definite exposure, no direct patient care from day 9 to 21; if rash develops, person is infective until 1 week after last lesion disappears
  - respiratory infections: a cold should not prevent work
  - gastroenteritis: no direct patient care until symptoms resolved

Risk factors for neonatal infection

Early infection
(i.e. occurring within 48 h of birth — likely to have been acquired in utero or during passage through the birth canal)

- Prolonged rupture of membranes
- Preterm rupture of membranes/preterm labour

- Fetal distress
- Chorioamnionitis
- Foul-smelling liquor
- Maternal infection, especially gastroenteritis, UTI
- Colonisation or previous baby with GBS.

Common organisms are GBS, and *E. coli* in the UK. Occasionally, there is systemic infection with *Listeria monocytogenes*, *Neisseria gonorrhoeae* or other organisms found on high vaginal swab (HVS).

Late infection
(i.e. occurring 48 h after birth — likely to have been acquired postnatally):

- Preterm delivery
- Congenital malformations with open skin or mucosal surfaces (e.g. spina bifida)
- Recurrent courses of antibiotics
- Invasive access, e.g. ETT, venous lines.

The commonest organisms causing acquired infection are *Staph. epidermidis* (>50%), *Staph. aureus*, *E. coli* and *Candida albicans*.

Types of neonatal infection

CONGENITAL INFECTION

It is a misconception to think only of *Toxoplasma*, rubella, CMV and herpes as congenital infections. This misconception has arisen partly because of doctors attachment to the acronym 'TORCH syndrome'. GBS, *L. monocytogenes*, *N. gonorrhoeae*, syphilis, enterovirus and varicella zoster are all infections which may be acquired before birth and therefore are truly congenital. Screening for congenital infections should be considered in:

- Malformations (see Table 13.2)
- Neonatal seizures
- Encephalopathy
- IUGR — usually if there is one other abnormality
- Micro/macrocephaly
- Thrombocytopenia
- Early jaundice with no blood group incompatibility
- Early-onset sepsis
- Hepatitis.

Many of the intrauterine infections give rise to congenital malformations. Table 13.2 shows the clinical features which may be seen in babies born following such infection and Table 13.3 the appropriate specimens which should be sent. Finally remember that congenital viral infections may present beyond the neonatal period with developmental delay or deafness.

Table 13.2 Association of clinical abnormality with congenital infection

Abnormality	Infection
CHD	Rubella
	CMV
	Mumps (endocardial fibroelastosis has been suggested but not proven)
Cataracts	Rubella (frequently associated with microphthalmos)
	CMV
Chorioretinitis	Rubella
	Toxoplasmosis
	CMV
	Herpes
	Varicella
	Syphilis
Microphthalmos	Rubella
	Toxoplasmosis
	Herpes
	Varicella
	CMV
Microcephaly	CMV
	Toxoplasmosis
	Rubella
	Varicella
	Herpes simplex
Cerebral calcification	Toxoplasmosis (punctate)
	CMV (periventricular)
	Rubella (rare)
	Herpes simplex (rare)
Purpura (usually appears on the first day)	CMV
	Toxoplasmosis
	Syphilis
	Rubella
	Herpes simplex
	Bacterial sepsis
Jaundice	CMV
	Toxoplasmosis
	Rubella
	Herpes simplex

Table 13.3 Appropriate specimens for the investigation of congenital infection

Specimen	Test
Urine	Viral culture — CMV
	Latex particle agglutination — GBS antigen

Table 13.3 *cont'd*

Specimen	Test
Throat swab	Viral culture CMV Enteroviruses
Neonatal serum (single specimen)	Rubella-specific IgM (occurs in 100% of cases of congenital rubella until 3 months of age). Absent rubella-specific IgG excludes infection Parvovirus B19 Syphilis (VDRL test) (FTA test — unreliable) Single specimen is unhelpful for herpes, HIV, toxoplasmosis
Paired neonatal sera	Diagnosis by documenting seroconversion by a rise in antibody titre Herpes[a] Varicella zoster[a]
Serology of both mother and infant	HIV[b] Toxoplasmosis[b]
CSF	Culture Herpes Enteroviruses Bacterial meningitis Syphilis Latex particle agglutination — GBS
Skin lesions	Virus isolation Herpes Enteroviruses Varicella zoster
Neonatal blood cultures	All bacterial infections
Stool cultures	Enteroviruses Echovirus Coxsackie virus

[a] Specific IgM not generally available.
[b] Passively acquired maternal IgG hinders the diagnosis. Comparison of antenatal booking sera and the current maternal sera may demonstrate recent infection by a rise in the titre. If HIV-infection is suspected, measure p24 Ag, HIV specific IgA and perform PCR for proviral DNA..

SUPERFICIAL INFECTION

Apparently trivial infections in the high-risk infant can rapidly lead to systemic sepsis. The following types of infections are frequently seen.

Conjunctivitis

Babies with conjunctivitis have purulent discharge, lid oedema, redness and conjunctival injection. The most important pathogens are *N. gonorrhoeae*, *Chlamydia trachomatis*, *Staph. aureus* and *Pseudomonas aeruginosa*. *Staph. aureus* is the most common.

Early conjunctivitis ('ophthalmia neonatorum')

- Purulent discharge within 48 h of birth is rare but frequently due to gonococcal infection. Discuss sample methodology with laboratory. Gram stain of eye swabs will show Gram-negative intracellular diplococci.
- May coexist with chlamydial infection.
- Urgent treatment is required for gonococcal infection with systemic cefotaxime, as penicillin resistance is not uncommon, together with local eye toilet. The obstetrician should be notified and appropriate swabs taken from the mother.

Purulent sticky eye after 48 h

- Take bacteriological swabs and *Chlamydia* scrapings after discussion with laboratory.
- Saline wash the eyes and treat with local antibiotics e.g. 0.5% neomycin ointment every 6 h. The use of chloramphenicol may interfere with any subsequent investigations for *Chlamydia*.
- Chlamydial infection is treated with 1% chlortetracycline ointment (four times per day for 1 month) plus oral erythromycin for 14 days to prevent risk of later pneumonitis. Refer mother and her partner(s) for treatment.

Purulent sticky eye with periorbital oedema. Swab, saline wash, and treat with both local (0.5% neomycin) and systemic antibiotics (flucloxacillin and gentamicin).

Sticky eye without purulent discharge. Culture discharge, give saline washes and observe.

Persistent sticky eye

- If no improvement occurs with standard treatment, stop treatment and repeat swabs for chlamydia.
- A persistent sticky eye is usually due to failure of the nasolacrimal duct to open. Non–pathogenic organisms (*S. albus*; diphtheroids) may then pool in the lacrimal sac and lead to secondary infection. Cleaning of the secretions and massage of the lacrimal sac are necessary to encourage patency. Only treat with antibiotics if there is evidence of acute infection.
- If this persists beyond 1 year, the nasolacrimal duct should be probed under general anaesthetic.

Skin sepsis

Superficial infected blisters are usually due to staphylococcal infection. Swab to confirm diagnosis. Keep area dry. If the infant is in an incubator, and humidification can be stopped, this should be done. A few localised spots can be treated by drying with an alcohol swab. More extensive lesions need treatment with topical fucidin. In the high-risk baby (e.g. preterm or requiring intensive care) take blood cultures and start systemic flucloxacillin.

Infection which is associated with infection of the deeper layers (usually signs of inflammation) may be due to a range of organisms, although *Staphylococcus* remains the most common. Staphylococcal abscesses can develop as breast abscesses or at the site of IV infusions, heel pricks etc. If possible, aspirate and send pus for culture before starting IV flucloxacillin and gentamicin.

Bullous impetigo (also known as neonatal pemphigus) is a staphylococcal skin infection resulting in blister formation. Scalded skin syndrome (also known as Lyell's or Ritter's disease) is due to a staphylococcal toxin and presents with erythema and epidermal separation on friction (Nikilsky's sign) and occasionally large fragile bullae which may shed to leave a raw area. Any part of the skin may be affected but mucous membranes are spared. In both conditions, Gram stain and culture of the bullous fluid will reveal *Staph. aureus*. Treatment is with IV flucloxacillin.

Paronychia

Single paronychia — use alcohol swabs. If there are multiple paronychia or evidence of local spread, treat with systemic flucloxacillin after taking swabs.

Umbilical infections

Local sepsis may be due to group A streptococcal infection or staphylococcal infection. With localised infection, swab with alcohol swabs. If there is evidence of spread, e.g. flare, or in the high-risk baby, use IV flucloxacillin.

Candida infection

Oral. White plaques will be present inside the mouth, which are difficult to remove, and may bleed when scraped. Rarely, infection can extend to cause oesophagitis or tracheobronchitis.

Swab and treat after feeds using nystatin suspension, 1 mL (100 000 units) q.d.s. for 14 days or miconazole oral gel, 1 mL q.d.s. for 5 days.

Perineal. Red satellite colonies are diagnostic. Swab and treat with nystatin cream (100 000 units g) q.d.s. If there is moderate dermatitis, use preparation with added hydrocortisone cream. Oral thrush should be simultaneously treated. With treatment failure, use 2% miconazole cream.

SYSTEMIC INFECTION

Signs and symptoms

The signs and symptoms of systemic infection, i.e. septicaemia, meningitis, pneumonia, UTI, osteomyelitis and gastroenteritis are non-specific and the cause is often not readily apparent. In the initial phase, the baby's symptoms may be very subtle. Often the nurse or mother will comment that the baby is 'off colour' or 'not himself'. Signs include: ● listlessness ● hypotonia ● pallor, mottled skin ● irritability ● temperature instability ● apnoea ● poor feeding ● jaundice ● vomiting and/or diarrhoea, bloody stools ● ileus ● tachypnoea ● grunting ● fits ● hypoglycaemia or hyperglycaemia.

Management of the baby with suspected systemic infection

History. Are there any risk factors (see above)?

Examination. Look for any localising signs (e.g. tense anterior fontanelle, umbilical flare, localised limb tenderness) and any circulatory compromise (decreased capillary return, hypotension).

Investigations. The site of infection is rarely clear in a newborn infant. Therefore, if infection is suspected, a full infection screen must be performed, including the following:

Full blood count
● Infection suggested by:
   — total WCC <4 or >20 × 10^9/L
   — neutrophil count <2 and >15 × 10^9/L
   — increase in immature (band) neutrophils
   — Ratio of immature neutrophils (e.g. band cells, mylocytes, metamylocytes) : total neutrophils (I:T)>0.2
● A single white cell count may be difficult to interpret, as the polymorph count is dropping during the first week of life. A rise in serial polymorph counts is very suggestive of infection (provided the child is not receiving systemic steroids).
● The total white cell count may be artificially elevated due to the presence of a large number of nucleated red cells in the early newborn period.
● Thrombocytopenia (<100 × 10^9/L) or falling platelet counts also suggest infection.

Blood culture
● Take at least 0.5 mL of blood.
● Use a peripheral vein or artery if possible. Avoid samples from IV or IA lines, unless taken during insertion, to reduce the chance of contamination.
● If central line sepsis suspected, take blood cultures from these in addition to peripheral cultures.

C-reactive protein
● Normal value <5 μg/mL.
● Takes 10–12 h to rise after onset of infection.

- A normal value 24 h post-onset of symptoms makes infection less likely.

Chest X-ray
Pneumonia can present in the absence of specific clinical signs.

Urine culture
- For the ill baby, who will commence antibiotics immediately after an infection screen, a suprapubic urine sample should be obtained.
- Bag urine should only be used where antibiotic treatment can be delayed until results are available, e.g. in the investigation of prolonged jaundice. If a specimen has been equivocal, discuss whether to carry out a suprapubic tap.
- Diagnose UTI if >10^5 organisms per mL (10^8/L) on culture.
- The presence or absence of white cells in the urine does not prove or disprove UTI.
- The presence of budding yeast forms as opposed to hyphae suggests disseminated fungal infection.

Lumbar puncture
- Only withhold if there are good grounds to believe that the infant will significantly deteriorate during the procedure; do not withhold because you do not think there is meningitis clinically — signs of meningism are rarely seen in the newborn.
- Send CSF sample for microscopy, culture, protein and glucose:
  — microscopy:
     > 20 polymorphs/mm^3 (i.e. 20 white cells per µL or 20 white
     cells × 10^6/L) — suspicious
     > 30 polymorphs — meningitis
     NB. can get organisms with no pleocytosis
     NB. IVH leads to increased neutrophils
     Bloody tap — allow 1 WBC to 500 RBC
  — protein: raised in meningitis and in newborn
     normal values: < 2.0 g/dL in term
                     < 3.7 g/dL in preterm
  — glucose: always compare to simultaneously taken true BG
     normal value CSF glucose >50% BG
     If CSF glucose <1 mmol/L or <30% of BG — strongly indicative of meningitis.
- If the child is drowsy and/or fitting, consider saving some CSF for metabolic investigations, e.g. to exclude non-ketotic hyperglycinaemia.

Blood gas analysis
- Is there metabolic acidosis?
- Does the infant need ventilatory support? (see Ch. 6)

Coagulation screen: Do if purpura, petechiae, bleeding from puncture sites, falling or low platelet count (Ch. 14).

Abdominal X-ray
- Do if any abdominal distension, blood per rectum.
- Is there ileus?
- Are there signs of NEC (see Ch. 9)?

Maternal high vaginal swab. Ask for this in suspected early sepsis if history of PROM, maternal pyrexia or diagnosis of early GBS infection possible.

Supportive management
- Consider early use of respiratory and circulatory support (Ch. 6) before systemic collapse occurs.
- Correct hypotension with 10 mL/kg aliquots of 4.5% HAS. Fresh frozen plasma can be given in the same dose and, although this corrects defective opsonisation, it is more expensive. If hypotension does not respond to plasma, IV dopamine at 5–20 µg/kg per min should be started early in illness.
- Transfuse if haemoglobin less than 12 g/dL.
- Correct fluid and electrolyte imbalance.
- Correct hypoglycaemia.
- Hyperglycaemia (Ch. 11) is often seen in infection but the use of insulin is very rarely justified and the risks of iatrogenic hypoglycaemia are very great. We commence insulin if the BG is persistently >10 mmol/L and there is ≥+++ of glycosuria.
- Granulocyte transfusion, granulocyte colony-stimulating factor, single volume exchange transfusion with fresh non-WBC-depleted blood and IV immunoglobulin are not in routine use in the newborn period, as none has been shown to reduce the overall mortality All may be considered on an individual basis in overwhelming sepsis. Discuss with your consultant first.
- Management of DIC is discussed in Chapter 14.
- Consider removing central venous lines, which may become colonised/infected with *Staph. epidermidis* in particular. Following such infections, bacterial endocarditis (right atrial and tricuspid valve) or fungal infection may complicate thrombus formation.

Antibiotic treatment. All babies in whom significant infection is suspected should be commenced on antibiotics until the results of cultures are available at 48 h. The antibiotic of choice will depend on the age of the baby, the infection suspected and any previous antibiotic treatment (Table13.4). Antibiotic doses are given in Appendix 4.

Table 13.4 Antibiotic guidelines in neonatal infection

Clinical situations	Risk factors	Possible organisms	Suggested regimes	Comments
'Early' onset sepsis/ ?RDS	PROM >24hrs Maternal infection — fever, leucocytosis etc. Maternal colonisation	GBS E. coli Other enterobacteria	Benzylpenicillin + gentamicin	If all cultures subsequently prove negative, antibiotics can be stopped after 48 hours if the baby is well Proven septicaemia is usually treated for 10 days
	Offensive or green liquor	Listeria monocytogenes	Benzylpenicillin + gentamicin	Convert penicillin to ampicillin following confirmation of diagnosis
Sepsis after >5 days	Presence of septic spots Umbilical flare Central venous line in situ	Staph. aureus Staph spp. Other gram +positive and -negative organisms	Flucloxacillin + gentamicin *	In proven S. epidermidis septicaemia secondary to long-line sepsis, change to vancomycin if symptoms not resolved by 48hrs
Pneumonia after prolonged stay in the neonatal unit	Ventilated Earlier course of antibiotics Last ET aspirate:	Not available, no growth or Staphylococcus	Flucloxacillin + gentamicin	
		Coliforms Pseudomonas aeruginosa	Cefotaxime Ceftazidime + gentamicin	
	Conjunctivitis /pneumonitis	Chlamydia	Erythromycin	

Table 13.4 *Cont'd*

Necrotising enterocolitis	Preterm Birth asphyxia Umbilical catheterisation	'Gut organisms' including anaerobes	Benzylpenicillin + gentamicin + metronidazole Or cefotaxime and metronidazole
Urinary tract infection	Commoner in males	*E. coli*/Other enterobacteria	Ampicillin + gentamicin
Meningitis	CSF Gram film:- Gram+ve cocci in chains Gram-ve bacilli Gram+ve bacilli No bacteria seen	GBS Coliforms Listeria monocytogenes	Benzylpenicillin and gentamicin Cefotaxime and gentamicin Ampicillin and gentamicin Cefotaxime and gentamicin
			Change according to culture and sensitivity results

* If new symptoms develop during treatment or signs do not resolve consider the use of cefotaxime as blind 'second line' treatment.

Duration of antibiotic therapy

- After 48 h of antibiotics, if all investigations are normal, the infant is now well and in retrospect infection seems unlikely, antibiotics should be discontinued.
- If investigations are normal but the infant remains unwell or continues to deteriorate, continue with antibiotics for a minimum of 5 days and consider repeating infection screen and removing any central lines. Carefully re-examine, including skin and bones, under hat and dressings, for possible infection source.
- If a pathogen is grown, treatment with IV antibiotics is usually for 7 days minimum (see specific infections below) except for *Staph. epidermidis* (5 days).
- If the mother has been given antibiotics prior to or during delivery, continue baby's antibiotics for at least 5 days if you suspect neonatal infection.
- Meningitis with a Gram-positive organism (except *Streptococcus faecalis*) — give antibiotics for 2 weeks.
- Gram-negative meningitis and *Streptococcus faecalis* infection — give 3 weeks antibiotics.

Management of baby at risk of intrapartum systemic infection

- Any baby showing signs of systemic infection should be managed as above
- Some units use benzylpenicillin alone as specific GBS prophylaxis for babies with no infection markers but who develop respiratory symptoms. Where there is a serious consideration given to the possibility of sepsis, gentamicin must be added (synergistic effect in GBS infection and essential in management of Gram-negative sepsis). In units using prophylactic benzylpenicillin, a blood culture, FBC and CRP should be performed before starting antibiotics.

PROLONGED RUPTURE OF MEMBRANES (ROM >24 H)

- Well term infant — *routine postnatal care*
- Well preterm infant — *FBC and blood culture, consider treatment if WCC or platelet count abnormal*
- Prolonged ROM **plus** offensive liquor **or** maternal pyrexia/signs of infection **or** respiratory symptoms **or** poor condition at birth — *admit to NICU, investigate* (full infection screen) *and treat* (IV penicillin and gentamicin; review at 48 h)

MATERNAL COLONISATION

- Intrapartum antibiotics >**4 h** pre-delivery and well term infant — *routine postnatal care*
- Intrapartum antibiotics <**4 h** pre-delivery and well term infant with <12 h ROM — *routine postnatal care*
- ROM >12 h or preterm infant **or** maternal pyrexia (>37.8°C) — investigate (FBC, CRP, blood culture) and treat (IV penicillin and gentamicin; review at 48 h)

PREVIOUS CHILD WITH GBS INFECTION

- No intrapartum antibiotics
- *Investigate* (FBC, CRP, blood culture) *and treat* (IV penicillin and gentamicin; review at 48 h)

CO-TWIN OF SUSPECTED INFECTED INFANT

- *Urgent investigation* (full infection screen) and treatment (IV penicillin and gentamicin; review at 48 h) — you must always treat **all** the other babies from a multiple pregnancy when you place one of the set on antibiotics in the first 48 hours after birth.

MOTHER WITH PERIPARTUM SIGNS OF SEPSIS

- *Investigate and treat* (IV penicillin and gentamicin; review at 48 h)

Management of specific proven systemic infections

As discussed above, the initial treatment of infection in the newborn infant is often empirical. Neither the organism nor the site of infection is usually known. However, the various investigations undertaken as part of the 'septic screen' may demonstrate the site of infection, and by 48 h an organism may have been cultured.

NEONATAL MENINGITIS

The classic signs of this disease in the older child (bulging fontanelle, photophobia, neck stiffness) are rarely seen in the newborn. A bulging fontanelle and opisthotonus are late signs with poor prognosis.

The organisms responsible are shown in Table 13.5. Suggested antibiotics are given in Table 13.4. Treat GBS meningitis for 2 weeks and *E. coli* and other Gram-negative

Table 13.5 Organisms causing neonatal meningitis

Organism	Percentage of all causes of neonatal meningitis
E. coli	40%
Group B Streptococcus	40%
Listeria monocytogenes	7%
Other streptococci	3%
Staphylococci (aureus and epidermidis)	3%
Klebsiella	2%
Proteus	2%
Salmonella, Pneumococcus, Haemophilus, Pseudomonas, Meningococcus, Candida, viral	3%

meningitis for 3 weeks. There is no evidence that intrathecal antibiotics improve outcome. If the infant responds to treatment there is no justification for further LP during treatment. Discuss with your consultant microbiologist whether it is necessary to perform an LP 48 hours after treatment is stopped.

The mortality from neonatal meningitis is at least 25% and a further 25% have disability. Complications are intracerebral abscess, acquired hydrocephalus and deafness. Babies who have meningitis should have serial cranial USS, to look for abscesses and ventricular dilatation, and a hearing test on discharge.

PNEUMONIA

Pneumonia occurs in the following situations:

- early-onset sepsis (usually GBS) when infection is acquired as a result of passage through the birth canal.
- as an acquired disease during the early weeks of life usually in an infant receiving neonatal intensive care
- as aspiration pneumonia
- as a complication of CLD.

The commonest organisms are GBS, *E. coli, Staph. aureus*, and viral infections. The diagnosis is rarely made from physical signs because most of these infants have other reasons for tachypnoea, recession and oxygen requirement. Microbiological diagnosis is rarely possible, as it is difficult to obtain specimens from the bronchial tree except in the ventilated infant. Microbiological proof is therefore usually obtained when there is coincident septicaemia. A CXR should always be performed, but again many of these infants will have coexisting lung disease making interpretation difficult.

Recommended antibiotics (Table 13.4) should be given for 5–7 days, except in *Chlamydia* infection where 2 weeks of erythromycin is required. There is little place for routine physiotherapy but frequent suction and physiotherapy may be necessary if secretions are a problem.

SEPTICAEMIA

Most infections will be sensitive to the empirical antibiotic regime (Table 13.4). Antibiotics should be continued for at least 7 days if septicaemia is proven. About 30% of newborn infants with septicaemia also have meningitis. There should be a low threshold for LP.

Interpretation of the growth of *Staph. epidermidis* in blood is not easy as this is a common skin commensal. If there is a pure growth within 48 h, especially in the VLBW infant, then it should be treated as a significant infection with a 5 day course of antibiotics (usually flucloxacillin and gentamicin). If symptoms do not settle, re-culture and start vancomycin. A culture of mixed organisms, unusual organisms, growth appearing after 48 h or obtained from a catheter tip should not be dismissed, but repeat blood cultures should be taken and the child reassessed in conjunction with the clinical picture, CRP and FBC results.

The mortality for blood culture proven neonatal infection varies considerably depending on the organism and the underlying condition of the infant.

URINARY TRACT INFECTION (see also Ch. 10)

UTI may be a primary infection or may be secondary to septicaemia with haematogenous spread to the kidneys. The commonest organisms are *E. coli* and other Gram-negative bacteria such as *Klebsiella* and enterococci.

The infant may present acutely with signs of generalised septicaemia, but commonly the presentation is in a non-specific way with vomiting, poor feeding, poor weight gain, prolonged or late onset jaundice, anaemia and mild fever.

The aminoglycoside in the blind empirical therapy (Table 13.4) will cover most organisms causing UTI, and within 48 h culture results should be available to direct further treatment. Treatment should be continued for at least 7 days. Treat with IV drugs initially to guarantee a rapid response and to prevent secondary septicaemia.

A repeat culture should be obtained post treatment to ensure eradication of the infection. If infection persists, there may be a resistant organism, renal abscess or obstructive uropathy. Following initial treatment, prophylaxis should be continued with nocturnal antibiotics (e.g. trimethoprim 2 mg/kg at night in the term infant; trimethoprim should not be used in the first month of life or in the preterm infant; cephradine 25 mg/kg at night is a suitable alternative) until the results of a renal USS and MCUG (see Ch.10) are known.

OSTEOMYELITIS AND SEPTIC ARTHRITIS

These infections, which often coexist, are rare in the newborn period. If a single site is involved, GBS is most common whereas *S. aureus* is more often responsible for widespread bone involvement. There may be localised redness, tenderness or oedema, or pseudo-paralysis of the affected limb due to pain.

The affected bone or joint must be X-rayed but the absence of changes does not exclude the diagnosis as these may take 7–14 days to appear. Obtain expert orthopaedic assistance to aspirate the affected joint or bone to provide a microbiological diagnosis. A skeletal survey and/or bone scan should be performed to look for other sites of infection. Initial treatment should be with systemic flucloxacillin and gentamicin until cultures are available. Antibiotics should be continued for 6 weeks.

Careful orthopaedic follow-up is essential as damage to the growth plate may lead to subsequent abnormal bone growth.

GASTROINTESTINAL INFECTIONS

Necrotising enterocolitis
See Chapter 9.

Neonatal gastroenteritis
This is rare in the immediate newborn period. It is likely to be contracted from the baby's mother or from non-sterile preparation of formula feeds. Most causes in the *UK* are viral, e.g. rotavirus and adenovirus although bacteriological causes, e.g. *Salmonella, E. coli* and *Campylobacter* can occur. Definitive diagnosis is made by stool culture or EM for virus particles. If the stools are persistently negative on culture, a non-infectious cause of diarrhoea, such as malabsorption secondary to CF or Hirschsprung's disease, should be considered.

Management
- Confirm diagnosis. Remember possetting and loose stools are a common occurrence in otherwise normal infants, especially breast fed infants. If the infant seems well and is gaining weight, there is no cause for concern.
- Barrier nurse.
- Prevent dehydration, which can occur rapidly in a newborn infant.
- There is no place for antibiotics except in proven *Salmonella* or *Campylobacter* infection. *Salmonella* should be treated with IV ciprofloxacin and *Campylobacter* with IV erythromycin.

- Parents should be warned that loose stools may continue for several weeks and that this is not a problem provided the child is gaining weight at the normal rate.
- Secondary lactose intolerance is relatively common and lactose-free milks are available. If diarrhoea persists even on a lactose-free milk, particularly if there is bloody diarrhoea and a family history of atopy, cows' milk protein intolerance should be considered.

Specific organisms causing infection in the neonatal period

VIRAL INFECTIONS

Cytomegalovirus

Forty percent of women with a primary CMV infection in pregnancy will pass the virus on to the fetus. The figure is lower during a recurrence of infection in pregnancy. Congenital CMV, occurs in about 0.3% of live births; 3% of these babies will have non-hearing handicaps attributable to cytomegalovirus whilst another 7% will be found subsequently to have unilateral or bilateral sensorineural hearing loss. Presenting signs in the neonatal period are shown in Table 13.2. Later complications include:

- sensorineural deafness
- cerebral palsy
- epilepsy
- global development delay
- blindness.

Infants may also become infected postnatally through breast milk or by CMV positive blood transfusion. These infections are characterised by systemic illness, pneumonitis or hepatitis.

The virus may be isolated from a throat swab or urine. Virus shedding in urine may persist for months after congenital or perinatal infection. Detection of CMV-specific IgM antibodies in a blood sample from the neonate or seroconversion between a first and second blood sample also indicates current infection.

There is no effective treatment for the infant with symptomatic congenital CMV. There should be careful neuro-developmental follow-up with particular attention to hearing loss which may develop over 1–2 years.

Enteroviruses

Examples of enteroviruses are polio virus, hepatitis A virus, Coxsackie viruses and ECHO virus. They are predominantly spread by the faecal–oral route, and while some of them do cause

GI symptoms, they can cause damage to other organs which they infect (e.g. polio virus can damage anterior horn cells and Coxsackie B virus can damage cardiac muscle).

Infection from the mother can be transmitted in utero but, more commonly, the baby acquires infection following birth. The following clinical patterns are recognised:

- fever
- meningoencephalitis — this is particularly seen with ECHO virus
- myocarditis — this is seen with Coxsackie B virus and there is a high mortality
- hepatitis — fulminant hepatic failure has been seen with ECHO virus
- DIC
- rash
- pneumonia
- vomiting
- diarrhoea
- pancreatitis.

Virus may be grown on tissue culture from faeces, throat swab, CSF or blood. Mother and infant should be isolated and the infant should be barrier-nursed. There is no specific antiviral drug available.

Hepatitis B virus

Hepatitis B can be transmitted perinatally from infected mothers to their babies. Transplacental passage is rare and transmission occurs either as a result of leakage from the maternal to the fetal circulation during labour or by direct ingestion of blood during birth. Horizontal transmission is also common during childhood in areas with a high prevalence of hepatitis B, e.g. Africa.

Early acquisition of hepatitis B infection is associated with persistent carrier status and later chronic active hepatitis. Consequently, all pregnant women should be offered screening (by measurement of (HBsAg) for hepatitis B infection. If a mother is found to be HBsAg-positive, her (HBeAg) and (anti-HBe) status should be assessed.

If the mother is HBsAg- and HBeAg-positive, more than 90% of infants will be infected, whereas if the mother is HBeAg-positive and anti-HBe-positive, the risk of the infant being infected is only about 10%. Serum which is both HBeAg- and anti-HBe-negative is of intermediate infectivity.

Neonatal management. This depends on mother's status:

- HBsAg-positive and HBeAg-positive vaccine and HBIG
- HBsAg-positive and HBeAg-negative and anti-HBe-negative (or not measured) — vaccine and HBIG

- active hepatitis B during pregnancy — vaccine and HBIG
- HBsAg-positive and anti-HBe-positive vaccine.

HB vaccine should be given as soon as possible after birth. Further doses should be given at 1 and 2 months with a booster at 12 months. Hepatitis B immunoglobulin (HBIG) 200 IU IM should be given within 24 h of birth at a different site to the immunisation. HBIG is supplied by the Public Health Laboratory Service (PHLS) and should be ordered well in advance of the birth.

There is no contraindication to breast feeding when a baby begins immunisation at birth and completes the immunisation course.

All immunised babies should have their HbsAG and anti-HBs status measured at 1 year to look for infectivity and effectiveness of immunisation.

Herpes simplex virus

Neonatal herpes simplex infection is a potentially lethal infection and has a significant morbidity in survivors. HSV type II accounts for 85% of neonatal infections. Infants born by vaginal delivery to women who have a primary HSV infection are at a high risk (50%) of developing significant infection. The risk to infants delivered vaginally to mothers experiencing recurrent infections is thought to be much lower (<8%). Caesarean section is indicated in primary maternal infection (this will decrease but not eradicate risk to the baby).

HSV infection can also be acquired postnatally — not necessarily from the mother.

Infants may present with congenital infection (Table 13.2), disseminated disease, local infection or encephalitis. The severity of the disease is not related to the gestational age at which exposure occurred:

- *Disseminated disease* presents at 4–5 days; 80% will have a vesicular rash. CNS involvement occurs in 60–75%. There is 80% mortality and high morbidity.
- *Localised infection* presents at 10–11 days with kerato-conjunctivitis or vesicular lesions on the presenting part or oropharynx. Progressive spread of the rash and repeated recurrence can occur up to 6 months of age.
- *Encephalitis* presents at 2 weeks often in combination with disseminated disease or superficial infection; 30% present with encephalitis alone. The presenting features can be very non-specific and the absence of a rash can make diagnosis difficult.

Babies with suspected HSV infection require isolation. Investigation includes:

- viral swabs from eyes/mouth/throat
- EM on any vesicular fluid obtained

- LFTs
- CSF examination including serology
- ophthalmological examination
- EEG
- cranial USS.

Treat with acyclovir 10 mg/kg IV t.d.s. for 14 days. Discuss longer term treatment with a virologist as this may have benefit in localised infection.

Babies born to mothers with a history of recurrent infection but no evidence of active lesions require no intervention. Babies delivered vaginally in the presence of active lesions should be isolated with their mother and prophylactic acyclovir (5 mg/kg IV t.d.s.) given for 10 days.

Breast feeding is contraindicated if herpetic lesions are present on the breast.

Human immunodeficiency virus

In Europe the risk of perinatal transmission of HIV infection is 15–20%. This incidence can be reduced by treating HIV-positive mothers during pregnancy and the baby after delivery with anti-retroviral drugs. Perinatal transmission is also reduced by delivering the baby via caesarean section. HIV-positive mothers should not breast feed as this doubles the risk of HIV transmission.

Positive encouragement to 'at risk' mothers to take up HIV screening is essential. Risk factors include:

- IV drug use
- prostitution
- previous residence or travel to Central Africa or Haiti
- sexual partners of HIV-positive or high-risk individuals, e.g. homosexuals, haemophiliacs.

HIV-infected babies are usually asymptomatic in the neonatal period. Diagnosis was previously difficult in the neonatal period as maternal HIV IgG antibodies can be detected until 18 months of age even in non-infected babies. Newer techniques such as PCR for proviral DNA in WBCs, testing for p24 antigen, using tests employing acid dissociation, and measuring virus specific IgA enable much earlier diagnosis. PCR will correctly identify 30–50% of HIV-infected babies at birth and almost all infected babies by 3 months of age. Virus-specific IgA develops over the first 3 months in HIV-infected infants. Diagnosis of HIV from intrauterine or perinatal transmission should only be made if two independent tests are indicative of infection and there is confirmation from a second blood sample.

If at 6 months the infant remains well and the three investigations described above remain negative, then HIV infection is very unlikely. However, the infant should be followed up until IgG antibodies are no longer present in two separate blood samples.

Neonatologists and general paediatricians should seek assistance in the management and counselling of families where HIV is being considered.

All infants should receive cotrimoxazole as prophylaxis against *Pneumocystis carnii*, from 1 month of age or once antiviral prophylaxis has stopped whichever is the later. Babies at risk of HIV infection should not receive BCG immunisation.

Prevention of transmission of HIV infection to staff and other patients.

Universal precautions to prevent transmission of any infection in clinical practice, e.g. hepatitis B and C, should be used at all times (Table 13.6).

Individuals who are put at risk of HIV following a used sharp injury, human bite/scratch or splash of body fluid to the eyes or mouth should be offered immediate prophylaxis against HIV infection.

Table 13.6   Routine prevention of transmission of infection to personnel in neonatal clinical practice

At resuscitation
- Wear gloves, plastic apron and gown
- Routine use of face mask and plastic glasses recommended
- Do not use mouth operated suction
- Decontaminate multi-use equipment e.g. bag and mask between patients

Routine handling of newborn infants
- Handle with gloves until cleaned of blood and maternal amniotic fluid
- Wear gloves only when dealing with blood or blood-stained products
- Thoroughly wash hands after soiling with vomit, urine or faeces

Invasive procedures
- Wear gloves for all invasive procedures
- Wear gloves when disconnecting/connecting infusion lines

Measles

Measles is infectious from 4 days before to 3 days after the onset of the rash. The incubation period is 2–10 days (mean 6 days).

Infection appearing in the first 10 days is considered transplacental and those after 14 days are probably acquired ex utero. The majority of babies are not infected despite maternal illness around the time of birth. The spectrum varies from mild illness with transient rash to a rapidly fatal disease.

A deep IM injection of human normal immunoglobulin (HNIG) 250 mg (1.7 mL) within 72 h of exposure prevents clinical measles. If given later (up to 7 days) it may still prevent or modify the illness. Passive immunisation is recommended for:

- exposed, susceptible pregnant women
- newborn infants at risk
- baby contacts in the nursery.

Immunoglobulin is of no proven value in established disease. Active immunisation should follow with live attenuated measles vaccine about 8 weeks later.

Parvovirus B19

One in three mothers infected with parvovirus B19 will pass the virus to the fetus. Fetal infection results in anaemia and hydrops both of which can improve spontaneously before delivery although transfusion is occasionally required.

Infection with parvovirus B19 can be confirmed by measuring B19 IgM.

Rubella virus

Maternal primary rubella infection during the first 12 weeks of pregnancy, almost invariably results in multiple congenital defects (Table 13.2). Infection between 13 and 16 weeks gestation reduces the risk to 20%. After 16 weeks gestation, the risk to the fetus is very low. Cardiac and eye defects are most likely to develop when maternal infection is acquired during the first 8 weeks of pregnancy, whereas hearing defects are more evenly distributed throughout the first 16 weeks of pregnancy.

Diagnose in the presence of rubella specific IgM. Rubella virus may also be isolated from throat swab or urine in most congenitally infected neonates.

There is no treatment for the infant affected with congenital rubella. Very close developmental and hearing follow-up is essential. Onset of sensorineuronal hearing loss may be delayed.

Varicella zoster virus

Acquired congenitally. Occurs within 10 days of birth.
- Babies born with a rash, or with early-onset rash, survive because maternal illness occurred long enough before birth for maternal antibodies to be produced and to cross the placenta.
- The high-risk group of babies are those born to mothers whose rashes appear less than 5 days before birth. This is because there is a lag before IgG is produced and crosses the placenta. In this group of babies the infection rate is 17% in term babies. Case fatality is up to 31%.

- Give (ZIG) 1.25 mL by deep IM injection to babies whose mothers develop rash in the 4 days before delivery or in the first few hours postpartum. Acyclovir should be given at the first sign of clinical infection. Mothers can barrier-nurse high-risk babies but should not breast feed them until no longer infectious.

Acquired postnatally: Begins 10–28 days after birth and is generally mild.

BACTERIAL INFECTIONS

Enterobaceriacae (i.e. *E. coli, Klebsiella* and *Proteus*)

E. coli, Klebsiella and *Proteus* are Gram-negative bacilli which are normal gut flora often described collectively as 'coliforms'. The VLBW infant receiving intensive care can become transiently colonised with *E. coli* at sites such as the mouth or umbilicus. Systemic infection, both early and late is indistinguishable from GBS.

    E. coli septicaemia and meningitis are associated with high mortality particularly in VLBW infants.

Listeria monocytogenes

Listeria monocytogenes is a Gram-positive coccobacillus. Infection is food-borne and a variety of foodstuffs including coleslaw, milk, soft cheeses, pate and 'cook -chill' foods, have been implicated in transmission.

    Listeria can result in miscarriage or stillbirth, early-onset or late-onset infection. Clinically, early-onset infection is usually indistinguishable from other causes of severe bacterial infection. There are, however, a number of clues that may suggest *Listeria* as the cause:

- the presence of meconium in the liquor of a preterm delivery or the observation that the liquor was green, pea-soup or foul-smelling
- abscesses on the surface of the placenta
- pinkish-grey granulomas on the skin of the newborn infant, 2–3 mm in diameter, or a less specific rash which may be salmon-coloured, erythemateous, papular, micropapular or petechial.

    Late-onset infection occurs between 7 and 21 days, usually with meningitis.

    The treatment of choice for *Listeria* is a combination of ampicillin and aminoglycoside IV. Cephalosporins are ineffective against *Listeria*. High-dose penicillin is effective in the short term so there is no need to start ampicillin before cultures are known.

Prognosis for early-onset listeriosis is poor, with up to 60% mortality, but the outcome for the late-onset disease is better than for other forms of bacterial meningitis.

Group B *Streptococcus (Streptococcus agalactiae)*

GBS is carried in the vagina and the GI tract of up to one third of pregnant women. However, carriage is 'unstable' so that a vaginal swab which yields GBS early in pregnancy is a poor predictor for carriage at the time of labour. Maternal carriage of GBS in the vagina has been associated with preterm delivery, preterm rupture of the membranes and stillbirth.

Early-onset neonatal infection occurs within the first 48 h, although 60% of cases are apparent within 6 h of birth. The incidence is approximately 0.5–1 per 1000 live births in the UK. There is a high mortality rate and there may be septicaemia and meningitis as well as pneumonia. Early infection can be almost completely prevented by giving intrapartum ampicillin to at-risk mothers at least 4 h before delivery (see p. 254).

Late-onset GBS infection is an epidemiologically distinct entity due to group III GBS and occurs after the first week. It may arise from maternally or nosocomially acquired organisms. It is less common than the early-onset variety, typically presents with meningitis and the mortality rate is lower. Late-onset disease is unaffected by maternal or infant chemoprophylaxis.

Diagnosis is by positive culture of blood or CSF. Rapid antigen detection, by latex particle agglutination, can also be performed on urine (sensitivity 88–96%) or CSF (sensitivity 67–80%).

The overall mortality is 20%, the highest mortality occurring in the very low birth weight infant with early onset infection. Following late-onset GBS meningitis, there is a risk of permanent significant neurological sequelae in 10–20% of survivors.

Syphilis

Congenital syphilis is now rare in the UK with less than 20 cases reported each year. Two-thirds of affected children have no clinical signs of congenital syphilis, and in those who do show signs, these most commonly develop 2–12 weeks after birth. The most frequent findings are failure to thrive, persistent snuffles, hepatosplenomegaly and an erythemateous rash, which may be macular or papular and affects the palms, soles, perianal and perioral regions. There may be radiological evidence of osteoporosis or periostitis even in the absence of clinically obvious lesions.

Serological diagnosis is not easy as maternal antibodies may be transferred across the placenta and persist for several months. Rising IgG antibody titres in the infant suggest congenital infection, as does the presence of specific IgM, although its absence does not exclude it.

If a mother is diagnosed as having syphilis during pregnancy, she should be treated with penicillin. Whilst this is highly effective, all infants of mothers who have been treated before or during pregnancy for syphilis should be tested serologically at birth and for up to 6 months thereafter. If syphilis is suspected in the infant, a LP should always be performed. Congenital syphilis should be treated with penicillin for a minimum of 10 days.

Tuberculosis

Tuberculosis is prevalent in almost all tropical developing countries and the incidence is increasing in developed countries *pari passu* with the increase in HIV infection. Infants born to mothers with active or open TB should receive immunisation with isoniazid resistant BCG and treatment with isoniazid. Isoniazid is continued until the mother is sputum negative and the baby has a positive tuberculin skin test. Babies should be isolated from their mothers until the mother has received 14 days of treatment.

Routine immunisation with BCG in the neonatal period is discussed on page 268.

OTHER ORGANISMS

Chlamydia

Infection can occur in utero and may increase the risk of preterm delivery. There are no reports of congenital abnormalities. If the mother has cervicitis, the risk of transmission to an infant exposed during vaginal delivery is 60%.

There are two clinical types of presentation in the newborn:

- conjunctivitis (p. 246)
- interstitial pneumonia.

Interstitial pneumonia has an insidious onset with a peak incidence at 6 weeks. Suspect if there is tachypnoea and cough in an afebrile child with eosinophilia, diffuse CXR changes and perhaps previous neonatal conjunctivitis. Detection of *Chlamydia trachomatis* IgM in blood or positive NPA culture is diagnostic.

Treat with IV erythromycin if the infant is seriously ill but most cases will respond to 2 weeks of oral therapy. The mother of an infected infant and her partner(s) must be investigated, counselled and treated.

Toxoplasma gondii

Humans acquire *Toxoplasma* either by direct contact with cat faeces or by eating contaminated vegetables or undercooked meat. The incidence of toxoplasmosis in pregnancy in the UK is approximately 2 per 1000; 5% of the babies from these pregnancies develop significant signs of infection and 25% have disease affecting the eye. The clinical features of severe congenital toxoplasmosis are described in Table 13.2.

If toxoplasmosis is suspected antenatally, fetal cordocentesis or amniocentesis should be performed to confirm the diagnosis. In the newborn, congenital toxoplasmosis may be suspected from the classic tetrad of hydrocephalus, epilepsy, punctate cerebral calcification and chorioretinitis. Serological diagnosis in the infant is not easy because passively acquired maternal IgG may be present in both infected and non-infected infants and only one-third of congenitally infected neonates produce a detectable IgM response. Therefore, if there is a strong suspicion of toxoplasmosis, serum samples should be investigated at 2 month intervals. The persistence of IgG beyond 10 months of age indicates congenital infection as maternal antibody will have been completely removed by this age.

Treatment of the mother with spiramycin using multiple courses from the time of diagnosis until delivery halves the incidence of congenital infection. Proven fetal infection after the first trimester is treated with sulphadiazine and pyrimethamine.

Even in the absence of clinical features, the infant who is definitely infected should be treated with spiramycin 100 mg/kg per day for 6 weeks, followed by 3 weeks of pyrimethamine 1 mg/kg per day and sulphadiazine 50 mg/kg per day. This 9 week regime should be repeated until the child is 1 year old. If the neonatal infection has not been confirmed but is suspected, treatment is controversial as the drugs used are potentially toxic.

Ocular disease should be followed up into adult life as there may be a relapsing and remitting course and acute exacerbation requires anti-parasitic and anti-inflammatory treatment.

Most infants born to infected women will have no problems. For infants with significant evidence of infection at birth, handicap is unfortunately likely. Those with ocular involvement may not present until later childhood.

Candida albicans

- Mucocutaneous candidiasis (see superficial infections above)
- Disseminated candidiasis

Suspect where sepsis fails to respond to antibiotics. It is more common in preterm infants who have received multiple causes of antibiotics and TPN via central or Silastic lines. Diagnosis is made by examining and culturing urine, blood and CSF for *Candida*. Urine will usually show budding yeast forms (active) rather than hyphae. Echocardiography may demonstrate vegetations on the tricuspid valve or a calcified mass within the right atrium.

Infants should be treated with either a combination of liposomal amphotericin and 5-flucytosine for 4–6 weeks or with fluconazole for 4 weeks. Liposomal amphotericin is less toxic, especially on the kidney, than plain amphotericin.

Mortality from disseminated candidiasis is high. Candidal meningitis is particularly associated with severe disability in survivors.

Immunisation in the UK

Preterm babies follow the same immunisation schedules as term infants.

SCHEDULE OF IMMUNISATION

Infants should be immunised at 2, 3 and 4 months after birth against pertussis, diphtheria, tetanus, *Haemophilus influenzae* type B (Hib), meningococcus type C and polio. Signed consent of the parents is required. It is our policy not to immunise with polio on the neonatal unit as it is a live vaccine with a small risk of transmission of illness to other very preterm infants in the nursery. We delay immunisation of babies on systemic steroids for 1 week after the course of treatment.

Contraindications

Vaccination should be delayed if the child has a significant pyrexial illness. Infections without fever, including upper respiratory tract infections, are not an indication to delay vaccination. If children are on oral or IV steroids, but not inhaled steroids, we delay immunisation. If there has been extensive local reaction (indurated erythemateous reaction involving most of limb into which it was injected) or generalised reaction — e.g. fever >39.5°C, anaphylaxis, collapse, convulsions within 72 h, prolonged inconsolable screaming, prolonged unresponsiveness — then this is an indication not to proceed with further doses of that vaccine.

Stable lesions such as periventricular leucomalacia or parenchymal haemorrhage are not contraindications to immunisation. Children with BPD should undergo full pertussis immunisation because of the significant risk should they acquire this infection.

BCG IMMUNISATION

Immunisation should be offered to all babies where either parent or their family originated in Asia, South-East Asia, Africa and the Middle East or where there is a family history of tuberculosis within the last 5 years. It can be offered at birth from 30 weeks gestation onwards, but do not give whilst the baby is receiving intensive care.

The dose of BCG is 0.05 mL for infants, given intradermally at the level of the lower insertion of the left deltoid muscle. This should lead to a branded area on the skin which completely disappears. No dressing should be used.

True immunodeficiency presenting in the newborn period

Congenital immunodeficiency diseases presenting in the neonatal period involve defects of polymorphoneutrophils, e.g. agranulocytosis and familial severe neutropenia. Defects of lymphocyte function are rarely detected in the newborn period because of passive immunity acquired from the mother.

FOURTEEN

Haematology

Normal physiology

The fetus is relatively polycythaemic, a physiological compensation against the hypoxic intrauterine environment. At term, 80% of haemoglobin is high-oxygen-affinity HbF. This extra Hb is no longer necessary to enhance oxygen carriage when the term infant is born and can breathe air. As a consequence, there is decreased erythropoiesis and Hb concentration falls after birth to its lowest level at 3 months. Although Hb concentration subsequently rises and reaches adult values by about 1 year, milk contains relatively little iron (see Ch. 15) and 'physiological' hypochromia and microcytosis are seen at 1 year.

Anaemia in the newborn

Anaemia can arise before birth, at birth or have a later onset in the neonatal period. The commonest causes of anaemia in the newborn in the UK are:

- *Antenatal*
  — intrauterine twin to twin transfusion; the larger twin is plethoric and the smaller anaemic
  — rhesus haemolytic disease; the advent of intrauterine transfusion means that few affected infants are now born in the UK very anaemic
  — intrauterine parvovirus infection
  — fetoplacental haemorrhage.
  Any cause of intrauterine anaemia, if severe enough, can result in cardiac failure and fetal hydrops (see below).
- *Intrapartum* — acute blood loss at the time of delivery. Initially the Hb concentration will be normal, but pallor, tachycardia and hypotension occur with significant haemorrhage (e.g. placenta praevia, vasa praevia, placental abruption, laceration of the placenta at caesarian section, bleeding from the umbilical cord, subaponeurotic haemorrhage, ruptured liver). However, similar signs may also be seen as a result of acute asphyxia.

- *Postnatal* — chronic anaemia of prematurity: a combination of haemolysis, repeated sampling and marrow suppression in small, sick infants. If repeatedly transfused, there is little stimulus for erythropoietin production.

These causes all give rise to normochromic, normocytic anaemias.

Rarer causes of neonatal anaemia include alpha-thalassaemia, red cell abnormalities (see 'Haemolytic anaemias', p. 273) and congenital neonatal hypoplastic anaemias (Blackfan–Diamond syndrome and Fanconi's anaemia).

When assessing the cause of anaemia in the newborn and its impact, the following should be considered.

History

- Overt blood loss (e.g. haematemesis, haematuria, blood in stools, blood from the umbilical stump) suggests coagulopathy (haemorrhagic disease of the newborn, haemophilia). Melaena alone suggests NEC (see Ch. 9)
- Dietary intake of iron is relevant beyond the first month of life. Prior to this, even the preterm baby is born with adequate iron stores. Congenital gut abnormality, previous surgery or NEC may explain malabsorption of iron.

Examination

- Conjunctivae for pallor. This is not reliable. Always confirm by measuring Hb
- Increasing oxygen requirement
- Jaundice
- Bruising or petechiae
- Systolic flow murmur
- Plot growth on a centile chart if anaemia is chronic.

Investigation and treatment

See individual diagnoses below.

Investigation if anaemic at birth

- FBC
- Blood group
- DCT
- Parvovirus IgM
- G6PD screen.

Management if anaemic at birth

See 'Blood transfusion' below and Chapter 3 for immediate resuscitation if anaemic and shocked at birth; see Chapter 9 for indications for exchange transfusion if anaemic and jaundiced at birth; see 'Hydrops fetalis' (p. 277) for management if anaemic and hydropic at birth.

Blood transfusion

INDICATIONS

Acute haemorrhage (see Ch. 3)

Whether to transfuse, and the rate and volume, depend on pulse and BP, not the Hb concentration, which will be normal initially. Take blood for FBC and cross-match if there is time, but otherwise give fresh O-negative CMV-negative uncross-matched blood if there is life-threatening haemorrhage.

Anaemia

Transfuse if:

- Hb < 12 g/dL if sick or ventilator-dependent
- Hb < 10 g/dL if stable but O_2-dependent
- Hb < 10 g/dL and surgery is urgently indicated. Do not transfuse if surgery is elective — defer operation and find and treat the cause
- Hb < 8 g/dL if baby in air and symptomatic (e.g. poor growth, slow to feed, tachypnoea)
- Cardiac failure is attributed to anaemia — give packed cells more slowly (see below) with furosemide (frusemide) 1 mg/kg IV midway through transfusion.

We do not use erythropoietin.

If anaemic at birth and Hb < 10 g/dL, an exchange transfusion should be considered rather than a top-up transfusion (see Ch. 9).

RATE AND VOLUME OF TRANSFUSION

For elective transfusion:

Packed cells:
Volume (mL) = weight (kg) × 4 × desired rise in Hb (g/dL).
Whole blood:
Whole blood (mL) = weight (kg) × 6 × desired rise in Hb (g/dL).

- In both cases, rate = 5 mL/kg per h with furosemide (frusemide) 1 mg/kg IV midway through transfusion.
- Aim for a final Hb of 16 g/dL in an O_2-dependent baby.
- Circulating blood volume is approximately 80 mL/kg body weight.
- Transfusions of more than 25 mL/kg are rarely indicated except in acute haemorrhage.

COMPLICATIONS

Always ask yourself: is this transfusion necessary?

- Transfusion reactions are extremely rare in the newborn.
- Following massive transfusion, hyperkalaemia, hypocalcaemia, acidosis, hypothermia and DIC are all risks.
- Transmission of infection is now probably the most serious hazard of trivial transfusion:
  — HIV screening of donor blood generally tests for antibody positivity and there is a variable latent period between viral infection in the donor and seroconversion. HIV antibody tests have a false-negative rate of up to 2% (i.e. blood is infected but the test is negative). Blood products (e.g. HAS, FFP) may be pooled from thousands of donors, increasing the risk further
  — hepatitis B and C are screened for
  — CMV can be transmitted by transfusion and cause life-threatening illness in the immunocompromised neonate. Therefore, use only CMV-negative blood, even if leucocyte-depleted blood is available. If blood transfusion is vital and no CMV-negative blood is immediately available, use a white cell filter
  — bacterial contamination can occur, or gain entry via the vascular access.
- In circulatory overload and pulmonary oedema, slow the rate of transfusion, give furosemide (frusemide) 1 mg/kg IV, and increase PEEP if on IPPV.

Haemolytic anemia

BACKGROUND

The classification of haemolytic anaemias is as follows:

Intrinsic red cell defects
- Abnormal membrane
  — spherocytosis (autosomal dominant)
  — elliptocytosis (autosomal dominant)
- Abnormal haemoglobin
  — sickle cell disease (autosomal recessive)
  — thalassaemias (autosomal recessive)
- Enzyme deficiency
  — G6PD (X-linked)
  — pyruvate kinase (autosomal recessive).

Extrinsic problems
- Immune (DCT usually positive)
  — Isoimmune — maternal antibodies affect fetal and neonatal red cells:
    i   ABO incompatibility

  ii Rhesus incompatibility
  iii other rare atypical antibodies.
- Mother had malaria during pregnancy.

INVESTIGATIONS

Initial investigations (see Ch. 9) are:
- SBR
- blood film
- DCT
- mother's and baby's blood groups.

The following investigations may be necessary.

Is there increased red cell destruction?
- FBC — low Hb
- Elevated unconjugated bilirubin
- Elevated urinary urobilinogen
- Reduced plasma haptoglobins.

Is there increased red cell production?
- FBC — polychromasia, macrocytosis due to reticulocytosis (>7% of red cells in the first 3 days of life or >4% thereafter).

Is the haemolysis mainly intravascular?
- Haemoglobinuria
- Schistocytes, burr cells or helmet cells
- Thrombocytopenia and abnormal clotting suggests DIC.

Why are the RBCs being destroyed?
Genetic cause
- RBC morphology — spherocytes, elliptocytes. Although spherocytosis is autosomal dominant, family history may be negative because of variable expressions. The osmotic fragility test may be normal in the newborn and spherocytes may not be present. Therefore, repeat at 3 months and consider testing parents
- Haemoglobinopathy — only the rare alpha-thalassaemias affect the newborn
- Enzymopathy — red cell pyruvate kinase assay, G6PD deficiency screen. Both may cause neonatal jaundice. In G6PD deficiency (X-linked), drugs may precipitate haemolysis (Table 14.1) and very rarely a girl may be homozygous.

Acquired
- Immune — usually positive DCT (although may be negative in ABO incompatibility). Determine blood groups and rhesus status of mother and infant.

Table 14.1 Precipitants of haemolysis in G6PD deficiency in the newborn

Drugs
  Chloramphenicol
  Nalidixic acid
  Nitrofurantoin
  Sulphonamides (including co-trimoxazole)
  Vitamins C and K (although not in prophylactic doses — see Ch. 15)

Most bacterial and viral infections

TREATMENT

See above for blood transfusion. See Chapter 9 for phototherapy and exchange transfusion.

Folic acid 0.25 mg/kg p.o. o.d. is given for 6 months if haemolytic anaemia is severe enough to justify phototherapy.

Haemoglobinopathies

Universal screening using cord blood is undertaken in some parts of the UK where there is a significant at-risk population.

SICKLE CELL DISEASE

Sickle cell disease does not cause problems in the newborn because HbF does not contain beta chains. It occurs in children whose families originate from Africa or the West Indies.

Possible screening tests include:

- prenatal diagnosis possible from fetal red cells or liquor fibroblasts
- neonatal diagnosis by Hb electrophoresis on cord or heelprick blood. Repeated at 3 months if positive for HbS.

BETA-THALASSAEMIA

Occurs in families from the Mediterranean and the Indian sub-continent. It is not a cause of neonatal jaundice, but homozygotes usually present by 1 year. Can also be screened for in the neonatal period.

The other haemoglobinopathies are all rare in the UK, but the alpha-thalassaemias may cause neonatal haemolytic jaundice, unlike the beta-thalassaemias and sickle disease.

Other red cell appearances

Rare abnormalities are:

- Target cells — asplenia syndrome (often associated with CHD)
- Heinz bodies (intracellular globin precipitate). These result in increased RBC rigidity and decreased RBC survival:
  — G6PD deficiency
  — haemoglobinopathies
  — asplenia syndrome
- Howell–Jolly bodies (intracellular DNA fragments)
  — haemoglobinopathies
  — asplenia syndrome
- Reticulocytosis. Implies an active marrow:
  — haemolytic anaemia
  — chronic bleeding (often accompanied by thrombocytosis)
  — response to iron.

Iron deficiency anaemia

BACKGROUND

This is the commonest cause of anaemia in neonatal follow-up clinics. Causes are:

- Dietary deficiency — commonest cause, particularly in families of lower socioeconomic class; also, infants weaned after 6 months, toddlers who dislike meat and vegetables, and ethnic minorities. Iron deficiency itself leads to anorexia
- Increased demand — prematurity, multiple births
- Previous blood loss — neonatal or antepartum haemorrhage, twin-to-twin transfusion, fetomaternal haemorrhage.

MANAGEMENT

- Take blood for Hb, ferritin and blood film (hypochromic, microcytic). Often there is associated thrombocytosis. Screen non-caucasian children for haemoglobinopathy at the same time.
- If iron deficiency anaemia is confirmed, give 2 mg/kg elemental iron per 24 h in three divided doses for 3 months. Warn that the stools will appear dark.
- Do not expect complete resolution until 3 months' iron therapy has been completed. Check Hb, iron, reticulocytes and film after 3 months (to confirm compliance and response). Appetite often improves with treatment.

- Continue iron for another 3 months after normal Hb levels are achieved. Transfusion is only rarely necessary (see above).
- If response to iron is poor, consider either poor compliance (iron may cause constipation or diarrhoea) or that anaemia is not due to poor dietary iron intake, e.g. malabsorption, chronic occult blood loss or haemoglobinopathy.

PROPHYLAXIS

If less than 33 weeks gestation at birth, start Sytron at 28 days age. If < 1500 g, give 0.5 mL p.o. o.d.; once > 1500 g, increase to 1.0 mL p.o. o.d. Continue until 1 year.

Hydrops fetalis

Hydrops fetalis may result from many causes (see Table 14.2) which are usually divided into:

- *Immunological.* Anaemia results from maternal isoimmunisation against rhesus or other red cell antigens, i.e. erythroblastosis fetalis. See Chapter 9 for rhesus haemolytic disease, management of jaundice and exchange transfusion. This condition is now extremely rare in the UK as a result of improved antenatal intervention.
- *Non-immunological.* In the UK, most cases of hydrops fetalis are non-immunological. In approximately 50% of these cases, no cause is found. Approximately 40% of cases will have another congenital abnormality.

Hydrops fetalis is more complex than simple fetal oedema, e.g. the severity of hydrops in rhesus haemolytic disease is not always in proportion to the haemoglobin concentration, and in analbuminaemia there is no hydrops. Although the causes of hydrops include heart failure, anaemia and hypoproteinaemia, there may be other ill-defined mechanisms.

ANTENATAL DIAGNOSIS

This is usually made by USS examination. The information provided by the scan may suggest a chromosomal anomaly or direct the clinician towards appropriate fetal therapy. Cordocentesis can provide a rapid karyotype, viral studies, haemoglobin and blood groups, and a route for IUT if appropriate.

PERINATAL CONSIDERATIONS

- There is a higher incidence of obstetric complications at delivery, especially vaginal delivery.
- Spontaneous, premature delivery may occur.

Table 14.2 Conditions associated with fetal hydrops (not necessarily causative)

Cardiovascular Structural congenital heart disease Arterial calcification SVT (mother with SLE or anti-Ro antibody) Any cause of cardiac failure in utero	*Chromosomal* Trisomies, triploidy, Turner's *Gastrointestinal* Congenital atresias Meconium peritonitis
Haematological Twin-to-twin transfusion syndrome Rhesus Isoimmunisation Fetomaternal haemorrhage Homozygous alpha-thalassaemia Severe fetal anaemia of any cause	*Genitourinary* Congenital nephrotic syndrome Urethral obstruction Polycystic kidneys
Lymphatic Congenital lymphangiectasia Cystic hygroma of the neck	*Infective* Parvovirus CMV Toxoplasmosis Syphilis
Respiratory Congenital diaphragmatic hernia Congenital cystic adenomatoid malformation TOF	*Skeletal* Osteogenesis imperfecta Asphyxiating thoracic dystrophy Thanatophoric dwarfism
Congenital tumour Teratoma Neuroblastoma Haemangioma	*Placenta/cord* Aneurysm of the umbilical artery Umbilical vein thrombosis Chorioangioma of the placenta

- Pulmonary hypoplasia is present in 90%, as a result of lung compression by pleural fluid.
- Intrapartum asphyxia is common.
- The placenta should be placed in formalin and sent to histopathology.

The neonatal team should ensure in advance of delivery that:

- fresh CMV-negative, O-negative blood is available, cross-matched against the mother
- full monitoring and exchange transfusion equipment is ready
- arterial BP and CVP transducers are set up and calibrated **BEFORE** the baby is born.

RESUSCITATION AND NEONATAL MANAGEMENT

Two experienced staff should be present.
1. The infant usually requires intubation (may be difficult because of oedema).

2. Ventilate initially with high pressures (e.g. PIP of 30 cm H_2O and PEEP of 4–6 cm H_2O).

3. Pleural effusions and ascites should be drained (see Ch. 21) in the delivery room if severe and compromising respiration.

4. Insert umbilical vein and artery catheters.

5. As the pulmonary oedema decreases, high inspired pressures and PEEP may obstruct the pulmonary circulation, and a reduction in pressure may paradoxically aid oxygenation. HFOV is an alternative strategy, taking care to avoid overdistension.

6. If metabolic acidosis is severe (pH < 7.1) consider correction. If circulatory support is required, inotrope infusion (dopamine or dobutamine) is preferable to plasma volume expanders. If considered necessary, sodium bicarbonate must be given slowly as the extracellular fluid space is already expanded and there may be incipient or overt heart failure.

7. If colloid is essential for hypoproteinaemia, use 20% albumin rather than 4% albumin because of the smaller volume required.

8. Exchange transfusion with semi-packed cells if anaemia is the cause of the hydrops. It may be necessary to complete the transfusion with a volume deficit if the CVP > 12 mmHg (16 cm H_2O). Aim for controlled reduction of CVP to 6 mmHg after ensuring the tip of the UVC is above the diaphragm on CXR.

9. Moderate fluid restriction for first few days (40 mL/kg/per day) and start diuretics furosemide (frusemide) IV 1 mg/kg b.d. until good urine output established.

10. Check coagulation daily, initially, as DIC may ensue.

INVESTIGATION OF NON-IMMUNOLOGICAL HYDROPS

- **Blood** — Urea, electrolytes and creatinine; Total protein, albumin and protein electrophoresis; LFTs; Bilirubin — conjugated and unconjugated; Osmolality; PCV; FBC; Film; Blood group and DCT; Hb Electrophoresis; TORCH screen and Parvovirus titre, including specific IgM; VDRL, even if negative on the mother; Karyotype; blood sugar.
- **Urine** — Albumin (congenital nephrotic syndrome).
- **Ascitic or pleural fluid**
  - Total protein and albumin
  - Lipid if enteral feeding was started before the fluid was obtained (chylous effusions)
  - Microbiology and lymphocyte count (raised in chylous effusions).
- **CXR**
- **ECG with rhythm strip**
- **USS of heart, liver and kidneys.**

NEONATAL OUTCOME

- In approximately 50%, no cause is found.
- Many of those detected by midtrimester USS will not be live-born, as some of the pregnancies may have been electively terminated, and others may be stillborn.
- Hydrops fetalis detected in the first and second trimesters may resolve by term, e.g. 45X (Turner syndrome).
- The mortality in different series ranges from 50 to 95%. Postmortem is essential.
- The recurrence risk is low, unlike isoimmune hydrops fetalis.

Polycythaemia

Definition: Venous or arterial haematocrit > 65%.

BACKGROUND

The causes of polycythaemia in the newborn are:

- delayed cord clamping
- IUGR
- macrosomic IDM
- twin-to-twin transfusion
- maternofetal transfusion.

The danger of a high Hb is that viscosity rises exponentially as haematocrit exceeds 65%. Poor capillary perfusion and cerebral ischaemia may occur.

CLINICAL DIAGNOSIS

- Plethora may be confused with cyanosis and true cyanosis may be detectable with a normal P_aO_2 if Hb is very high.
- Most infants are asymptomatic and need no intervention.
- Some show features of hyperviscosity (cerebral irritability or seizures, PPHN, respiratory distress, hypoglycaemia, cardiac failure, renal vein thrombosis) or jaundice.

MANAGEMENT

1. Measure the PCV on a free–flowing venous sample which has been centrifuged at 3000 rpm for 10 min.
2. Take blood for Hb, glucose and bilirubin estimation.
3. If PCV > 70% and symptomatic, perform partial (dilutional) exchange transfusion. Infuse 20 mL/kg plasma or normal saline via a peripheral vein whilst removing 20 mL/kg blood from a peripheral arterial line; perform over 30 min; infuse 10 mL before beginning first withdrawal.

4. Give sufficient IV fluids to optimise hydration and monitor haematocrit 6-hourly.

Platelets and coagulation

AETIOLOGY OF ABNORMAL BLEEDING

Potential mechanisms of abnormal bleeding are given in Table 14.3.

Thrombocytopenia

In the perinatal period, classification of thrombocytopenia by time of presentation is most useful.

Fetus

- Passive transfer of maternal antiplatelet antibody:
  1. Immune thrombocytopenia (ITP)
     — may be due to maternal ITP or SLE–associated IgG antiplatelet antibodies
     — antibodies cause neonatal disease in approximately half the infants of affected mothers

Table 14.3 Causes of abnormal bleeding in the newborn

Abnormality of the platelets
Thrombocytopenia
Decreased production
  Specific megakaryocyte failure, usually following congenital viral infection
  Placental insufficiency (PIH, IUGR, diabetes)
  Perinatal hypoxia/ischaemia
  Inherited forms or associated with syndromes (e.g. thrombocytopenia and absent radii syndrome)
Increased destruction
  Immunological (maternal ITP or neonatal ATP)
  DIC, usually due to infection or NEC
  Kasabach–Merritt syndrome (giant haemangioma)
  Wiskott–Aldrich syndrome (eczema, prone to infection, thrombocytopenia)
Normal platelet count
  Abnormal platelet function
  Von Willebrand's disease

Abnormality of clotting factors
Decreased or abnormal production
  Vitamin K deficiency and liver disease both deplete factors II, VII, IX, X
  Haemophilia A and Von Willebrand's disease (factor VIII)
  Haemophilia B (factor IX), i.e. Christmas disease
  Antagonism — heparin
  Consumption — DIC

Abnormality of vascular endothelium (often leads to DIC)
Endothelial damage as a result of asphyxia or profound shock
Infections, especially GBS

    — fetal thrombocytopaenia can be diagnosed from cordocentesis, but there is a risk of bleeding
    — caesarean section is of unproven benefit, but maternal steroid or immunoglobulin treatment may help
    — the risk from maternal ITP is increased if maternal platelet count is low or she has had a splenectomy
    — neonatal thrombocytopaenia can occur with normal maternal platelet count.

2. Alloimmune thrombocytopenia (ATP)
    — the commonest form occurs when a fetus with platelets positive for the PLA1 antigen is carried by a PLA1-negative mother
    — consider if there is thrombocytopenia from birth in an infant whose mother has a normal platelet count and no past history of thrombocytopenia
    — there is a 75% risk in future pregnancies.

- Congenital infection (CMV, rubella, herpes)
- Severe rhesus disease
- Chromosome abnormalities
- Rare syndromes and inherited thrombocytopenias.

Neonatal (< 72 h of age)
- Placental insufficiency (PIH, IUGR, IDDM)
- Perinatal hypoxia/ischaemia
- Sepsis — with or without DIC; thrombocytopenia associated with low-grade bacteraemia from indwelling catheters
- ATP
- Maternal autoimmune (ITP, SLE)
- Congenital infection (CMV, rubella, herpes)
- Rare syndromes and inherited thrombocytopenias
- Thrombosis (renal vein, aorta).

Neonatal (> 72 h of age)
- Sepsis — with or without DIC; thrombocytopenia associated with low-grade bacteraemia from indwelling catheters
- NEC
- Maternal autoimmune (ITP, SLE)
- Congenital infection (CMV, rubella, herpes)
- Rare syndromes and inherited thrombocytopenias.

Clotting problem
- Haemorrhagic disease of the newborn (vitamin K deficiency, usually breast-fed or liver disease)
- Haemophilia and other inherited coagulopathies only rarely present in the neonatal period (excessive bleeding from umbilical stump, circumcision, surgical incision).

INVESTIGATION

The interpretation of some common coagulation tests is summarised in Table 14.4. Laboratories use their own controls or normal ranges but most clotting times are longer in newborn infants, particularly the very preterm (Table 14.5).

Bleeding time. Useful but rarely performed. Normally < 8 min. Prolonged in thrombocytopenia and von Willebrand's disease. In the latter, family history may be negative but diagnosis is confirmed by low factor VIII activity, low factor VIII antigen level, and decreased platelet aggregation.

Prothrombin time (PT). Principally assesses extrinsic pathway and is prolonged by deficiencies of factors II, V, VII and X, and fibrinogen.

Table 14.4 Interpretation of common coagulation tests

	PT (extrinsic)	PTT (intrinsic)	TT (fibrinogen)
Vitamin K deficiency Liver disease	Prolonged	Normal	Normal
Haemophilia A Haemophilia B Von Willebrand's disease	Normal	Prolonged	Normal
Heparin (reptilase time normal)	Prolonged	Very prolonged	Prolonged
DIC (raised FDPs, thrombocytopenia)	Prolonged	Prolonged	Prolonged

Table 14.5 Coagulation tests in the newborn

	APTT (s)	PT (s)	TT (s)	Reptilase time (s)	FDP (mg/mL)
Child	35–45	12–16	10–12	18–22	0–7
Preterm	35–100	13–23	12–28	18–30	0–10
Term	35–70	13–16	10–18	18–24	0–7

Partial thromboplastin time (PTT). Principally assesses intrinsic pathway and is prolonged by heparin and deficiencies of factors II, V, VIII, IX, X, XI and XII.

Thrombin time (TT). Assesses final common pathway and is prolonged principally by abnormalities in the amount or activity of fibrinogen, i.e. heparin, FDPs, hypofibrinogenaemia. The TT with reptilase is usually normal in the presence of heparin and much improved in DIC.

MANAGEMENT

Depends on the cause but the following are important guides.

Thrombocytopenia

- In the face of acute illness, active bleeding or in a preterm infant < 32 weeks, platelet transfusion can be used to keep the platelet count above 30×10^9/L after investigation.
- Platelet transfusion is of more value where there is decreased production rather than increased consumption. A poor incremental count 30 min after the end of transfusion is helpful in diagnosing rapid consumption.
- Platelet transfusion is indicated in any thrombocytopenic disorder if there is active bleeding, or prior to surgery (but not bone marrow biopsy). Platelets are not cross-matched but a donor from the same ABO group is used.
- No treatment has been shown convincingly to alter morbidity or mortality in an infant born to a mother with ITP:
  — platelet transfusion: only a very transient response and not recommended unless there is active bleeding
  — oral prednisolone 2 mg/kg per 24 h for 5 days
  — human immunoglobulin 0.4 g/kg per 24 h by IV infusion for 5 days.
  The latter two treatments are usually only considered if platelets are < 30×10^9/L, or in a preterm infant at increased risk of intracerebral haemorrhage.
- In neonatal ATP, the mother possesses antibodies against the antigenically different fetal platelets. The antibodies cross the placenta and lead to consumption of the fetal platelets. Because the maternal IgG antibodies have a half-life of about 6 weeks, the problem persists after birth. The commonest incompatibility is when the fetal platelets are PLA1-positive (which is rare) and the mother is PLA1-negative (the commonest phenotype in the population). This arises because the father is PLA1–positive and this gene is dominant. The situation is analagous to rhesus incompatibility of red cell antigens. Neonatal ATP can be treated by giving maternal platelets which are not destroyed, since they are PLA1-negative.

Abnormality of clotting factors

- All infants should be given vitamin K as prophylaxis against haemorrhagic disease of the newborn (see Ch. 15).

- If there is active bleeding and the exact diagnosis is unclear, give 1 mg vitamin K IV slowly and FFP 10 mL/kg IV over 30 min after blood is taken for investigation.
- DIC implies a triad of thrombocytopenia, abnormal clotting times and elevated FDPs. There is simultaneous overactivity of thrombosis and fibrinolysis with consumption of platelets and clotting factors, abnormal bleeding and sometimes an associated microangiopathic haemolytic anaemia. Treatment of DIC remains controversial. Platelets and FFP should be given as sparingly as possible. If haemorrhage is significant, give 10 mL/kg FFP IV, 20 mL/kg platelets and discuss with haematologist the use of cryoprecipitate IV. Sepsis or profound shock are the commonest causes of DIC.
- If bleeding in a newborn infant does not respond to vitamin K, and DIC is not present, consider one of the congenital deficiencies of coagulation factors. All are rare but specific assays of individual clotting factors can confirm the diagnosis. In haemophilia A, factor VIII concentrate is currently preferred to cryoprecipitate because of the lower risk of HIV infection. The level of factor VIII in the affected child's blood is < 20% but does not require treatment unless there is clinical bleeding.

FIFTEEN

Nutrition

Background physiology

Nutritional requirements vary with gestation, birthweight and clinical condition. Average daily requirements are given in Table 15.1. However, adequacy of nutrition is best judged by demonstrating normal growth and development. Breast milk is always the best feed for newborn infants, term or preterm (although supplements are needed for preterm infants — see below), even if only given for a short time. Benefits include anti-infective properties, less allergenicity, faster tolerance, less gastroenteritis and NEC, and possible developmental advantage. Infants who require tube feeding should have their feeds increased gradually (Table 15.2). Small sick infants may require slower introduction of milk depending on tolerance.

Enteral feeding at term

The well term baby should be put to the breast or bottle as soon as possible after birth and allowed to demand feed.

BREAST FEEDING

Breast-fed babies often feed more frequently than bottle-fed babies and may feed up to 12 times per day initially but usually settle into a pattern of roughly 3–hourly feeds (compared with an average of 4-hourly for bottle-fed). The mother alternates which breast she offers to the baby first. Most of the milk is obtained within 7 min of starting but many babies suckle for longer.

Table 15.1 Average daily nutritional requirements

Age	Water (mL/kg)	kcal/kg	Protein (g/kg)	Na+	K+ (mmol/kg)	Ca2+	PO4 3- (mmol/kg)
Infant > 2.5 kg at birth							
1 day	60–90	115	2.2	2–3	2–3	1.5	1.5
2 days	90–120	115	2.2	2–3	2–3	1.5	1.5
10 days	120–150	105	2.0	2–3	2–3	1.5	1.5
3 months	140–160	105	2.0	2–3	2–3	1.5	1.5
Infant < 2.5 kg at birth							
<1 month	60–150	110–165	2.9–4.0	1–8	2–5	2–6	2–5

Table 15.2 Gradual increase in feeds for infants who require tube feeding

Postnatal age	Fluid Intake (mL/kg per 24 hrs)	
	< 2.5 kg	> 2.5 kg
Day 1	60	40
Day 2	90	60
Day 3	120	80
Day 4	150	110
Day 5	150–200	150

Problems with breast feeding

The atmosphere in the postnatal ward and home is the key. It helps if the mother is relaxed, if the baby suckles early, and if mother and infant have free and easy contact. Fixed schedules and unnecessary supplementary feeds can and often interfere with the natural process. Assessment by a nursing expert of the adequacy of the mother's supply of milk, the feeding position and technique, and the suckling efforts of the baby is invaluable. Clearly, if the mother is uncertain, tense, depressed, frightened or in pain, the problem may lie in the supply. It is most unlikely that the breast is biologically unable to perform its task. Alternatively, a lethargic or irritable baby may not be sucking effectively. Some babies have to be encouraged whilst others are so lively they would test the patience of a saint. With support and encouragement, most mothers who wish to are able to breast feed. A feeding problem may be a symptom of the mother's mood or a sign of a disorder in the infant.

Contraindications to breast milk

These include:

- HIV-positive mother or a mother with active TB in the UK
- Maternal chickenpox starting within 4 days of birth. The mother may express and commence breast feeding when all the lesions are crusted.
- Galactosaemia (standard term formula also contraindicated)
- Maternal medication — drugs that are contraindicated during breast feeding include amiodarone, antineoplastic drugs, bromocriptine, chloramphenicol, cimetidine, clemastine, cyclosporin A, dapsone, ergot and ergotamine, gold salts, indomethacin, iodides, lithium, high-dose oestrogens, phenindione, all radioisotopes, tetracyclines, thiouracil, high-dose vitamins A and D, and sulphonamides (in jaundiced infants) (see Appendix 4).

In phenylketonuria, part breast feeding can be continued together with part low phenylalanine formula. Discuss with paediatric dietician.

Maternal drug abuse is not necessarily a reason not to breast feed. However, we strongly recommend that mothers who are using crack cocaine or taking > 20 mg methadone/day should not breast feed. Consider whether the mother's HIV status should be checked. Breast feeding should not be stopped abruptly as this may lead to acute withdrawal. If the mother is using crack cocaine or > 20 mg methadone /day, breast feeding should be avoided.

NB. Analgesics, anticonvulsants and antihistamines are not contraindications to breast feeding but may cause drowsiness in the infant and delay establishment of feeding. Oral steroids and antithyroid drugs do not contraindicate breast feeding, but the infant should be followed carefully for growth and clinical signs of side-effects. Maternal thyroxine will not harm the baby, provided the mother is euthyroid, but may interfere with neonatal screening tests for hypothyroidism.

Severe maternal mental illness is a reason for the mother not to feed at all, either by breast or by bottle.

BOTTLE FEEDING

The bottle-fed term baby should take 150–180 mL/kg per 24 h in 5–6 feeds by the end of the first week, i.e. about 100 mL per feed (28 mL = 1 fluid ounce). Standard term formula provides about 67 kcal/100 mL and babies require around 100 kcal/kg per day — hence 150 mL/kg per day (see Tables 15.1 and 15.3). For powdered milks the key to producing the correct mixture and the recommended calorie density is filling the scoop. It is all too easy to give extra for good measure, but this produces a feed with an electrolyte load (especially sodium) which some infants cannot handle. The resulting hypernatraemia can be potentially dangerous if the infant becomes dehydrated by gastroenteritis. Some companies have developed 'step-up' or 'follow-on' formulas for infants over 6 months of age, partly to guarantee the iron which is not provided by early use of doorstep milk. Casein based formulas are marketed as more satisfying. There is no research to support the need for either of these formulas in infants born at term.

In breast- or bottle-fed babies, waking for a night feed may stop anytime from 6 weeks to 1 year.

WEANING

In the UK, it is recommended that a weaning diet is not introduced until 4 months. In practice, most mothers begin to wean before that time. However, milk should continue to be a major component of the diet for a growing infant. Doorstep milk should

Table 15.3 Composition of various milks (all per 100 mL of milk)

Milk	Energy (kcal)	Protein (g)	Casein: whey	CHO (g)	Fat (g)	Na (mmol)	K (mmol)	Ca (mmol)	P (mmol)
Mature term breast milk	70	1.3	1:2	7	4.2	0.65	1.5	0.9	0.5
Preterm breast milk	67	1.8–2.4	N/A	6	4	2.2	1.8	0.6	0.5
Preterm EBM + fortifier	80	2.5–3.1	N/A	9	4	3.1	–	1.8	1.4
Donor bank milk	46	1.1	N/A	7.1	1.7	0.7	–	0.9	0.5
Cow's milk	67	3.4	3:1	4.6	3.9	2.2	3.9	3	3
Whey based term formula	65–68	1.5	1:1.5	7.0–7.3	3.6–3.8	0.8	1.4–2.2	0.9–1.5	0.9–1.1
Casein-based term formula	65–69	1.5–1.9	4:1	7.2–8.6	3.1–3.6	0.8–1.1	1.6–2.2	1.2–2.1	1.2–1.8
Follow-on (>6 months)	70	1.8	3.5:1	7.2	4.6	1.0	2.2	2.2	1.6
LBW formula	80	2.0–2.4	1:1.5	7.0–8.5	3.5–4.9	1.3–2.0	1.8	1.8–2.7	1.1–1.7
LBW follow-on	74	1.8	1.5:1	7.5	4.1	1.0	1.9	2.0	1.3

not be given until 12 months as the major source of milk, as this may cause occult GI bleeding. Artificial infant formula should be used if extra milk is required.

Enteral feeding of the LBW infant

BREAST VERSUS ARTIFICIAL MILK

There are many constituents of human milk which cannot be duplicated in formula milk and research has shown that breast feeding protects the term infant against infection and possibly against atopy in exclusively breast-fed infants. For term infants, breast milk is the preferred feed. The choice is less clear-cut for the preterm infant. Human milk production has evolved as a feed for term infants and so, not surprisingly, it is less than perfect for preterm infants. Even though preterm milk is more appropriate for preterm infants than term milk, it is still less than optimal to satisfy the preterm infant's increased protein, energy and electrolyte requirements (see Table 15.3). Moreover, although the initial protein content of preterm expressed breast milk (EBM) may be satisfactory, this drops over the first few weeks to an inadequate level. However, human milk may protect preterm infants from NEC and enhance absorption of dietary calcium and fat, especially palmitic acid.

For these reasons, it is generally accepted that neither unsupplemented breast milk nor term formulas alone are suitable for feeding infants <2.0 kg (Table 15.3). There are two options:

- If the mother wishes to express, and she should be encouraged to do so, the LBW infant can be fed with this preterm EBM provided it is fortified.
- If the mother chooses not to express, or is unable to sustain expression, the infant should be fed a low birthweight (LBW) formula. These provide more protein, calcium, phosphorus and calories (Table 15.3).

Breast milk fortification

Previously, EBM has been supplemented with various combinations of calories, e.g. Duocal (carbohydrate and fat), calcium and phosphorus, term infant formula (1 scoop to 100 mL EBM) or hydrolysed protein formula (e.g. Pepti-Junior). None of these is ideal. More recently, commercial breast milk fortifiers (BMFs) have become available (e.g. Eoprotin, Nutriprem breast milk fortifier). We use BMFs for all infants <1.8 kg if the mother is expressing more than 50% of the infant's requirement. Enteral feeding is started with EBM, but once an intake of 150 mL/kg per 24 h is reached, BMF is added.

BMF must *never* be added to infant formula. A LBW formula is used to top-up the volume requirement. BMF is stopped once the infant reaches 2.0 kg in weight or when full breast feeding is established, whichever occurs first.

The advantages of breast milk are particularly important for the preterm infant and are apparent even when breast milk is given for only a short time, so expression should always be encouraged even if breast feeding is not the mother's ultimate choice. Long-term expressing of milk is difficult to achieve. Milk production may be enhanced by:

- providing privacy for expression when mother visits the NNU
- having breast pumps available for home loans
- allowing the baby to suckle on the breast after expression
- maternal treatment with metoclopramide or domperidone (rarely necessary).

In the past, if the mother did not provide EBM herself, donor banked breast milk (containing human term EBM) was used to feed preterm infants. The nutritional quality of this donated milk is generally poor (Table 15.3), and with the anxiety that HIV might be transmitted, there are few banks in operation.

WHAT VOLUME OF MILK TO GIVE?

See Table 15.2. Infants with CHD or CLD may have higher energy requirements but further volume increase is undesirable. Their feeds may need to be concentrated further after discussion with a dietician.

WHICH PRETERM FORMULA? WHAT IS THE OPTIMAL COMPOSITION?

The optimal composition of preterm formula

Protein

The casein:whey ratio in term human milk falls from 10:90 in the first days of lactation to 45:55 in mature milk. Growth rates of term infants do not differ between those fed whey-predominant formulas and those receiving casein-predominant formulas. Theoretically, whey predominant formulas are advantageous in that they have a finer curd, leading to faster gastric emptying rates and bowel flora which are more comparable to breast fed infants. Human and bovine caseins are structurally different and this affects curd formation. There have been anecdotal reports of milk curd plugging in association with neonatal bowel obstruction. The dominant proteins in the whey fraction are lactalbumin, immunoglobulin A and lactoferrin. Lactoferrin has been shown to have bacterisostatic activity and so to enhance iron absorption.

Animal versus vegetable protein. Over 90% of the formula milk market uses cow's milk protein; most of the remainder is derived from soy protein. Humans can be allergic to both. All breast milk fortifiers contain cow's milk proteins. Recent research has shown that milk derived from soy beans has increased amounts of phyto-oestrogens, chemicals which bind to and stimulate oestrogen receptors. In animal experiments these have been associated with decreased fertility. No short-term feminising effects have been seen in male human infants, but longer–term studies are needed.

There is no justification for routinely feeding preterm infants with semi-elemental formulas (designed with term infants in mind), such as Pepti-Junior, in which the nitrogen requirement is provided as peptides rather than whole proteins. However, such protein hydrolysates may be indicated when restarting feeding after NEC or surgery.

Carbohydrate. Both human milk and cow's milk contain the disaccharide lactose (galactose and glucose), whereas soy-derived infant formula milks usually contain glucose polymer (glucose and no galactose). The latter is only of benefit if there is lactose intolerance, most commonly secondary to gastroenteritis. Alternatively, Galactomin 17, a cow's milk formula wihout lactose, can be used in this situation. Energy supplements such as Duocal (a combined fat and carbohydrate source) contain glucose polymer. Such additional energy supplements should not be used unless protein intake is adequate and they are not suitable for routine use in preterm infants as they increase weight gain by adipose tissue deposition but without increase in linear growth.

Lipid. Recent nutritional research has focused on LCPs derived from essential fatty acids (EFAs in the diet). The two families of LCPs are created by elongation and desaturation of the parent EFAs, linoleic acid and alpha-linolenic acid (the n6 derivatives and the n3 derivatives, respectively).These fatty acids are important components of cell membranes, especially in the brain and eye. The amounts of EFA and LCP in breast milk vary with postnatal age and maternal diet. Formula milks have always contained EFAs but, until recently, no LCPs. Very preterm infants have smaller stores of LCPs and less ability to elongate and desaturate linoleic acid and alpha-linolenic acid. Hence, preterm infants fed formulas without LCPs may be disadvantaged. Most major preterm formulas now contain added LCPs. Research continues to determine whether the apparently beneficial effects of LCPs on development and vision are permanent, and to investigate the optimal combination of LCPs with which to supplement cow's milk formulas.

Other factors. Breast milk also contains urea, uric acid, ammonia, creatine, creatinine, free amino acids, nucleic acids and nucleotides, polyamines, carnitine, hormones, growth factors, amino sugars and amino alcohols. Should formula contain all these too? The 'breast is best' or 'mother nature knows' argument may be flawed for two reasons. First, breast milk is a 'dialysate' of whatever is in the maternal blood (e.g. drugs) and therefore those substances will appear in breast milk whether beneficial, harmful or incidental to the baby. Second, evolution is geared to early survival; factors which improved survival millions of years ago may be irrelevant now, or indeed may shorten life span (e.g. breast milk contains more cholesterol). Once we have reproduced another generation, evolution is not interested in whether we live to 50 or 80!

WHEN SHOULD ENTERAL FEEDING START?

As soon as possible. If TPN is required because the infant is too ill to tolerate full enteral feeds, minimal enteral feeding (MEF) with small, nutritionally inconsequential volumes of milk should be started. Ideally this should be mother's own EBM. Studies have shown that MEF is associated with maturation of GI motility, better gastric emptying, more rapid introduction of full enteral feeding, improved growth and less preterm bone disease. MEF seems to enhance gut hormone production and exert a trophic influence. Studies have not shown an increased incidence of NEC or pulmonary aspiration with MEF and indeed, if EBM is used, this may protect against NEC. However, in the subgroup of babies who are very growth-restricted, especially those with absent or reversed end-diastolic Doppler flow velocities in the umbilical artery antenatally who are at particular risk of NEC, we withhold all feed for at least the first 48 h.

HOW LONG TO CONTINUE WITH SPECIAL FEEDS?

There is no scientific answer to this. We generally stop BMFs in breast-fed babies or change to a term formula in bottle-fed babies once a weight of 2.0 kg is reached. We continue a BMF or preterm formula longer if further catch-up growth is possible. Remember that to provide the same energy as 150 mL/kg of LBW formula, the baby would have to take 180 mL/kg of term formula and this would still provide 20% less protein. Therefore, even > 2.0 kg, EBM + BMF or LBW formula should be continued if:

- the rate of weight gain is poor
- the baby was SGA with a lot of catch-up growth to make,
- the baby has greater energy needs and less capacity for this volume (e.g. CHD, CLD, short gut).

'LBW FOLLOW-ON' FORMULAS ('POST-DISCHARGE' FORMULA)

These have been marketed to bridge the gap between LBW formula and term formula (Table 15.3). They provide more protein, energy, minerals and vitamin D than term formula and early trials have shown a benefit in growth and bone mineralisation. Further trials are required before firm recommendations can be made. These formulas may have a role in some infants who fail to thrive or who have increased requirements or poor feeding (e.g. infants with CLD). These milks are not available on tokens or prescription and are twice as expensive as standard formulas.

WHAT ROUTE? HOW FREQUENT?

Wherever possible, the enteral route should be used. Continuous and intermittent feeding have been the subject of a number of studies, but the best conducted of these studies showed no significant difference in weight gain. The risk of aspiration is perhaps less with continuous feeding. In our unit, NG feeds are started continuously. Once full feeds are reached (150–180 mL/kg per day), hourly bolus feeds are commenced and the interval gradually increased to 3–4 hourly. The pre-feed residue aspirated from the stomach gives an indication of whether the feed is tolerated. Bile- or blood-stained aspirates should always lead to cessation of feeding and a search for the cause. Prior to extubation of ventilated infants, feeding is stopped and the stomach emptied.

Transpyloric (nasojejunal tube) feeding was used more widely in the past than it is now. Because the stomach is empty, theoretically, the risk of pulmonary aspiration with vomiting is lower. However, transpyloric feeding is associated with less efficient fat and nitrogen absorption, increased risk of NEC and increased mortality, and we no longer use this route. Cup feeding is an alternative to tube or bottle feeding but there are no randomised controlled trials comparing weight gain or time to establish full feeds.

WEANING THE LBW INFANT

The Department of Health advice for term infants is to introduce solids at 4 months. For the preterm infant, should this be 4 months after birth or after EDD? A rule of thumb is to count 4 months from the midpoint between actual and expected date of birth. The Department of Health also advises that for preterm infants, solids should not be introduced before 5 kg. However, if a previously settled baby begins to wake early for feeds, is not settled after feeds, or starts to wake at night again, then introduction of baby rice mixed with formula or EBM can be considered sooner.

SUMMARY

If well enough to tolerate full enteral feeding, VLBW infants should be given 150–200 mL/kg per day of fortified EBM or a LBW formula. Otherwise MEF should be started as soon as possible, except in IUGR babies with abnormal Doppler studies (Ch. 2). Consider TPN. Stopping BMF or changing to a term or 'LBW follow-on' formula should be considered at 2.0 kg.

The preterm infant is particularly vulnerable to impaired growth at a time when brain development is rapid. The concept of nutritional 'programming' of long-term development during this critical window is important and as much attention should be paid to aggressive nutrition of the high risk infant as to other aspects of neonatal intensive care.

Iron and vitamin requirements of the preterm baby

Deficiencies can occur because of compromised intrauterine stores, delayed nutrition and rapid postnatal growth.

Iron

- All preterm infants should receive an intake of 2 mg/kg per day up to a maximum of 15 mg/day throughout the first year.
- The practice in Nottingham is that iron supplements are started at 4 weeks of age in all infants born < 33 weeks gestation as follows:
  - *unfortified breast milk, fortified breast milk, LBW formula or term formula*: 0.5 mL Sytron (2.75 mg iron) once daily until 1.5 kg; then 1.0 mL once daily until 1 year. Although these recommendations are more than sufficient for infants receiving certain LBW formulas, it allows for a standard single safe prescription for all infants
  - *LBW follow-on formulas*. May not need iron supplementation
  - *TPN*: If still largely TPN-dependent by 6 weeks, consider adding 100 micrograms/kg per day of iron to the aqueous solution.

Vitamin A

- 700–1500 IU/kg per day is recommended.
- Amount in TPN is low.

Vitamin B$_{12}$. Amounts from fortified breast milk or LBW formulas are sufficient.

Vitamin C. Amounts from fortified breast milk or LBW formulas are sufficient.

Vitamin D

- 400 IU/day is recommended.
- Large doses of Vitamin D are not required for metabolic bone disease of prematurity (see below) unless there is evidence of Vitamin D deficiency (extremely rare).

Vitamin E. Minimum requirements are met from human and formula milk and there is little evidence to support further supplementation.

Vitamin K. Human milk is very low in vitamin K — see below.

Folate. A recommendation of 25–50 micrograms/kg per day can be achieved from fortified breast milk or LBW formulas.

Vitamin supplementation

- 5 DoH vitamin drops = 0.15 mL once daily (660 IU vitamin A, 20 mg vitamin C, 280 IU vitamin D)
- The practice in Nottingham is that vitamin supplements are given to all all infants born < 33 weeks gestation once on full enteral feeds as follows:
  - *unfortified breast milk or term formula:* 50 micrograms folate and 10 drops DoH vitamins once daily until discharge. After discharge, 5 drops DoH vitamins once daily and stop folate
  - *fortified breast milk or LBW formula:* 5 drops DoH vitamins once daily until discharge
  - *LBW follow-on formulas:* No vitamin supplementation.

UK Department of Health recommendations for all term infants

- 5 drops DoH vitamins once daily from 6 months in breast-fed infants
- 5 drops DoH vitamins once daily started when formula intake falls below 500 mL/day
- Continue until 5 years.

Vitamin K

All infants should be given vitamin K as a prophylaxis against haemorrhagic disease of the newborn. Babies are more at risk if they are given oral vitamin K rather than parenteral vitamin K, if they are breast-fed, or if they have liver disease. An epidemiological study has shown a statistical association between neonatal vitamin K injection and subsequent risk of malignancy. Although other studies have failed to confirm this, a small but increased risk of leukaemia cannot be excluded. However, the risk of haemorrhagic disease is certain; that of cancer is not. Our present policy is to give IM vitamin K only to infants on the neonatal unit (1 mg if >1.5 kg birthweight; 0.5 mg if <1.5 kg) and infants of mothers receiving anticonvulsants. This injection is never given on the labour suite because of the danger of inadvertent administration of syntometrine. All other infants receive 1 mg vitamin K orally. Further 0.5 mg doses are given to breast-fed infants at 1 week and 1 month after birth, unless they have had IM vitamin K.

An alternative regime is to give Konakion MM (a new mixed-micellar oral preparation licensed for healthy neonates of 36 weeks gestation and older) 2 mg orally soon after birth and repeat at 4–7 days. Exclusively breast fed babies receive a third 2 mg oral dose at 1 month.

Folic acid

Folic acid 0.25 mg/kg p.o. o.d. is given for 6 months if haemolytic anaemia is severe enough to justify phototherapy. Start as soon as enteral feeding is established.

METABOLIC BONE DISEASE (OSTEOPENIA OF PREMATURITY)

In all infants there is a postnatal fall in plasma calcium (lowest 24 h after birth) which enhances PTH production, which acts on:

- bone, causing resorption
- kidney, causing production of active vitamin D (1,25-dihydroxyvitamin D), reabsorption of calcium and phosphate wasting in urine.

In susceptible infants, these changes may lead to:

- reduced bone mineralisation and hence density
- reduced linear growth
- fractures of ribs or long bones.

Pathogenesis of MBD

- Calcium deficiency is rare.
- Phosphorus deficiency is common.
- Vitamin D deficiency is probably not a common cause — preterm infants with MBD usually have high levels of 1,25-dihydroxyvitamin D which fall with mineral supplementation.

Infants at greatest risk:

- < 33 weeks (75% of in utero calcium accretion occurs in the final trimester)
- breast-fed (phosphorus deficiency)
- prolonged TPN (phosphorus deficiency)
- chronic diuretic therapy or diarrhoea (excessive losses in urine or stools).

Investigations suggesting MBD

- Hypophosphataemia (< 1.2 mmol/L) after 7 days of age
- Hypercalcaemia (> 2.7 mmol/L) is indicative of phosphate depletion
- ALP rises in most infants over the first 3 weeks but levels > 1200 IU/L suggest MBD

- Osteoporosis, rickets and fractures may be seen on X-rays
- Urinary calcium:phosphate ratio > 1 after 3 weeks of age (high tubular phosphate reabsorption in MBD).

Management

Monitoring. Weekly calcium, phosphate and ALP measurements in all infants < 33 weeks.

Prevention
- Fortify EBM for all infants < 2 kg and ensure phosphate intake of 2 mmol/kg per day
- Vitamin D supplements (400 iu) to all infants < 33 weeks.
- Calcium 2 mmol/kg per day and phosphate 2.5 mmol/kg per day in long term TPN.

Treatment of established MBD
Infants < 33 weeks with ALP > 1000 IU/L or phosphate < 1.2 mmol/L after 10 days require supplementation.

- Enteral feeds — 1 mmol/kg per day potassium acid phosphate.
- TPN — discuss additional Ca and phosphate with pharmacist to ensure solubility and watch for nephrocalcinosis.
- Stop oral potassium acid phosphate once ALP < 1000 IU/L.
- If ALP remains high and plasma phosphate > 1.8 mmol/L consider calcium supplements.

Parenteral nutrition (TPN)

Intravenous nutrition is not physiological and carries the acute complications of infection, hyperglycaemia and metabolic acidosis, and cholestasis and hepatitis with long-term use. There are also theoretical concerns that the lipid fraction of TPN can increase the risk of neurotoxicity with jaundice and worsen lung disease. However, there will be babies with such severe lung or gut disease that significant enteral feeding is not feasible and TPN should be considered early. Nevertheless, enteral feeding aids the maturation of gut enzymes, hormones and absorption and even if minimal enteral feeding is insignificant in terms of calories, it is important for its trophic effects on the gut and in preventing cholestasis.

ROUTE OF TPN

Parenteral nutrition should always be given through a long line with the tip site confirmed radiologically to be in a central vein or the right atrium. TPN solutions are hyperosmolar and irritant and, although they can be given via a peripheral vein in extreme circumstances, this should only be a short-term measure. Because most infants of birthweight < 1 kg will require TPN, a Silastic long line should be inserted within 48 h of birth before the peripheral veins are damaged.

COMPONENTS OF TPN

Almost every unit has a different regimen for TPN. However, there are some general principles which are set out below. Many units use TPN customised by their own pharmacy and we give details of our own regimen in Table 15.4. However, if your pharmacy does not prepare TPN, you can give adequate TPN using the commercially available preparations in Table 15.5.

Nitrogen

An amino acid solution is used to provide the nitrogen needs normally met by dietary protein. We use Vaminolact, which has an amino acid profile similar to human milk and provides both essential and non-essential amino acids. The full regime provides 0.4 g nitrogen/kg per 24 h (2.5 g protein/kg per 24 h). Some units give up to 3.5 g protein/kg per 24 h.

Energy

The regime we recommend (Table 15.4) provides 100 non-nitrogen kcal/kg per 24 h once the full amounts are reached, 60% from carbohydrate and 40% from fat.

Carbohydrate

Glucose is used as the carbohydrate source (glucose and electrolytes are added to the Vaminolact by our pharmacy). Neonates need a minimum of 4–6 mg glucose/kg per min (6–9 g/kg per 24 h, equivalent to 60–90 mL 10% dextrose/kg per 24 h) but can usually tolerate more. However, very immature infants may have poor glucose tolerance and develop hyperglycaemia following the regime in Table 15.4, which provides 10–15 g glucose/kg per 24 h (7–10 mg/kg per min). As a result of this insulin resistance, less energy reaches the cells and there is often glycosuria with an osmotic diuresis.

Fat

We use Intralipid 20% (i.e. 20 g fat/100 mL), which contains both phospholipids and triglycerides, to provide energy and EFAs. Hydrolysis of triglycerides releases fatty acids which are carried in the circulation bound to albumin. Theoretically, these can compete with bilirubin for albumin binding sites. Again, very immature infants may not tolerate IV fat emulsions well (the liver is the principal site of uptake of fats from the circulation) and as a result the plasma may become lipaemic. However, provision of fat is essential in TPN — extra glucose is not a substitute — and

Table 15.4 Standard TPN regime. This allows a graded introduction of full nutrition over 4 days and assumes the infant is already receiving a fluid intake of 150 mL/kg per 24 h. For infants in the first few days of life, when fluids are gradually being increased (see Table 4.2), only the 'Day 1' regime should be used until 150 mL/kg per 24 h is reached. If an older infant is subsequently fluid restricted, the Day 4 final regime can be administered in as little as 120 mL/kg per 24 h

	Day 1	Day 2	Day 3	Day 4
Protein (g/kg per 24 h)	1.0	1.5	2.0	2.5
Nitrogen (g/kg per 24 h)	0.16	0.23	0.33	0.4
Carbohydrate (g/kg per 24 h)	10	12	14	15
Fat (g/kg per 24 h)	1	2	3	4
Energy (kcals/kg per 24 h)	50	68	86	100
Sodium (mmol/kg per 24 h)	3	3	3	3
Potassium (mmol/kg per 24 h)	2.5	2.5	2.5	2.5
Calcium (mmol/kg per 24)	1.9	1.9	1.9	1.9
Phosphorus (mmol/kg per 24 h)	1.5	1.5	1.5	1.5
Volume (mL/kg per 24 h)	150	150	150	150

the aim is for approximately 40% of calories to come from fat. Therefore, IV lipid should not be discontinued lightly. There is great variation between neonatal units in the amount of fat given to neonates, varying from 2 to 4 g/kg per 24 h. Some units monitor plasma triglyceride levels, titrating the fat in TPN to keep plasma triglycerides < 2.7 mmol/L. There is no evidence that any benefit from reduction of lipid outweighs the disadvantage of reduction in energy supplied to the infant.

With modern blood gas and analytical chemistry equipment, there is no need to stop lipid infusions for 6 h before blood sampling. Intralipid may be infused continuously over the 24 h.

Table 15.4 TPN — regimen using only commercially available components. The full regime is given — the infant should build up to this gradually over 4 days, starting with about one third of these amounts on the first day. The total volume of fluid given must be adjusted to the daily requirements in Table 15.2, ultimately aiming for 150 mL/kg per day. As the full regime below gives about 125 mL/kg per 24 h, the deficit must be made up with 5% dextrose or water

Vamin 9 glucose (Pharmacia)	30 mL/kg per 24 h
This provides:	
Nitrogen	0.28 g/kg per 24 h
Non-protein energy	12 kcals/kg per 24 h
Glucose	3.0 g/kg per 24 h
Sodium	1.5 mmol/kg per 24 h
Potassium	0.6 mmol/kg per 24 h
Magnesium	0.045 mmol/kg per 24 h
Calcium	0.075 mmol/kg per 24 h
Chloride	1.5 mmol/kg per 24 h
Dextrose	14 g/kg per 24 h (70 mL/kg per 24 h of 20% solution = 56 kcal/kg per 24 h)
Sodium chloride	1.5 mmol/kg per 24 h
Peditrace (Pharmacia)	1 mL/kg per 24 h
KH2PO4	2.5 mL/kg per 24 h
Solivito N (Pharmacia)	0.5 mL/kg per 24 h (see text for reconstitution)
Intralipid 20% (Pharmacia)	20 mL/kg per 24 h (4 g fat/kg per 24 hrs; 40 kcals/kg per 24 h)
Vitlipid N Infant (Pharmacia)	4 mL/kg per 24 h

Vitamins

Solvito N comes in a vial as powder for reconstitution. A vial should be dissolved in 5 mL water for injection and 0.5 mL/kg of this solution provides the total daily needs of water-soluble vitamins.

Vitlipid N Infant 4 mL/kg added to Intralipid provides the total daily need of fat-soluble vitamins. Note that all infants receiving TPN should also receive IM vitamin K as described above.

Minerals

Peditrace mineral solution of 1 mL/kg is added to the glucose solution to provide the total daily requirements of zinc, copper, manganese, selenium, fluoride and iodide.

In addition, the following are added to each 24 h of the regimen:

- 50% magnesium sulphate — 0.2 mmol Mg/kg
- 10% calcium gluconate — 1.9 mmol Ca/kg
- 21.6% sodium glycerophosphate — 1.5 mmol PO_4/kg
- 20% potassium chloride — 2.5 mmol K/kg

Further sodium chloride is prescribed if more than the 3.0 mmol Na/kg per 24 h (provided by the sodium glycerophosphate) is required. This provides a calcium:phosphate ratio of 1.7:1 (mg:mg).

Of these minerals, only the prescriptions of sodium and potassium are likely to need altering, depending on plasma electrolyte measurements. Some units substitute acetate for chloride as non-metabolisable base to reduce metabolic acidosis.

Drugs

Drugs should not be added routinely or infused with TPN. The IV long line should be used only for TPN, broken into as infrequently as possible and only with an aseptic technique. An alternative cannula should be inserted for drugs and blood products unless using a double-lumen catheter.

COMPLICATIONS

Infection

Long line infection may present with apnoeas and bradycardias, metabolic acidosis, hyperglycaemia or thrombocytopaenia.

- If there is proven line infection (positive culture of the same organism from the line and from peripheral blood), remove the long line and send the tip for culture. Start IV antibiotics depending on the sensitivity of the organism and do not insert a fresh long line for 48 h.
- If placement of a new line will be very difficult technically, occasionally the line must be left in and antibiotics given via the line. However, it is often preferable to remove the line and place a central line surgically 48 h later.
- If there is a positive culture from the line only, do not remove unless infant deteriorating. Many lines/hubs become colonised but there is no bacteraemia.
- If the infant is septic but the line is not to blame, leave the line in and continue full TPN.

Cholestasis

Risk factors are increasing prematurity, infection, duration of TPN and absence of enteral feeding. If TPN is continued, cirrhosis may ensue.

Jaundice

Preterm infants who need TPN also commonly develop unconjugated jaundice. There are no reports of an increased incidence of kernicterus since the widespread introduction of TPN. The theoretical risks are probably overstated and full TPN should be continued unless exchange levels are approached.

Thrombocytopenia

This may be the first clue to long line sepsis. If not proven, continue full TPN unless the platelet count is $< 10 \times 10^9/L$.

Hyperglycaemia

Initially, a temporary trial of a regimen with less glucose is reasonable (see Table 15.4). However, this reduces the energy supplied and growth will not be sustained. If reintroduction of the full regime once again causes significant hyperglycaemia or glycosuria (true laboratory BG > 10 mmol/L or urinalysis showing +++ of glycosuria), a human-soluble insulin infusion should be started at 0.05 unit/kg per h and BG monitored at least 4-hourly initially.

Insulin must never be given for glycosuria in the absence of hyperglycaemia (i.e. reduced renal threshold).

Lung disease

It is not proven that IV lipid causes CLD, nor is it proven that decreasing IV lipid reduces oxygen requirements in CLD.

Metabolic acidosis

This is often seen in infants receiving TPN, but TPN may not be the cause. These infants are usually ill and often ventilated and they badly need nutrition. TPN should be continued and the acidosis corrected with sodium bicarbonate.

Never add bicarbonate directly to TPN in the same line, as chalk will precipitate!

MONITORING TPN

Urine. Dipstick for glucose daily.

Blood tests. Test daily until stable on maximum TPN regimen, then thrice weekly: FBC, U & E, BG.

Weekly: LFTs including albumin and bilirubin, calcium, phosphate, triglycerides (when on full lipid amount).

Monthly: Selenium, copper, zinc, manganese.

TRANSITION FROM PARENTERAL TO ENTERAL NUTRITION

1. Minimal enteral nutrition (as little as 0.5 mL milk 4-hourly) throughout TPN decreases cholestasis and decreases the time to establish full enteral nutrition.
2. Do not start to decrease TPN until the infant is tolerating 2 mL/kg per h of milk (unless fluid-restricted, when TPN can be made more concentrated).
3. Then, for every 0.5 mL increase in milk intake, decrease Vaminolact/glucose solution by 0.4 mL and Intralipid by 0.1 mL.
4. Do not stop TPN until the infant is receiving 75% of daily requirements by the enteral route.

SIXTEEN

Surgical problems

Cleft lip and palate (CLP)

These occur in 1 in 1000 births and follow a polygenetic inheritance. Many are now identified antenatally and referral is made to a CLP team for counselling. This team, which includes an orthodontist and a plastic surgeon, will provide specialist help after birth and during the preoperative period. All infants with CLP should be referred to the CLP team straight after birth. Many hospitals have key workers (a nurse or speech and language therapist) who will visit parents and help with advice about feeding and treatment. Parents may be greatly reassured by being shown photographs of other similarly affected children pre- and post-operatively.

CLEFT LIP

A cleft lip may be repaired immediately after birth, or more commonly at around 3 months, as earlier correction may not produce the best long term facial growth. The cleft may be bilateral.

CLEFT PALATE

Cleft palate is usually found in association with cleft lip, although it may be isolated. The infant should be examined to exclude other anomalies, e.g. micrognathia in the Pierre–Robin sequence, or midline brain malformations, e.g. holoprosencephaly. Feeding difficulties are related to the size of the defect and specialist help should be sought from the cleft palate team. A dental plate and strapping may assist feeding in infants with severe bilateral clefts and the use of special teats may be required. Many infants successfully breast feed.

The palate is usually repaired at around 9–12 months of age. Later surgery to the dental arch or nose may be necessary. Speech therapy may be helpful to improve the nasal quality of speech. Cleft palate patients have an increased incidence of otitis media and glue ear.

Lesions in the mouth, pharynx and neck

Ranula

- Cystic mass in the floor of the mouth near the frenulum of the tongue caused by obstruction of the sublingual salivary duct.
- Surgical excision may be necessary.

Branchial cyst/sinus

Remnants of the embryological branchial pouches may persist as a fistula opening onto the skin at the anterior border of sternomastoid, which may discharge clear mucus. A cyst may develop if the cutaneous opening becomes occluded and presents more commonly beyond the neonatal period.

Sternomastoid tumour

Usually not present at birth, develops at 2–8 weeks (see Ch. 19).

Preauricular pit/sinus

- Arises anterior to the tragus of the ear.
- Extends from the skin surface to the cartilage of the external auditory canal.
- Most are asymptomatic.
- If pit becomes infected, excision is indicated.
- Must be referred for hearing assessment.

Midline neck masses

- Rare in newborn infants; occasionally goitres may be present at birth (Ch. 11).
- Thyroglossal duct cysts present in later infancy.

Cystic hygroma

- A multilocular cystic malformation of the lymphatic system.
- Cysts may be small or very large and occur in the lateral neck, mediastinum and axilla.
- May obstruct the airway or enlarge due to haemorrhage or infection.
- Extension into the thoracic inlet may produce stridor, cyanosis or difficulty in feeding.
- Treatment is usually by excision, which may be difficult. Injection of the cysts with sclerosing agents has been tried with limited success.
- Some regress considerably after birth.

Oesophageal atresia and tracheo-oesophageal fistula

The incidence is 1 in 4000 births. Between 50 and 70% of infants have other congenital anomalies, commonly the VACTERL association (other gut atresias, vertebral anomalies, cardiac, renal and limb defects). Oesophageal atresia may be suspected antenatally by presence of polyhydramnios and absence of the fluid-filled stomach on USS, or postnatally with choking and cyanosis due to inability to swallow saliva or milk.

- Diagnosis is confirmed by inability to pass size 10 NG tube into the stomach and aspirate acid gastric contents (note that NG tubes frequently coil in the throat, so a wide–bore tube is used and the aspirated secretions tested using litmus paper; Ch. 3).
- CXR reveals the gastric tube in the oesophagus; if air is seen in the stomach or bowel, a fistula between the trachea and the lower oesophageal segment is present (TOF — present in 85% of cases).

MANAGEMENT

- Keep nil by mouth.
- Nurse head up, with Replogle tube in the oesophageal pouch on continuous suction to minimise aspiration into the lungs from the pouch.
- Give IV fluids, antibiotics and parenteral vitamin K preoperatively.
- An echocardiogram should be performed preoperatively to exclude cardiac anomalies and to establish on which side the aortic arch is sited in order that the surgeon may perform a thoracotomy from the opposite side.
- Note that if the infant has respiratory distress requiring intubation, due to immaturity or aspiration, it may be impossible to adequately ventilate the lungs in the presence of a TOF because of progressive abdominal distension and eventually perforation. Ligation of fistula may be required as an urgent procedure, or in some centres, where the baby is unstable or very preterm, gastrostomy in combination with fast rate CMV or HFOV has been used — seek help urgently.
- Primary anastomosis of the oesophagus with ligation of an associated TOF is the treatment of choice. A trans-anastomotic NG tube is sited through which the infant can be fed enterally. The tube should be securely fixed so that it does not fall out until the anastomosis is healed.
- If necessary postoperatively, it is usual to ventilate using muscle relaxants to avoid having to replace the ETT. This

should be done only by a skilled intubator, who should avoid head flexion (puts tension on anastomosis).

- It is usual to site an extra pleural chest drain with the tip close to the site of the oesophageal anastomosis (the presence of bubbles or saliva in the chest drain suggests a leak at the anastomosis site).
- A contrast swallow is routinely performed before allowing oral feeds.
- Later complications include stenosis at the primary anastomosis site.

If the gap between the two ends of the oesophagus is too long, primary closure is not possible. A gastrostomy is fashioned to permit enteral feeding. The upper oesophageal pouch must be continuously aspirated until either an oesophagostomy is performed or an attempt at primary closure is made when the infant has grown and the upper oesophagus has stretched. Colonic interposition between the two ends of the oesophagus may be required. Gastro-oesophageal reflux is very common in babies with oesophageal atresia due to abnormal oesophageal motility and there is a consequent risk of aspiration pneumonia.

Isolated TOF (H type)

- Rare — occasionally presents in the newborn period with choking and coughing during feeds.
- Diagnosis is by contrast radiography or bronchoscopy and oesophagoscopy.
- Treatment is by surgical repair, usually through a neck incision.

Laryngotracheo-oesophageal cleft

This is a very rare condition presenting at birth with respiratory distress on feeding, hoarse voice, weak cry, stridor and cyanosis.

Intestinal obstruction

Many are diagnosed before birth during investigation of polyhydramnios or at routine anomaly assessments. USS may suggest the level of obstruction if there are dilated, fluid filled loops of bowel.

1. At birth a NG tube should be passed and the gastric contents aspirated.
2. Admit to the neonatal unit.
3. Commence IV fluids and replace aspirates with normal saline.
4. Perform supine and erect (or lateral decubitus) X-rays.

5. The need for further appropriate radiological investigations may then be assessed during discussion between the paediatric radiology and surgical teams.
6. Management will be surgical, with primary anastomosis where possible. Defunctioning ileostomy or colostomy will be required in some cases depending on individual circumstances such as the level of obstruction, weight and gestational age and degree of illness in the infant.

NB. Green staining of the liquor at delivery may be due to bile and not the more usual meconium; this may be an early clue that intestinal obstruction is present.

DUODENAL OBSTRUCTION

This may be complete, as in duodenal atresia, or partial, due to an annular pancreas or duodenal web. Duodenal atresia is commonly associated with Down syndrome.

- Presentation is with vomiting and feed intolerance. In 85% of cases, obstruction is distal to the entry of the bile duct into the duodenum, so NG aspirates or vomitus may be bilious.
- Abdominal distension is not a feature, but the epigastrium may be full due to gastric distension and there may be visible gastric peristalsis.
- Plain X-ray shows double bubble of air in the stomach and first part of the duodenum. Some air may be seen distally if duodenal obstruction is partial or there is a 'Y'-shaped pancreatic duct.
- Treatment is surgical.

MALROTATION AND VOLVULUS

Normal rotation and fixation of the small and large bowel during fetal life secures the bowel to the posterior abdominal wall on a long diagonal from the left upper to the right lower quadrant. If there is failure of these processes, the bowel has an abnormally short mesentery and may twist on itself, obstructing the vascular supply; necrosis of the bowel quickly develops (volvulus).

Acute midgut volvulus

- Presents with bile-stained vomiting.
- Abdominal distension and tenderness are present in 50%.
- As bowel ischaemia increases, the infant becomes dehydrated and shocked.
- Plain radiographs may show a gasless abdomen (high obstruction) or dilated bowel consistent with a more distal intestinal obstruction.

- The less acutely ill infant with bile-stained vomiting should have an upper GI contrast study to demonstrate the position of the D-J flexure. Normally this is to the left of the midline.
- *Volvulus is a surgical emergency* and laparotomy should be performed once the shocked infant has been resuscitated.

INTESTINAL ATRESIAS

Atresias of the small and large bowel may be single (85%) or multiple (15%) and occasionally are familial. Atresias of the jejunum or ileum are more common than atresia of the colon. There is a low incidence of associated anomalies, but up to half of babies are of low birthweight.

- Infants present with bilious vomiting, abdominal distension and failure to pass normal amounts of meconium in the first 24 h.
- The lower the level of obstruction, the greater the degree of abdominal distension.
- Jaundice is common.
- Bowel loops may be visible and respiratory distress may develop due to splinting of the diaphragm.
- Diagnosis is usually confirmed by a lower GI contrast study, which may identify the level of obstruction and demonstrate a microcolon (which occurs due to failure of the colon to distend before birth in the presence of a high obstruction).
- Treatment is surgical.

MECONIUM ILEUS

Obstruction of the gut due to inspissated meconium is associated with CF in 90% of cases. In contrast, only 20% of infants with CF present with meconium ileus. Intestinal obstruction presents within 24–48 h.

- Suggestive symptoms include abdominal distension, failure to pass meconium and bilious vomiting.
- In complicated meconium ileus, atresia, volvulus or perforation may occur and presentation is usually immediately after birth.
- Plain radiographs show dilated intestinal loops of varying size, relative absence of air-fluid levels, a soap-bubble appearance of the gut contents and calcification if there has been perforation some time before birth.
- A soluble contrast enema may wash out obstructing plugs of meconium and confirm the diagnosis. In 40% of cases, repeated enemas may clear the obstruction and avoid laparotomy.
- Other patients require ileostomy to decompress the obstructed bowel with later re-anastomosis.
- Pay particular attention to fluid balance and give broad-spectrum antibiotics.

- Whilst awaiting a diagnosis of CF, we commence prophylactic flucloxacillin. Pancreatic enzyme supplements are used if there is a suspicion of malabsorption. If the diagnosis is confirmed, both are required.

Over 80% of cases of CF are homozygous for the Δ-F508 gene deletion. Confirmation of the diagnosis by the demonstration of at least two elevated sweat chlorides is required at 6 weeks post term age.

HIRSCHSPRUNG'S DISEASE

Incidence is 1 in 5000 births; the male to female ratio is 4:1. Associated anomalies may include Down syndrome and CHD. There is an increased risk of Hirschsprung's disease in siblings.

Congenital aganglionosis of the intestine is the result of arrested fetal development of the myenteric nervous system. The usual cranial to caudal migration of neuroblasts may be halted anywhere between the pylorus and anus, but is usually in the sigmoid colon or rectum. The proximal bowel has a normal myenteric nervous system and is distended. The distal bowel has absence of ganglion cells in the intermuscular and submucosal plexuses. In addition, thickened non-myelinated cholinergic nerve fibres are seen.

Presentation

- Failure to pass meconium within 48 h of birth in a term infant should arouse suspicion of Hirschsprung's disease.
- Infants may present more acutely soon after birth with bilious vomiting, abdominal distension and failure to pass meconium.
- Less commonly, they present with signs of shock and sepsis due to associated enterocolitis.

Diagnosis

- Radiographic evidence of distal intestinal obstruction with multiple dilated bowel loops is suggestive.
- Diagnosis is confirmed by rectal suction biopsy.
- Barium enema may be helpful, particularly to rule out other causes of intestinal obstruction, but it does not always reliably demonstrate a transition zone between normal and aganglionic bowel in the newborn period.

Management

- If necessary, resuscitate with IV fluids, aspiration of gastric contents and IV benzylpenicillin, gentamicin and metronidazole.
- Acute obstruction may be relieved by colostomy with a definitive pull-through operation between 6 and 12 months of age.
- Alternatively, wash out the rectum twice daily and perform early pull-through at 3 months avoiding colostomy.

Prognosis

Long-term prognosis is good with low incidence of incontinence, but there is a tendency to chronic constipation. Mortality is low due to early diagnosis. Half of the cases are diagnosed in the neonatal period and most by 2 years.

MECONIUM PLUG AND NEONATAL SMALL LEFT COLON SYNDROME (MICROCOLON)

Either may present with evidence of colonic obstruction, similar to that seen in Hirschsprung's disease. In 50% of infants with neonatal small left colon syndrome, there is a maternal history of diabetes.

- Plain radiographs demonstrate intestinal distension with air-fluid levels.
- A contrast enema shows dilated colon proximal to a tapered transition zone which is usually at the splenic flexure in small left colon syndrome and can be anywhere in the colon in meconium plug syndrome. The soluble contrast enema is therapeutic.
- Suction biopsy to rule out Hirschsprung's disease is recommended since the clinical presentation is similar.

OTHER CAUSES OF OBSTRUCTION

Rare causes of intestinal obstruction include pyloric atresia, internal herniae, Meckel's diverticulum and intestinal duplications which may be cystic or diverticular.

Anorectal anomaly

Antenatal suspicion may be raised by signs of intestinal obstruction, but anorectal problems are more usually detected at birth, as an imperforate or malplaced anus, by the midwife whilst attempting to measure rectal temperature. The perineal area must be inspected as part of the neonatal screening examination. It is important not to miss imperforate anus in a female infant who may pass a nappy full of meconium via a rectovaginal fistula.

Anorectal anomalies occur in 1 in 500 births and are more common in males. The abnormality may be classified as low, intermediate or high in relation to the level of the puborectalis portion of the levator ani muscle. In high or intermediate lesions, 85% of males have recto-urinary fistula and 75% of females have a rectovaginal fistula. Other gut atresias may be present. GU tract malformations occur in 60% of infants with high anorectal anomalies, but in only 15–20% of infants with low anomalies.

Male infant

- Careful examination of the perineum is carried out for an external opening anywhere from tip of penis to usual anal site.
- A high anomaly is suspected if there is absence of gluteal fold (flat bottom appearance), in the presence of a sacral anomaly or if no external sphincter contracture can be elicited.
- An invertogram — lateral abdominal X-ray with the baby inverted, with a lead marker or paper clip taped over the presumed site of the external sphincter — may be performed at 24 h when air has had time to descend into the pelvis.
- Fistula injection of contrast or USS of the perineum may help to define anatomy.
- Investigations should be planned by discussion with the paediatric surgeon and radiologist.

Female infant

- Anomalies that do not communicate via a fistula are rare so invertograms are rarely helpful.
- Careful inspection of the perineum will usually reveal three orifices: urethra, vagina and fistula which may be into the vestibule or onto the external skin surface.

MANAGEMENT

- High lesions usually require a defunctioning colostomy and later a pull-through procedure.
- Anoplasty is usually possible with low lesions.
- All infants with anorectal agenesis should have renal USS and MCUG to screen for renal malformations and VUR.

PROGNOSIS

Continence is achieved following anoplasty in infants with low lesions, although constipation may be problematic. Results in those requiring more complex surgery depend on the level of the anomaly; 75% of patients with intermediate lesions and 65% of those with high lesions are continent.

Anterior abdominal wall defects

EXOMPHALOS

Occurring in about 1 in 5000 fetuses, this is a defect of the umbilicus through which the abdominal contents herniate. The gut is covered by a sac comprising an inner layer of peritoneum and an outer layer of amnion. Diagnosis usually made during antenatal USS examination. Note that exomphalos may cause an increased αFP concentration in amniotic fluid. Associated abnormalities occur in 40% of fetuses, including trisomy 13, 18 and 21, Beckwith–Wiedemann syndrome and other congenital midline anomalies. Fetal karyotyping is recommended.

1. Delivery should be by vaginal route unless there are maternal reasons for surgical delivery, preferably in a neonatal surgical centre.
2. Immediately following delivery, a Replogle tube should be passed to decompress the stomach and limit air passing into the bowel which may hinder attempts at surgical repair if the defect is large.
3. The baby and exomphalos should be placed in a sterile plastic bag, feet first up to the armpits, to limit fluid and heat loss and to prevent accidental rupture of the sac.
4. Perform a cardiac USS looking for anomalies.
5. Primary closure on the first day of life can be achieved in most cases. If the defect is very large, a staged procedure using a Silastic silo to contain the viscera is employed. The viscera may be gradually reduced over 3–10 days. In exceptional cases where the defect occupies most of the anterior abdominal wall, or the infant is too unstable for surgery, a non-operative policy with application of mercurochrome or povidone iodine solution will allow the sac to epithelialise. This requires prolonged hospitalisation and there is a large residual ventral hernia.
6. Prognosis is dependent on the size of the defect and the severity of associated anomalies.

GASTROSCHISIS

This is the herniation of the bowel through a defect in the anterior abdominal wall, usually to the right of the umbilicus. There is no peritoneal sac so the bowel floats freely in the amniotic fluid exposed to fetal urine and occasionally meconium, and the bowel wall becomes thickened. The incidence of coexisting anomalies is low compared with exomphalos. However, intestinal atresia secondary to intrauterine volvulus may occur in 15%. There has been an increased incidence in the UK since the mid-1990s; it is particularly common in young teenage mothers. The diagnosis is usually made antenatally, and progressive bowel distension occurring in the second trimester appears to be a poor prognostic sign.

1. The baby and bowel should be placed in a sterile plastic bag at delivery, as for exomphalos (it is our practice to give a wrapped bowel bag to the mother prior to delivery in case she should deliver precipitously at a maternity unit other than the regional surgical centre, as it is critical to prevent infection in the exteriorised bowel).
2. A Replogle tube should be passed to deflate the bowel at birth and IV fluids commenced.

3. Colloid may be necessary to resuscitate the baby prior to surgery as there are often large volume losses from the exteriorised bowel.
4. Primary closure is possible in most cases; only rarely will a silo be required.
5. Motility of the thickened gut is abnormal and prolonged TPN is usually required before establishment of full enteral feeds.
6. Despite what may be a protracted neonatal stay, the long-term prognosis is excellent, unless significant amounts of bowel are excised following volvulus.

Diaphragmatic hernia

The commonest hernia is the posterolateral Bochdalek hernia caused by failure of fusion of the diaphragmatic leaflets. Incidence is 1 in 2000. Left-sided hernias are more common (85%). For reasons that are not known, right-sided hernias are associated with GBS infection. The defect may vary in size from 1 cm diameter to complete absence of the hemidiaphragm. Associated anomalies seen in 15–25% of infants include CHD, chromosomal abnormalities, particularly trisomy 13 and 18, CNS malformations and pulmonary sequestration.

Prognosis is not related to the size of the defect alone, but rather to the degree of pulmonary hypoplasia on the ipsilateral and contralateral sides and to the responsiveness of the pulmonary hypertension that occurs secondary to the abnormal pulmonary vascular bed. The pulmonary arterioles are reduced in number and size and have a hypertrophied smooth muscle layer, producing pulmonary hypertension (Ch. 6).

PRESENTATION AND PREOPERATIVE CARE

Antenatal diagnosis is now usual and polyhydramnios is common.

Delivery should take place in a centre with neonatal intensive care and surgical facilities. At delivery, a skilled resuscitator should be present. The baby should be intubated and ventilated immediately following birth. Avoid mask ventilation in order to minimise gas in the gut. As soon as possible pass a NG tube and aspirate frequently. Early paralysis of ventilated infants is necessary to keep the bowel decompressed and reduce the risk of PPHN. Transfer the baby ventilated to the neonatal unit.

Postnatal presentation depends upon the degree of pulmonary compromise. Severe lesions may present with a difficult or failed resuscitation; less severe lesions with tachypnoea, recession or cyanosis. In either, there may be asymmetry of chest shape, with reduced air entry on the affected side and a scaphoid abdomen. In left-sided lesions, the heart sounds are easily heard on the right. The rarer hernia through the anterior foramen of Morgagni presents as a surprise finding on CXR in infants or children with respiratory symptoms.

Investigations. Obtain CXR and AXR. Initially the hemithorax may be opaque, but as air is swallowed, gas-filled loops of bowel or stomach become visible. The mediastinum is shifted to the opposite side. USS may help to differentiate CAM. In the presence of dysmorphic features, an urgent karyotype may be warranted.

Preoperative care. The infant should be stabilised before surgical repair is attempted. This may take several days and the repair undertaken as an elective procedure. The transitional circulation remains labile and pulmonary hypertensive crises may occur before, during or in the first few days after surgery (Ch. 6).

ECMO. The role of ECMO in the management of these babies is controversial. Generally, ECMO does not have a role in stabilising infants who are unventilatable from birth, in whom the pulmonary hypoplasia is so severe that gas exchange cannot take place.

Surgical repair is usually via an abdominal approach, with repair or patching of the diaphragm.

POSTOPERATIVE CARE

- Postoperatively there will always be a pneumothorax on the side of the lesion unless pulmonary hypoplasia is minimal. Do not drain without consulting the surgeon, as reducing the volume of air will cause mediastinal shift to the side of the lesion and circulatory compromise!
- Colloid infusions will be required as the postoperative pneumothorax fills with fluid over the next few days.
- Surgical repair can be undertaken on ECMO, but may be associated with significant postoperative haemorrhage and difficulty weaning from the ventilator.
- Prolonged ventilator support or inspired oxygen is required in approximately one-third of infants. Negative pressure ventilation may be helpful if more than 7 days of postoperative respiratory support is required.

PROGNOSIS

- Following antenatal diagnosis, about 40–50% babies will survive (lower than postnatally because of the presence of associated abnormalities). Approximately 50–60% of live-born infants who present with symptoms in the first few hours survive. Survival may be increased to 70–80% with the use of ECMO in selected patients.

- Lung growth, in terms of alveolar number, occurs over the first postnatal year and it is important to minimise the period of long term positive pressure ventilation.
- Some children are wheezy. Mildly reduced peak flow has been demonstrated in children 7–19 years post-surgery.
- Where one lung is severely hypoplastic, chest asymmetry and scoliosis may develop.

Genitourinary problems

POSTERIOR URETHRAL VALVES

Antenatal diagnosis is by the presence of an enlarged trabeculated bladder. VUR usually coexists and renal dysplasia may develop. If bladder outflow is almost totally obstructed, oligohydramnios with pulmonary hypoplasia develops (Potter's sequence).

- Postnatal presentation of less severe urethral valves causing partial obstruction is with signs of sepsis, a palpable bladder or weak or intermittent urinary stream.
- Diagnosis is by MCUG under antibiotic cover.
- Treatment is ablation by diathermy.
- Long term follow-up should be maintained to monitor renal function if the bladder is dysfunctional or VUR is present.

BLADDER EXTROPHY

Very rare (1 in 40 000 births). There is deficiency of the anterior wall of the bladder, resulting in exposure of the bladder, urethra and ureteric orifices. The pubic bones are splayed and the hips may be dislocated.

- Primary closure is usually attempted in the newborn period to protect the upper renal tract.
- Complications of bladder reconstruction include hydronephrosis due to bladder outlet obstruction, UTI and incontinence.
- Further surgical procedures are usually required to improve continence and cosmetic appearance.

HYPOSPADIAS

This proximal placement of the urinary meatus occurs in 1 in 500 boys. It may be accompanied by chordee (causing curvature of the shaft, best assessed during erection). The meatus may be seen along the ventral surface of the penis or on the perineum.

- Parents should be reassured that their son will be able to pass urine normally and have normal sexual function.
- The parents should also be warned not to have the child circumcised.
- Early referral to a paediatric urologist or plastic surgeon experienced in hypospadias repair should be made.

EPISPADIAS

This is very rare (1 in 100 000 births). The urethra opens on the dorsal side of the penis. There may be incontinence of the sphincter mechanism. In females, a patulous urethra may be displaced anteriorly and also be associated with incontinence.

CIRCUMCISION

Circumcision is **contraindicated** in any child who has an abnormality of the penis such as hypospadias or epispadias since the skin may be required during the repair operation.

Circumcision is performed routinely within some cultural groups. Consideration should be given in individual cases to requests by parents for circumcision by a paediatric surgeon rather than a religious elder in order to minimise the risk of complications such as infection and bleeding. Ideally, circumcision should be deferred until the infant is out of nappies. Other complications include meatal ulceration or stenosis, post circumcision phimosis and penile necrosis.

TESTICULAR TORSION

Twisting of the cord structures interrupts blood flow to the testis and epididymis. If the baby is born with a firm, enlarged testis that may or may not be tender, there is no potential to salvage the testis, so immediate surgery is not indicated. In contrast, a testis that is normal at birth and then undergoes torsion should be immediately explored. It is a matter of debate whether the contralateral testis should be fixed by orchidopexy to prevent torsion, or left untouched to avoid vascular damage secondary to surgery.

TESTICULAR TUMOUR

A solid testicular swelling may represent tumour such as teratoma or rhabdomyosarcoma. Measure αFP and examine carefully for other evidence of malignant disease.

UNDESCENDED TESTES

The testis may be palpable in the inguinal canal. Examine the scrotum. If it is small and contracted, it is unlikely the testis has been contained in the scrotum in utero. If the scrotum is well developed and the testis palpable in the inguinal canal, it is probably retractile and can be eased gently into the scrotum by palpation.

- If both testes are not palpable, investigate as per ambiguous genitalia (Ch. 11), unless very preterm.
- If one testis is still undescended at 1 year, referral to a paediatric surgeon is recommended.
- There is an increased risk of abnormal spermatogenesis and malignant change in testes that are not placed in the scrotum before the age of 5 years.

HYDROCELE

This is a swelling in the scrotum that cannot be separated from the testis. The examiner's fingers can be opposed above the swelling as distinct from an inguinal hernia. The swelling transilluminates. A communicating hydrocele may empty on gentle compression of the scrotum. Reassure parents that most resolve spontaneously. Referral to a paediatric surgeon is recommended at 1 year if not resolved.

INGUINAL HERNIA

An intermittent swelling in the groin best felt when the baby is crying. It is common in preterm boys who have been ventilated. Ensure the testis is within the scrotal sac to avoid mistaking retractile testis for a hernia. Inguinal hernia is rare in girls and presents as a bulge in the labia majora. If a mass is palpable it may represent an ovary. Consider testicular feminisation if bilateral gonads are palpable in the labia. If the hernia is irreducible, assume that strangulation is imminent. Refer to the paediatric surgery team for immediate assessment and repair.

- If the hernia is reducible, repair should be arranged before the baby is discharged from the Neonatal Unit.
- In very tiny infants a period of weight gain is optimal before surgery. Vigilance is essential so that strangulation does not occur.
- Infants with BPD may have surgery under spinal anaesthesia.

Perioperative care

PREOPERATIVE CARE

Consent

This should be obtained by the surgeon who is to do the operation. On occasions it will be necessary for a member of the neonatal team to talk to parents about a procedure, e.g. when collecting a baby from a referring hospital. It is important to ensure that you obtain a telephone number where a parent can be contacted by the surgeon so that he or she can speak to them before surgery.

Medical issues

- All babies should receive parenteral vitamin K according to the local dose schedule (Ch. 15).
- Check with the surgeon whether blood for transfusion should be ordered.
- Check a FBC and electrolytes, and correct any deficiency. We usually ensure that the haemoglobin is >10 g/dL.
- All notes, prescription charts and X-rays should accompany the child.
- Discuss with the anaesthetist who is to establish IV or IA access (if no infusion in progress).

POSTOPERATIVE CARE

General management

- After any surgical procedure and transfer of the infant back to a cot in the neonatal unit, check temperature and plasma glucose immediately.
- The baby should be carefully examined and a general assessment made of fluid balance, skin perfusion, BP, oxygenation and pain control. The examination should be recorded in the medical notes. Check that IV and IA lines are functioning.
- If a central venous line or ETT has been inserted in theatre, check position on CXR. Read anaesthetic charts and operation notes to establish estimated blood loss, GI tract fluid losses and replacements given. Note anaesthetic drugs, analgesia and reversal agents administered.

Fluids

- Correct hypovolaemia with blood or colloid.
- Record NG tube and drain losses and urine output and reassess fluid balance after 6 h and regularly thereafter.
- Give maintenance crystalloid according to the age of the baby (although many units restrict fluid for 24 h after surgery); we replace NG tube losses with normal saline.
- Check U&E, creatinine and blood gas 6 h postoperatively and adjust fluids accordingly. A metabolic acidosis may indicate hidden fluid loss, e.g. fluid-filled loops of bowel associated with paralytic ileus. If there is clinical evidence of hypovolaemia, give colloid 10 mL/kg and reassess.
- It is usual to discontinue TPN during the first postoperative day if the infant is unstable, e.g. acidotic, since it may not be well

tolerated. It should be recommenced on the following day if at all possible, unless full enteral feeds are to be given. This is particularly important in preterm infants who have few energy stores. Even if the establishment of full enteral feeds is not possible, minimal enteral nutrition should be commenced as soon as possible.

Respiratory

If ventilated or in oxygen, measure ABG on readmission and regularly thereafter. Following some procedures, a period of ventilation may be requested. Ensure that the ventilation is the least necessary to achieve normal blood gases (Ch. 6) and that if muscle relaxants are used, they are effective.

Haematology

Check FBC and haematocrit within 12 h of surgery or sooner if indicated by heavy blood loss or pallor.

Analgesia

Check what analgesia was given during the procedure (on the anaesthetic sheet).

Ensure adequate pain relief (assess by posture, irritability, grimace, cry and tachycardia). We use a diamorphine infusion for moderate to severe pain (Ch. 6) or rectal paracetamol following minor procedures.

Antibiotics

- The surgeon will specify when antibiotics are to be given. Where there has been GI surgery we use triple antibiotics (benzylpenicillin, gentamicin and metronidazole).
- Ensure the infant is passing urine before giving further doses of aminoglycoside and check levels around every fourth dose.

Parents

Ensure parents are given an explanation of the operation findings and procedures performed.

SEVENTEEN

The eye

Examination

Early detection of eye disease and intervention may be of great importance for the development of normal binocular vision. The eye is inspected as part of the routine screening examination performed soon after birth. More detailed examination, usually with pupillary dilatation, should be reserved for an ophthalmologist. The simple process outlined below will identify most lesions apparent in the neonatal period:

1. Inspect the lid and globe for external abnormality and signs of infection.
2. Ensure the cornea is bright and clear.
3. Look for a red reflex using a direct ophthalmoscope.
4. Assess visual fixation — most term infants will fix and follow a brightly coloured object, a light or a face.

Refer to an ophthalmologist for a more detailed examination and indirect ophthalmoscopy following dilatation of the pupil if:

- any abnormality is detected on such an inspection (see below)
- there is
  - a constant squint
  - a family history of eye disease
  - any suspicion of congenital infection (CMV, toxoplasmosis, rubella)
  - a suspicion of a systemic abnormality associated with eye defects
- Screening for retinopathy of prematurity is indicated (see below).

DISORDERS OF THE EYELID AND ORBIT

Gap in lid margin (coloboma) — usually upper and nasal
- Associated with Goldenhaar's syndrome.
- Surgical repair on cosmetic grounds.

Cryptophthalmos — unilateral or bilateral absence of a palpebral fissure and formed globe. No treatment is possible.

Fused lids (blepharophimosis)
- Normal <26 weeks, partial or complete. Will open without intervention
- Occasionally requires surgery in more mature babies.

Ptosis — weakness of superior rectus muscle
- Usually congenital and needs no investigation
- Surgery if amblyopia develops or for cosmetic reasons
- May be due to tumour in the eyelid or Horner's syndrome (small pupil).

Dermoid cyst. Usually in outer part of the upper lid. Remove for cosmetic reasons.

Capillary haemangioma (strawberry naevus). Increases in size in the first year, and then there is spontaneous involution. Surgery (laser ablation) is performed if it interferes with the visual axis.

Anterior protrusion of the eye (proptosis)
- Traumatic haemorrhage
- Orbital tumours (haemangioma and lymphangioma)
- Due to shallow orbits (craniostenosis and Crouzon's disease [craniofacial dysostosis]).

DISORDERS OF GLOBE SIZE

Congenital glaucoma (buphthalmos)
- Unilateral or bilateral
- Usually sporadic, occasionally recessive
- May be associated with systemic abnormalities
- Presents as an enlarged weeping eye with corneal opacity and photophobia
- Urgent referral for surgery is required, usually goniotomy.

Microphthalmia. This is associated with congenital infection and other systemic abnormalities. It requires investigation, but there is no curative treatment.

CORNEAL OPACITIES

Generalised

Birth trauma. Causes splitting of Descemet's membrane which allows fluid into the cornea, causing opacification.

Congenital glaucoma. As 'birth trauma' above.

Sclerocornea. Developmental abnormality (no treatment).

Anterior chamber cleavage syndrome. Incomplete formation of the structures bordering the anterior chamber.

Mucolipidosis type IV. Other metabolic causes are *very* unusual at birth.

Localised

Birth trauma

Congenital glaucoma

Dermoid tumours. The surface is irregular, unlike sclerocornea. Opacity spreads from the limbus.

Corneal ulceration. This is very rare and is usually caused by gonococcal or *Pseudomonas* infection. Use broad-spectrum antibiotic, e.g. ciprofloxacin.

ABNORMALITIES OF THE IRIS, PUPIL AND LENS

Absence (aniridia). This is frequently dominant with significant sequelae. Sporadic cases are associated with a chromosomal deletion (aniridia, hemihypertrohy, Wilm's tumour complex).

Cleft in inferior or inferonasal iris (coloboma). May be dominant. It is associated with a choroidal coloboma, frequently bilateral, which will affect the otherwise good prognosis.

Eccentric pupil (corectopia). May be dominant. It is associated with glaucoma or subluxation of the lens, otherwise good prognosis.

Unequal pupils (anisocoria)
- Usually idiopathic abnormality with no associations and good prognosis
- Horner's syndrome
- Third cranial nerve lesion.

Albinism
- May be generalised (recessive) or ocular albinism (X-linked recessive)
- Lacking melanin pigment in the iris and retina
- Albinos develop macula hypoplasia, poor acuity and nystagmus.

Cataract. This may be an isolated finding with variable inheritance (usually dominant). It may be found in a variety of other conditions (although in many it may develop after birth):

- intrauterine infection (e.g. rubella)
- metabolic disorders (e.g. galactosaemia)
- chromosomal abnormalities (e.g. trisomy 13, 18, 21, Turner's syndrome)
- with other ocular abnormalities (e.g. microphthalmia)
- various other syndromes.

Surgical advice is necessary.

Leucocoria (a white reflex from behind the pupil). This signifies a serious problem such as:
- retinoblastoma
- cataract
- coloboma of the choroid
- persistent hyperplastic primary vitreous
- cicatricial retinopathy of prematurity
- infection — *Toxoplasma*, CMV, herpes simplex
- Norrie's disease and incontinentia pigmenti.

RETINAL ABNORMALITIES

Most retinal pathology requires urgent ophthalmological referral. Investigation and treatment will then usually be directed by the ophthalmologist. Other pathology may comprise the following.

Retinal haemorrhage. Localised haemorrhages may occur following facial congestion, trauma or hypoxia. They may be rounded (under the internal limiting membrane) or flame-shaped (in the nerve fibre layer). They disappear spontaneously, usually without sequelae.

Congenital toxoplasmosis. Choroidoretinitis presents as a white destructive lesion with surrounding dark pigment proliferation. The disease process has usually ceased by birth but the eye may be blind if the macula is involved.

Retinopathy of prematurity

ROP develops as a proliferative retinopathy following retinal ischaemia mainly in very premature infants. It is more common and more likely to be severe in the most immature survivors born before 26 weeks gestation, in whom as many as 14% will need treatment. The precise aetiology and clinical predisposition are poorly understood beyond this but hyperoxia seems to be a potent cause of retinal vasoconstriction and should be avoided in the first weeks after very preterm birth (keep P_aO_2 7–10 kPa). Swings in perfusion, oxygenation and hypocarbia, which may also cause vasoconstriction, should also be avoided if possible. During recovery from retinal ischaemia (probably after the first month) allowing the child to be relatively hypoxic may be equally harmful: as children recover from severe lung disease, higher P_aO_2 values are accepted in line with values found in babies without lung disease.

In clinical practice, ROP is confined to very immature or very small babies and screening is aimed at the early detection of advancing disease in these groups. Screening is performed by an experienced ophthalmologist using indirect ophthalmoscopy via an aspheric lens under cycloplegia. With early detection and treatment, blindness due to ROP seems to be largely preventable.

It is critical that neonatal units establish fail-safe protocols for the identification of at-risk babies and ensure their referral for screening at the appropriate time.

- It is the responsibility of the neonatal staff to ensure that screening is commenced at the correct time.
- Once commenced, it is the responsibility of the ophthalmologist to continue the screening process.
- Communication between clinical neonatal staff and the ophthalmologist accepting responsibility for screening is thus of great importance.

Cycloplegia is induced with cyclopentolate 0.5% (or homatropine 1%) and phenylephrine 2.5%.

Screening criteria are infants born <31 weeks *or* <1501 g birthweight:

- Births <26 weeks gestation — commence at 6 weeks and then 2-weekly until 36 weeks gestational age equivalent or active progression has ceased.
- Births >25 weeks gestation — commence at 6 weeks and repeat at 36 weeks gestation if normal at first exam; 2-weekly otherwise as above.

The importance of ensuring that screening appointments are not missed must be stressed. Disease which requires intervention should be treated rapidly following identification (usually within a week at the latest). *Babies who have not completed their screening programme and are discharged home or back to referring neonatal units must be identified and measures taken to ensure that the process is completed.*

Progression of ROP is classified according to an international staging scheme:

- Stage 1 — Flat demarcation line between pink, normally vascularised posterior retina and white unvascularised ischaemic peripheral anterior retina
- Stage 2 — Demarcation line extends up into vitreous in a ridge

- Stage 3 — New vessels elevated into vitreous cavity from ridge, with or without vitreous haemorrhage
- Stage 4 — Traction retinal detachment (extra-foveal or involving the fovea)
- Stage 5 — Complete retinal detachment

'Plus' is added to each grading if there are dilated and tortuous retinal vessels in the posterior retina, iris vessel engorgement and rigidity or a vitreous haze, and implies active progressive disease.

Furthermore, the surface area of the retina is classified into three zones:

- *Zone 1* — a radius of 30° from the optic disc
- *Zone 2* — a circle from the peripheral of the nasal retina around the anatomic equator of the eye
- *Zone 3* — the residual crescent of temporal retina

If the worst stage that develops is 1 or 2, the process will generally resolve without major sequelae. Higher stages are termed 'threshold' disease if there are at least five contiguous clock hours or eight cumulative clock hours of disease in zone 1 or 2. Threshold disease requires treatment with laser or cryotherapy to halt progression. There is accumulating evidence that laser treatment is associated with better outcomes than cryotherapy and earlier treatment (of stage 2 'plus' disease) may improve outcomes further. 'Posterior disease' is where the retinal vascularisation is halted in the central retina near the macula (zone 1) and is a feature of the most immature babies, whose retinal vascularisation is minimal at birth. Laser treatment may be most effective for these cases.

Refraction errors may follow resolved ROP that has not progressed to stage 4 disease, and regular ophthalmological follow-up is usually indicated for babies who have received treatment.

FURTHER READING

Royal College of Ophthalmologists & British Association of Perinatal Medicine (1995) Retinopathy of prematurity: guidelines for screening and treatment – report of a joint working party. London: Royal College of Ophthalmologists and British Association of Perinatal Medicine.

EIGHTEEN

Neonatal skin

Background

The skin is the interface between the infant and his carers, both visually and microbiologically. You must be familiar with the wide range of common blemishes which the parents may be concerned about and the much smaller number of significant lesions which require further investigation and treatment. The best source of information about neonatal skin disorders is a colour atlas.

Infants born before the last trimester usually have an absence of subcutaneous fat and the skin may be covered by fine lanugo hair which is usually shed in the last 2 weeks of gestation. The preterm infant has a thin poorly keratinised stratum corneum which renders the infant's skin more vulnerable to the passage of water, drugs and bacteria and more susceptible to trauma. Transepidermal water loss is high leading to high, evaporative heat losses (see Ch. 3). However, with increasing postnatal age, there is the rapid development of an effective epidermal barrier, so that by about 2 weeks of postnatal age, even the most preterm infant has an insensible water loss through the skin comparable to that of the term infant. Sweating occurs in term infants from birth in response to a warm environment, and palmar sweating can be measured as a response to pain or stress in term infants. However, sweating is absent in infants below 36 weeks gestation at birth but will appear in most infants by about 2 weeks of postnatal age. Fragile preterm infant is easily damaged by the fixation of monitoring probes or ECG electrodes and desquamation can occur following the removal of adhesive tape used to secure IV cannulae. Because the skin of the newborn infant is thinner, all drugs and topical agents pass through it more easily and may lead to toxic systemic levels. Infants lying in pools of cleansing solutions containing antiseptic or alcohol may suffer local burns or reach sedative levels of alcohol in the bloodstream.

In the term infant, the skin is often covered with vernix caseosa derived from sebaceous glands and from cells which have been shed. Vernix may be particularly marked in a post-mature infant. The skin of term or preterm infants may appear very pink in the first few days after birth due to vasomotor instability.

Routine skin care in the newborn

- Excess vernix may be wiped off, the scalp and the face cleaned, particularly of blood, but the baby should not be bathed immediately because of the risk of evaporative heat loss.
- Infant skin is more vulnerable to irritants than adult skin and therefore infants should be cleaned with warm water and non-medicated, non-perfumed soap.
- Sites of trauma that may serve as an entry site for infection (e.g. fetal scalp electrode puncture marks) should be observed daily. There is no indication for routine topical antibiotics.
- The umbilical cord will usually slough off within a week. Delayed separation of the cord is a genuine but neither specific nor sensitive sign of immune deficiency. There is no indication for the routine use of antibiotic powders or sprays. Umbilical granulomas can be treated with a silver nitrate swab. Wear gloves to avoid getting black hands and cover skin around the umbilicus with liquid paraffin to prevent burning.

Nappy rash

This is usually a contact dermatitis, but secondary infection may occur. Risk factors are:

- neonatal skin is thin and susceptible to irritants
- poor hygiene and prolonged contact with urine and faeces
- urea-splitting organisms cause ammoniacal dermatitis
- secondary *Candida* infection
- change from breast feeding to formula feeds.

Most infants in the UK now wear disposable nappies, and therefore contact dermatitis with detergents is rare.

MANAGEMENT

- Use disposable nappies and change frequently to keep the area clean and dry.
- Expose to air whenever feasible.
- Apply emollient (e.g. zinc and castor oil cream) after every change.
- Apply topical nystatin ointment (for *Candida* infection) four times a day until 7 days after the last lesion has cleared.
- Apply 1% hydrocortisone 6-hourly for 1 week if the above measures are ineffective.
- Preterm infants can develop severe perineal excoriation, particularly if they are under phototherapy or have

malabsorption. These infants are best nursed prone in the incubator with their perineum completely exposed.

If napkin rash is resistant to the above measures, consider rarer causes such as psoriasis, contact dermatitis from fucidin cream, and acrodermatitis enteropathica (due to zinc deficiency).

Normal variants

MILIA

Term infants, especially those who are breast-fed, may develop multiple white or yellow cysts approximately 1 mm in diameter. They:

- are common on the nose and cheeks
- occur in almost half of normal term infants and may be widespread
- are due to blocked sebaceous follicles and require no treatment.

NEONATAL ACNE

- Due to sebaceous gland hyperplasia.
- Can be treated with 0.5% salicylic acid in aqueous cream.
- Associated with other self-limiting maternal hormone effects:
  — gynaecomastia
  — secretion of breast milk ('witch's milk')
  — withdrawal vaginal bleeding.
- If severe or prolonged, suspect a virilising syndrome.

MILIARIA

- One of the commonest neonatal rashes.
- 1–2 mm pink papules most common over the forehead, trunk and back.
- Appear to be induced by warm environments.
- No treatment is indicated.

ERYTHEMA TOXICUM

- An extremely common fleeting maculopapular rash.
- Occurring in half of normal term infants typically around the third to fourth day.
- May appear to have a white *or yellow* centre with blotchy macular erythema surrounding this.
- The cause is unknown and it disappears by the end of the first week.
- No treatment is required.

If the papules proceed to form pustules and there is concern about infection, the pustule can be pricked with an orange (25 g) needle and the contents smeared onto a glass slide. When stained, these will show copious éosinophils.

HARLEQUIN COLOUR CHANGE

The change comes on abruptly, with one side of the baby appearing pale and a sharp midline demarcation from the other side of the baby which remains pink. Alternatively, the upper part of the body may become paler than the lower half. It is attributed to vasomotor immaturity, is of no significance and rarely persists beyond the first week.

LIVEDO RETICULARIS

This is sometimes also known as cutis marmorata (marble skin). There is a common pattern seen in the newborn, again attributed to vasomotor instability, it is of no significance.

SUCKING BLISTERS

These may be present at birth, usually on a hand or wrist, and they are due to the fetus sucking in utero. They may develop on the midline of the upper lip a few days after the onset of feeding. No treatment is necessary.

Common naevi

The lay term for a naevus is a birthmark. Histologically, a naevus is a benign lesion which contains only normal tissue (i.e. no malignant tissue), but the proportions of the constituent elements are different from a normally developed organ. For example, a pigmented naevus contains an excess of melanocytes, whereas a haemangioma contains an excess of vascular elements.

Mongolian blue spots

These are found in 90% of non-caucasian infants. Despite the name, they are not confined to Mongolian children or even Chinese children but are found in children from the Indian subcontinent, Africa, the Caribbean and the Mediterranean. The lumbosacral region and buttocks are most commonly involved. The lesions may be greyish-blue or bluish-black in colour and are irregular in shape varying from 2 to 10 cm in diameter. A benign Mongolian spot is never elevated or palpable. They may fade as the child gets older and are of no consequence. If the lesion is elevated or associated with a hairy patch, this should be assessed in the newborn period by a dermatologist as there is a risk of malignant change in such giant, hairy naevi.

Melanocytic naevi

These are much rarer at birth than in later childhood when various brown spots and freckles are extremely common.

Capillary haemangioma (port wine naevus)

This is a circumscribed defect of dermal capillaries. It may be seen in two forms. At its mildest, it may appear as a salmon patch or 'stork mark' which is most commonly seen on the eyelids, forehead and nape of the neck. These are of no consequence, are extremely common and usually fade as the child becomes older.

If the lesion is more extensive and deeper in colour, it is known as a port wine stain. These are present at birth, often on the face, and usually continue to grow with the infant and may become darker. All three sensory divisions of the trigeminal nerve area may be involved, but only involvement of the ophthalmic division of the fifth nerve is accompanied by neuro-ocular involvement (Sturge–Weber syndrome). If the ophthalmic area is involved, 60% will have involvement of vessels on the ipsilateral side of the brain and there are risks of seizures, mental retardation and glaucoma. Truncal lesions associated with spinal vascular anomalies may lead to limb hypertrophy (Klippel–Trenaunay–Weber syndrome). Parents should not be misled that a port wine stain will disappear. An honest answer is to say that with the advent of laser treatment and improved cosmetics, the stigma can be greatly reduced.

Cavernous haemangioma (strawberry naevus)

These are less common than capillary haemangiomas and again can be relatively minor or very significant. Small 'strawberry marks' are found in 1 in 10 infants during the neonatal period, more common in girls and preterm infants, and although they usually increase in size over the first few years of life, they mostly disappear completely. They do not require treatment unless they are causing problems with bleeding (usually those on the scrotum or perineum and occluded by a nappy) or interfering with vision or swallowing.

The larger cavernous haemangioma may be extremely unsightly, particularly if on the face, and may be several centimetres in diameter. These may be extremely vascular and haemorrhage or ulceration may occur. Further complication is the Kasabach-Merritt syndrome in which thrombocytopenia and high output cardiac failure occur as a result of the large arterial-venous communications. Kasabach-Merritt syndrome justifies treatment with systemic steroids. Most of these larger lesions will also involute with time but they may not disappear completely. A paediatric dermatologist can advise on the place of laser therapy.

APLASIA CUTIS (CONGENITAL ABSENCE OF SKIN)

This is seen most frequently in the midline of the posterior scalp; it is 1–2 cm in diameter and devoid of hair. This is usually idiopathic but may also be associated with in utero chickenpox infection and trisomies. The lesion usually heals slowly, but plastic surgery may be required.

PIGMENTATION ABNORMALITIES OF SKIN

Café-au-lait spots

These may occasionally be apparent at birth as an isolated anomaly. The hyperpigmented café-au-lait spots of neuro-fibromatosis are rarely present at birth but they may be preceded by depigmented patches, visible at the newborn check, which subsequently disappear and are replaced by pigmented patches during the first year. Neurofibromatosis should be strongly suspected in any newborn infant with more than three café-au-lait spots (especially if any of the spots are larger than 3 cm) and particularly if there is a positive family history.

Albright's syndrome

In the newborn period there may be large irregular pigmented areas up to 10 cm in diameter. The bony lesions and endocrine disorders appear later.

Peutz–Jegher syndrome

Multiple hyperpigmented macules may be present at birth, especially around the nose and mouth and on the mucous membranes of the mouth. Bowel problems only develop later.

Giant hairy naevus (bathing trunk naevus)

This lesion is present at birth and may be very extensive. The lesion is darkly pigmented with a large amount of hair and a hard consistency. There may be other areas of pigmentation on the remaining skin. Surgical removal is extremely difficult and over 10% of these lesions progress to malignant melanoma.

HYPOPIGMENTATION

Albinism

This is an autosomal recessive disorder in which the skin is very pale, the hair is blond and the iris is translucent and may appear pink. The fundus is very pale. The newborn infant may present with coarse nystagmus and photophobia, and advice must be given that the infant should be protected from ultraviolet light.

Piebaldism

This is also known as partial albinism with some areas of pigmented skin and some pale areas. A white forelock is seen in

Waardenburg's syndrome (congenital deafness) and in some types of long segment Hirschsprung's disease (which may lead to neonatal intestinal obstruction).

Vitiligo

Patchy areas of decreased or absent pigmentation. Lesions are only occasionally present at birth and usually develop later in childhood.

Tuberous sclerosis

Depigmented ash leaf macules are rarely present in the newborn period but may be seen with the aid of a Wood's lamp. Infants with tuberous sclerosis may also have café-au-lait spots.

Blisters, vesicles and bullae

Blistering occurs more readily in the neonate. Some of these disorders are infective and respond to treatment, whereas others have important genetic implications and may be fatal so that early diagnosis is important.

HEREDITARY CAUSES

Non-scarring

Autosomal recessive epidermolysis bullosa lethalis. This may be very severe and lead to miscarriage, stillbirth or a very ill neonate. The bullae heal poorly, infection is a real risk, and the mouth, oesophagus and other mucosal surfaces may be involved. However, despite the name, the condition is not uniformly lethal. (Autosomal dominant epidermolysis bullosa simplex does not develop in the newborn period but in the older child when the skin is subject to trauma. Lesions heal without scarring.)

Cockayne–Weber's syndrome. Bullous eruption of hands and feet.

Incontinentia pigmenti. This is a rare disorder, probably X-linked dominant, in which only female infants survive to birth. In the newborn period there may be bullae which precede the characteristic pigmented warty linear lesions which appear around the first month of age.

Scarring

Autosomal dominant epidermolysis bullosa dystrophica. Again, this disorder usually presents in older childhood when the skin is subject to trauma, but it does heal with scarring. Nails may also be affected.

Autosomal recessive epidermolysis bullosa dystrophica. This may present at birth and may be generalised or localised. Infection is a risk and the oesophagus may be involved. The nails and hair may be affected and due to scar formation, pseudo-webbing of the fingers may occur.

INFILTRATIVE DISEASES

Urticaria pigmentosa. This may present at birth as a generalised bullous eruption which may be localised, diffuse or systemic (bones, liver, spleen, lymph nodes and GI tract are involved). Pigmentation may not appear until 6 months of age.

Langerhans' cell histiocytosis. This may present in the newborn period with a skin rash which may resemble chickenpox, or there may be multiple purple papules which involve the palms and soles. Further investigation should include skin biopsy, liver function tests, clotting studies, skeletal survey and CXR.

INFECTIONS (see also Ch. 13)

Bacterial infections
- Staphylococcal infection
  - Bullous impetigo — sometimes confusingly called 'neonatal pemphigus'
  - Scalded skin syndrome — this is also known as Lyell's or Ritter's disease.
- Listeriosis
- Congenital syphilis.

Viral infections
- Congenital varicella zoster
- Congenital herpes simplex (type II).

DRUG REACTION

Toxic epidermal necrolysis. This is clinically similar to scalded skin syndrome but the mucous membranes may also be involved. There are no bacterial organisms on Gram stain or culture of blister fluid, unless the lesions have become secondarily infected. There may be a drug aetiology.

TRAUMA

Sucking blisters may occur on the fingers, lip and forearms and require no treatment.

Non-bullous skin infections (see also Ch. 13)

- Superficial skin sepsis due to staphylococcal infection
- Paronychia
- Umbilical infection due to group A *Streptococcus* or *Staph. aureus*
- *Candida*
- Congenital rubella and CMV.

Ichthyoses

These are characterised by increased keratinisation leading to dry skin with scaling.

Sex-linked ichthyosis. This affects only males and onset is in the first few weeks of life. There are large pigmented scales on the trunk and there may be corneal opacity.

Congenital non-bullous ichthyosiform erythroderma. This is an autosomal recessive disorder which may present as a collodion baby (see below). Alternatively, the baby may be born as a harlequin fetus (i.e. covered in markedly thickened plates of skin with deep red fissures between these 'armour plates'). Skin rigidity may limit respiration.

Congenital bullous ichthyosiform erythroderma. This is autosomal dominant and bullae may appear within days of birth. These bullae eventually are replaced with hyperkeratotic areas.

Collodion baby. The baby is born encased in a shiny membrane and this membrane may be shed, sometimes after several recurrences, after a number of weeks to reveal an underlying ichthyosis. In the milder form, it may be the result of placental insufficiency or post-maturity and when the covering dries and peals normal skin subsequently develops.

Ectodermal dysplasia

Most cases are male, suggesting X-linked recessive inheritance. The skin is smooth and dry due to absent or reduced sweating and in the newborn this may lead to hyperthermia.

Acrodermatitis enteropathica

- Due to zinc deficiency.
- Erythematous rash affects the hands, feet, face and genital or perianal area.
- There may also be scaling and even blisters evolving into crusts and pustules.
- There may also be a glossitis or stomatitis.
- Diarrhoea and failure to thrive.

Infantile eczema

This is extremely common in infancy although less so in the immediate newborn period. In 70% of cases there is a family history of atopy. Infantile eczema may also be a feature of cow's milk protein intolerance in a formula-fed infant, and in those with a very strong positive family history of atopy, the infantile eczema may be exacerbated by a breast-feeding mother who is eating dairy products. The treatment of infantile eczema usually involves only aqueous cream and, for the more severe lesions, 1% hydrocortisone. This should be used sparingly, as topical corticosteroids are easily absorbed across newborn skin.

NINETEEN

Orthopaedics

Congenital anomalies involving the musculoskeletal system

These includes limb malformations, malformation of the digits and arthrogryposis multiplex congenita (see Ch. 4).

Deformations

The various congenital postural deformities are listed in Table 19.1. Only a few of the main ones will be considered here. Their importance stems from the fact that they are common and, with early treatment, are usually easily correctable, because growth is proceeding rapidly and the tissues are still relatively plastic.

Table 19.1 Musculoskeletal deformations present at birth

Site	Deformation
Skull	Dolichocephaly (flattening from side to side)
	Plagiocephaly (asymmetry)
	Brachycephaly (occipital flattening)
	Depressions in skull
Face	Potter's facies
	Nasal and oral deformities
	Mandibular asymmetry
	Retrognathia
	Midline cleft palate (Pierre–Robin anomalad)
	Facial nerve palsy
Neck	Sternomastoid 'tumour'
Upper limbs	Dislocation of the shoulder
	Radial nerve palsy
Body	Pigeon chest
	Pectus excavatum
	Postural scoliosis

Table 19.1 *cont'd*

Site	Deformation
Lower limbs	Dislocation of the hips
	Bowing of the long bones
	Genu recurvatum
	Foot deformities (talipes equinovarus, calcaneovalgus and metatarsus varus)
	Sciatic and obturator nerve palsies
Whole body	Arthrogryposis multiplex congenita
	Generalised compression (as in Potter sequence)

NB. Not all cases of the conditions noted here are always due to mechanical factors (e.g. cleft palate and arthrogryposis).

CONGENITAL STERNOMASTOID TORTICOLLIS ('TUMOUR')

- A unilateral condition, present in approximately 1 in 300 births.
- Often there is associated plagiocephaly and invariably the jaw is tilted away from the affected side.
- Contracture of the sternomastoid may be demonstrated by turning the chin towards the shoulder on the affected side. Normally the head may be rotated so that the chin points over the back of the shoulder. When significant contracture is present, the chin will not turn as far as the front of the shoulder.
- As granulation forms in the damaged muscle, a tumour develops and is usually first palpable at about 2 weeks of age.
- Stretching the damaged muscle is the only useful treatment, consisting of passive gentle stretching which the mother may be taught to do. This is usually taught by the physiotherapist. Early presentation is rare and some sources recommend delaying physiotherapy for the first 4 weeks or so after birth. Most present at 4–6 weeks and may be commenced on physiotherapy straight away.
- Very occasionally, a tenotomy and neck collar may be required later in the first 1–2 years.

CONGENITAL POSTURAL SCOLIOSIS

- A single, gentle spinal curve, not to be confused with the usually more angular scoliosis due to malformation of the spine.
- Occurs in approximately 1 in 1000 births.
- If the spine is not examined routinely for lateral flexion, the condition is easily missed until the infant sits.

- Examination is best carried out by lifting the laterally lying infant from the bed with a hand under the baby's side just under the rib cage. This is then repeated on the other side.
- If suspected, X-ray the spine in full lateral flexion to each side.
- Referral to and follow-up by the orthopaedic team are required.

CONGENITAL DISLOCATION OF THE HIP (CDH)

- Approximately 1.5% of all newborn infants have either dislocation of the hip (10%) or hips that are dislocatable (90%) at birth.
- CDH is 4 times more common in girls than in boys, and 10 times more common following breech presentation. Examination should also be particularly careful if there is a family history of CDH or if other deformities such as talipes are apparent.
- While many of these hips will stabilise without treatment, some will not and others may destabilise or become dysplastic later in infancy.
- Early diagnosis and treatment of all cases offer the safest and most satisfactory outcome.
- Examine every baby's hips for dislocation at the neonatal screening examination. The hips should also be carefully examined at 6–12 weeks but in addition the hips should be assessed at each clinical assessment until the child has a stable gait at 18–24 months of age.
- If the initial screening for CDH is being undertaken by a relatively inexperienced examiner, it is essential that suspect hips be checked again on the same day by a more experienced colleague.

Examination

The examination technique is described in Chapter 3 (p. 54). Experience in hip examination may be acquired through use of a teaching simulator such as the 'Baby Hippy'.

Static and dynamic US examination of the hips offers a useful adjunct to diagnosis and follow-up surveillance during the first 6 months. It may also be used for back-up screening of infants at high risk of CDH. With further experience, it may prove safe to observe without splinting a proportion of newborn infants with hip instability whose static US morphology falls within normal limits.

Radiological examination is of limited value in the first 3 months but then becomes progressively more useful, for the assessment of the acetabular shape and status of the upper femoral epiphysis (95% present by 9 months of age).

Management

Most neonatal services have developed their own system of screening and referral and you should be aware of local practice. Where this is unclear, the following has been a safe method of management for some time:

- Dislocatable hips usually resolve after 4–6 weeks. Treat with a plastic over-nappy abduction splint (the Aberdeen splint), which may be removed by the mother when changing the nappies. If the hip is still unstable at 6 weeks, continue treatment until 12 weeks or consider orthopaedic referral.
- Dislocated hips should be treated for 6 weeks in a metal abduction splint such as a von Rosen splint, although some doctors now favour the Pavlik harness, followed by a similar period in an Aberdeen splint. Pressure should never be used to achieve abduction because tension of the adductor muscle may lead to ischaemic necrosis of the femoral head. Abduction should not exceed 80° and enlocation may be checked by USS examination in the splint.
- If there is a limitation of abduction at any time, seek orthopaedic advice. If the hip is still unstable at 3 months, perform USS or X-ray (single adducted AP film of hips) and seek orthopaedic advice.
- All cases should be followed up with clinical and radiological examination at 6–9 months. Where hips were dislocated at birth or remained unstable for longer than the initial period of splinting, it is prudent to follow up until a stable gait has been achieved.

The parents

Explain that the hip joint is lax because the baby has been tightly curled up in the womb, and the ligaments softened by pregnancy hormones. Explain that this is quite a common finding, that the baby is not abnormally formed in any way, is not in pain, and that, with early treatment with the legs kept wide for a few weeks, full recovery is the rule. Also explain that there will be no reason why the child should not be entirely normal. It is essential to ensure that the parents are not unnecessarily worried or distressed and also that they know how to handle the baby and splint.

CLUB FOOT

Foot deformities affect approximately 1 in 250 babies; there are three main types:

- Talipes calcaneovalgus — commonest variety; may be associated with CDH
- Talipes equinovarus or 'club foot'

- Metatarsus varus — may be acquired during the early weeks, if the infant is nursed prone with the weight of the leg resting on the forefoot; this should be avoided as the deformity is often difficult to treat and tends to give rise to problems when shoes are worn.

In mild deformities, the infant can move its foot into the neutral position, and gentle manipulation overcorrects the deformity; treatment is unlikely to be required.

Where such correction is not achieved, institute treatment at once. This may range from passive exercises, to strapping or splinting in overcorrection, to surgery. All severe cases should be photographed and referred to an orthopaedic surgeon as the ligaments of the feet tend to tighten up within a day or two of birth, making correction more difficult.

Each hospital should have a system for early referral to an orthopaedic surgeon for more serious deformities.

TWENTY

Death

Sensitive caring and supportive management of death benefit the family and may help to avoid later misunderstandings or distress. Whenever possible, the death of a baby should be planned, managed and consultant-led after extensive discussion with the family.

Death on the labour suite

Babies may die soon after birth. This may be a very preterm infant or an infant with a severe congenital anomaly such that a decision has been made in advance, in concert with the parents, not to intervene. Alternatively, resuscitation may have been abandoned in the face of poor response or overt severe abnormality. In these circumstances, the parents should be asked if they wish to hold their baby, but they may be in such profound shock that this is not possible. They may find it is only possible after some time has elapsed. Parents deserve sympathetic care and as much time as they need to come to terms with this loss. Senior advice should be sought. Do not ask for postmortem permission immediately (but see immediate investigation on p. 349). Liaise with the midwives and revisit. Discuss follow-up with obstetric colleagues and offer a joint meeting.

Whenever possible, infants with severe congenital anomalies not compatible with survival should be admitted to the neonatal unit so that the death of the baby can be managed by the whole neonatal team.

Death on the neonatal unit

There are a number of guiding principles:

- The needs of individuals differ. Therefore staff must be sensitive to the requirements of families regardless of race, colour, nationality or religious beliefs.

- The dying baby and the family should be cared for by a team of nurse, paediatrician and, if they wish, religious advisor to coordinate their care.
- Parents should be fully involved at all times in the decisions about caring for their dying baby.
- The legal requirements regarding documentation of death should be dealt with smoothly and be supported by written information, to minimise stress for the parents.
- Brain death criteria do not apply to deaths in the newborn period *although the diagnosis may be established in term infants from the age of 2 months (see Ch. 12).*

On neonatal units, approximately one-third of deaths follow withdrawal of active treatment. When a baby is deteriorating despite full intensive care, this knowledge must be shared with the parents. If the parents, having understood the seriousness of what has been said, respond by saying that they continue to want everything to be done, then this is an important factor to be taken into account in planning future treatment. On the other hand, the parents may feel the continuation of intensive care is inappropriate, distressing and hopeless. Most parents do not respond at either of these extremes but make it clear that they understand the situation and know we will endeavour to make the right decisions for their baby whilst sharing with them all that is happening. In this way, the whole of the team caring for the baby and the family will move together over a period of time to a point where they are all in agreement that the baby is dying and that the continuation of intensive care is no longer appropriate. 'Caring for life' then needs to become 'caring for death', which is not the same as withdrawal of all care entirely.

WHEN NOT TO RESUSCITATE AND WHEN TO STOP (see also Chs 1 and 3)

The Royal College of Paediatrics and Child Health acknowledge five situations where the witholding or withdrawal of curative treatment might be considered, three of which apply to the newborn:

- The 'no chance' situation — the child has such severe disease that treatment only delays death without alleviating suffering.
- The 'no purpose' situation — the degree of physical or mental impairment will be too great.
- The 'unbearable' situation — in the face of progressive and irreversible illness, further treatment over and above what the child is receiving is more than can be borne.

The other two situations (brain death and permanent vegetative state) do not apply to the newborn.

Examples from neonatal practice include:

- non-resuscitation of a baby at birth with a congenital abnormality that is incompatible with survival
- non-resuscitation of a baby born at 23 weeks gestation or less when parents accept that survival without serious impairment is extrememly unlikely
- withdrawal of artificial ventilation from a baby with profound brain damage

Death on the neonatal unit can often be anticipated to some extent and withdrawal planned during the day when there are sufficient staff to support the parents. Hopefully, death is anticipated at least enough to allow you to:

- call both parents
- try to explain the situation to both parents together, not separately
- call the chaplain if the parents wish
- ask about baptism; in extreme circumstances, a lay person can baptise a child by following the order of service as printed
- nominate a key worker (nurse, doctor or chaplain) who can guarantee uninterrupted time with the parent.

If the baby dies before the parents arrive, try to intercept them so that they can be given the news in a private room rather than on the open ward. There is no easy way to tell parents that their child has died but some useful guides are given below:

- The environment in which the news is given is very important. It should be quiet, private and with sufficient chairs for the whole family. Ideally, there should be no pagers or telephones in the room
- It is reassuring to say that the child did not suffer
- The parents should decide when and how other family members should be told. Generally, parents should tell the other children and there is little to be gained by delaying this or using euphemisms. Siblings must grieve as well as parents.

If a decision is taken to electively discontinue treatment, the parents must be asked whether they wish to be present at the time of discontinuation of ventilation and whether they wish to hold the child afterwards. If parents are resident on the unit, it may be appropriate to transfer the baby to the parents' accommodation while still ventilated. The procedure for discontinuing treatment is as follows:

- Discontinue all infusions.
- Remove the NG tube, ETT, peripheral arterial and venous cannulae and apply a pressure dressing to avoid blood leakage.

Both doctor and a nurse should be present when the ETT is removed.

- Do not remove chest drain, central venous or umbilical catheters, transanastomotic or gastrostomy tubes, urethral catheters; clamp all such tubes.
- Dress or swaddle the child and take a photograph for the parents; give the child to the parents and ask whether they wish to be alone or accompanied.

Checklist of who to inform of a neonatal death

- GP
- Consultant paediatrician (and arrange bereavement counselling in 6 weeks)
- Consultant obstetrician, postnatal ward and community midwife
- Referring hospital if in utero or postnatal transfer
- Health visitor
- Pathologist if there will be a postmortem
- Coroner, if relevant (see below)
- Clinical geneticist, if relevant
- Hospital administration, to avoid further appointments being sent.

Counselling

The parents can be given a 'memory box' containing items such as a lock of hair, photographs, clothing, cot labels etc. Parents should be reassured that they can view the body again at any time in the chapel of rest.

Bereavement is a long process with several phases and the family require continued support. All parents should be given a follow-up appointment with a consultant paediatrician, even if the baby died on the labour suite, not more than 6 weeks after the death and sometimes sooner. At follow-up, the parents' questions can be addressed, any conclusions from the autopsy communicated and a check made that the grieving process is occurring. The feelings of any siblings should also be discussed.

Certification of death

The most senior doctor present should write in the notes:

- the discussions with the parents leading up to the withdrawal of intensive care

- the time of death
- the examination performed to certify death
- the causes of death as completed in the death certificate (unless a coroner's postmortem will be performed in which case a death certificate should *not* be completed).

DEATH CERTIFICATES

There are different death certificates for neonatal (< 28 days old) deaths and older children. The body cannot be released, buried or cremated until the death certificate has been completed and this should not be deferred pending the outcome of a postmortem, unless this is a coroner's postmortem. Cremation forms are separate from death certificates. If the parents wish the baby to be cremated, a doctor who has cared for the baby in life and seen the body after death should complete the cremation form as soon as possible.

Postmortem requests

Neonatal postmortem rates as high as 80% can be achieved by a sensitive approach involving senior staff. The postmortem acts as an important audit of clinical care, imaging and diagnosis during life and may alter the diagnosis sufficiently to influence subsequent counselling. In cases where there are no unexpected finding, the postmortem is still of value as it helps parents and staff to know that nothing has been missed and that nothing more could have been done.

The request for a postmortem should be undertaken by a senior doctor and not be broached immediately after death.

If for medical interest, explain the reason to the parents. They may be reassured to know that the postmortem incisions are not visible when the child is dressed and that it does not delay their funeral arrangements. The finding may alter couselling of future pregnancies. Written consent should be obtained. This must be from the mother if the parents are not married. If the parents do not wish to consent to a full postmortem, they should be asked whether they would consider limited postmortem of the relevant organs or biopsies of specific organs.

If the case is reported to the coroner (cause of death unknown, no medical practitioner attended the death, death duuring operation or before recovery from anaesthesia, suspicious circumstances), the parents have no control over the decision regarding postmortem. We should usually speak with the coroner's officer when death follows a history of violence or 'accident' in pregnancy or perinatal asphyxia, even though the immediate cause of death is known. If the baby died at home or with the parents while 'rooming in', warm the parents that they may be interviewed by the police, that this is routine and does not imply suspicion of the parents.

Immediate investigation of an infant who dies unexpectedly on labour suite, the neonatal unit or postnatal ward

- Blood by cardiace puncture for bacterial culture.
- Blood by cardiac puncture to be spun, separated and the serum saved.
- Throat, ear and rectal swabs for viral and bacterial culture.
- SPA of urine for a metabolic screen.
- A punch skin biopsy from the axilla, placed in sterile saline and sent for fibroblast culture.
- Skeletal X-ray survey can be done at the time of postmortem.
- If an IEM is suspected, see Chapter 11 for appropriate investigations.

Death at home

In some circumstances, a baby may be transferred home to die. It is crucial that this is carefully planned, that the parents are not left in any doubt about what to expect, and that the parents know they can bring the baby back to the hospital at any time if they cannot cope. The local ambulance service, the GP and the local A&E department should all be sent written, signed confirmation that the infant is not to be resuscitated if this has been agreed with the parents. The parents should be given a supply of oral morphine to be administered to the baby if they feel the baby is distressed. It is very important that parents are reassured that their baby will not be allowed to suffer. The baby should be fed on demand.

Neonatal organ and tissue donation

At present in the UK no transplant teams are using organs or tissues from neonatal donors and it is therefore not appropriate to approach parents for this purpose. Neonatal corneas have been used in the past but this has now ceased.

TWENTY ONE

Procedures

Before performing any procedure for the first time, always observe it at least twice and then perform under supervision. Never have more than three attempts without getting a colleague to come and help. If this is not possible, at least have a break.

Airway-opening techniques

HEAD TILT, CHIN LIFT

- These should be performed before starting mask ventilation. The head should be tilted back gently to a neutral position (Fig. 21.1) and the chin lifted forward taking care not to compress the floor of the mouth.
- A folded towel placed under the neck and shoulders may help to maintain the neutral position.

ORAL SUCTION

- Use a 10FG (black) suction catheter for a term baby or where there is meconium. A 6FG (green) or 8FG (blue) catheter should be used for preterm infants.
- The pressure should not exceed 100 mmHg (13.3 kPa).
- Beware inserting the catheter too far and producing reflex vagal bradycardia.

Bag and mask/mask and Y-piece ventilation

- A mask which is big enough to cover the face from the bridge of the nose to below the mouth should be chosen (Fig. 21.2). A good seal must be obtained around the infant's face.
- When using a mask and Y-piece, the oxygen flow rate should be set at 5–8 L/min.
- When using a bag and mask system, use a 500 mL bag with a blow-off valve set at approximately 45 cmH$_2$O and an oxygen

Correct position

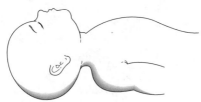

Too flexed

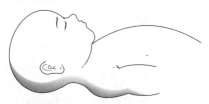

Too extended

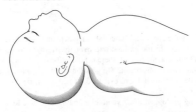

Fig. 21.1 Head tilt, chin lift. (Reproduced with permission from Resuscitation of Babies at Birth. Royal College of Paediatrics and Child Health, Royal College of Obstetricians and Gynaecologists, BMJ Publishing Group, 1997.)

flow rate of 5 L/min. The oxygen flow rate should be increased as indicated up to a maximum of 10 L/min.

- When a mask and Y-piece or bag, valve and mask system attached to a reservoir bag is used then the baby will receive the full concentration of oxygen delivered to the circuit. If no reservoir is used, the maximum concentration of oxygen provided will be approximately 40–60%.

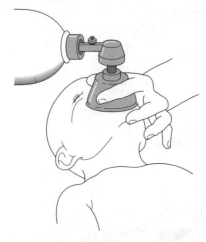

Fig. 21.2 Mask ventilation. (Reproduced with permission from Resuscitation of Babies at Birth. Royal College of Paediatrics and Child Health, Royal College of Obstetricians and Gynaecologists, BMJ Publishing Group, 1997.)

- Observe the chest wall for equal movement and auscultate both lung fields (in the axillae) and over the stomach to confirm equal bilateral air entry. If there is poor inflation, check that the airway is not obstructed. Re-position the head, making sure that the neck is not overextended. If necessary, perform oral suction.
- During prolonged mask ventilation, pass a NG tube to deflate the stomach.
- For details of ventilatory rates and pressures, see IPPV below.

Endotracheal intubation

Equipment
- ETT
  — size 3 for babies ≥32 weeks gestation
  — size 2.5 for babies <32 weeks gestation
- Straight-bladed laryngoscope
- Bag and valve system or Y system attached to pressure manometer to attach to ETT
- Suction equipment.

Procedure

1. Preoxygenate the baby using mask ventilation.
2. Hold the laryngoscope in the left hand and insert it into the right-hand corner of the baby's mouth so that the tip of the blade lies in the oesophagus.
3. Use the laryngoscope blade to sweep the tongue across to the midline.
4. Gently lift the laryngoscope forwards and upwards until the larynx and vocal cords come into view. Cricoid pressure either by an assistant or by using the little finger of the left hand may be helpful.
5. Hold the ETT with the right hand and gently insert it into the right-hand corner of the baby's mouth. Make sure not to obscure the view of the vocal cords.
6. Advance the tip of the ETT through the vocal cords for 1–2 cm. Some ETTs have a black marker to make identification of this distance easier. Approximate lengths of ETTs at the lips for infants of 1, 2 and 3 kg, respectively are 6.5, 7.5 and 9 cm.
7. Remove the laryngoscope. Attach the ETT to either a Y-piece and pressure manometer system or to a bag and valve system.
8. For details of ventilatory rates and pressures see IPPV below.
9. Observe chest movement and auscultate over both axillae and over the stomach to assess the correct position of the tube.
10. Fixate the ETT.
11. Once the baby is stable, organise a CXR to check the ETT position.

Important points

- No longer than 30 s should be spent in trying to intubate an infant before recommencing mask IPPV, for a minimum of 1 min.
- Never attach an intubated baby directly to either the wall oxygen supply or any supply of oxygen which is not connected to some type of pressure limit valve.

Intermittent positive pressure ventilation (IPPV)

- At delivery, the first 5 breaths should be held for 2 s to establish a functional residual capacity. If using a bag system, give the breaths as slowly as possible compressing the bag with the fingers for 1–2 s. The infant should then be ventilated at a rate of 30 breaths/min.
- The initial PIP will depend on the reasons the baby is being ventilated e.g.
  — 30 cmH$_2$O for first 5 breaths during resuscitation

immediately following delivery. Once the chest wall is moving, the inflation pressure may be reduced to 15–20 cmH_2O
— 20 cmH_2O for the previously spontaneously breathing infant being ventilated for RDS
— 16 cmH_2O for the infant being ventilated for apnoea
— the previous PIP for the infant requiring reintubation for a blocked ETT.

- When using a bag system compression with:
  — one finger and thumb $\cong 20$ cm H_2O
  — two fingers and thumb $\cong 25$ cm H_2O
  — three fingers and thumb $\cong 30$ cm H_2O
  — four fingers and thumb $\cong 35$ cm H_2O.

External cardiac massage

External cardiac massage must be started if HR is <60/min.

Procedure
1. There are two techniques (Fig. 21.3):
   — the chest is encircled with both hands so that the fingers lie behind the baby and the thumbs are opposed over the sternum
   — two fingers are used over the sternum.
2. The thumbs or fingers should be positioned 1 cm below the inter-nipple line.
3. Compress sufficiently hard to reduce the sternum to spine distance by half, at a finger rate of 120/min and a ratio of 3 ECM to 1 ventilation, i.e. 40 cycles/min.
4. ECM should continue until the heart rate is >80 bpm and increasing.

Blood sampling

CAPILLARY

Capillary heel prick blood can be used for blood gas, FBC and electrolyte estimation. An automated device should be used to prevent inserting the lancet too far and damaging the bone.

Equipment
- Alcohol swab
- Petroleum jelly
- Automated device with a sterile lancet.

Procedure
1. Clean heal with alcohol swab.

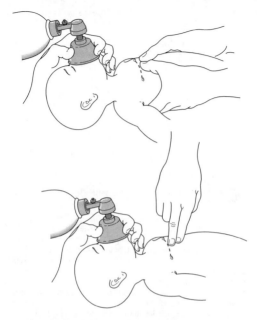

Fig. 21.3 External cardiac massage. (Reproduced with permission from Resuscitation of Babies at Birth. Royal College of Paediatrics and Child Health, Royal College of Obstetricians and Gynaecologists, BMJ Publishing Group, 1997.)

2. Smear a small amount of petroleum jelly onto the heel.
3. Prick the edge of the plantar surface of the heel beyond the lateral and medial limits of the calcaneus (Fig. 21.4).
4. Wait 20 s and then gently massage the heel to improve blood flow.
5. Avoid excessive squeezing which will increase the haematocrit and potassium values.
6. When sampling is complete, prevent further bleeding by compression with cotton wool for at least 30 s. Do not use Elastoplast.

VENOUS

The ideal site for venous sampling is the dorsum of the hand. If possible, avoid larger veins, e.g. the long saphenous, and those in

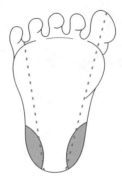

Fig. 21.4 Site for capillary blood sampling. Use plantar surface of heel (shaded areas).

the antecubital fossa as these may be required for long line insertion. If it is difficult to visualise the vein, use a cold light source held beneath the hand or foot to light up the veins.

Equipment
- Alcohol swab
- 21 g butterfly needle with the plastic tubing removed and if necessary the butterfly wings shortened. (Do not use a needle from which the hub has been removed as there have been reports of these becoming fully embedded within the baby.)

Procedure
1. Clean site with alcohol swab.
2. Insert butterfly needle bevel uppermost into vein.
3. Allow blood to drip out into bottles.
4. If collecting blood for blood culture drip the blood into a 2 mL syringe from which the plunger has been removed and which is attached to a 25 g needle. Immediately inject into blood culture bottle using a sterile technique. Other techniques for obtaining blood cultures include direct aspiration of blood from the hub of a freshly inserted IV cannula or direct aspiration via a butterfly needle from a large vein.
5. On completion of sampling remove the needle and compress the site with a piece of cotton wool for at least 1 min. Do not use Elastoplast.

SINGLE ARTERIAL PUNCTURE

Suitable sites are the radial and posterior tibial arteries. The dorsalis pedis can be used but is technically difficult and should be left to an experienced person. The femoral and brachial arteries are end arteries and should not be used. If more than a single ABG sample is anticipated then an arterial line (see p. 362) should be inserted in preference to performing a stab sample.

Equipment
- Alcohol swab
- 25g needle or heparinised butterfly needle
- Heparinised capillary tube or 2 mL syringe.

The equipment used will depend on the amount of blood required. For an ABG alone it may be easier to fill a heparinised capillary tube directly from the hub of the needle. If several blood samples are required, a syringe will be needed.

Radial artery. Located in the lateral third of the flexor aspect of the wrist.

Posterior tibial artery. Positioned behind the medial malleolus. Best located when the foot is gently dorsiflexed or in the neutral position.

Dorsalis pedis artery. Located between the first and second metatarsals. Best accessed with the foot partially plantarflexed.

Procedure (radial artery)
1. Clean site with alcohol swab.
2. Visualise the artery using a cold light source or palpate for arterial pulsation.
3. Confirm that the ulnar artery (located in the medial third to half of the flexor aspect of the wrist) is present by occluding the radial and ulnar arteries, causing the hand to blanch. Release the ulnar artery. The colour should return to the hand. Alternatively use a cold light source to visualise the two arteries.
4. Hold the wrist slightly extended with palm facing upwards. Take care not to over-extend as this compresses the artery.
5. Insert needle just proximal to the wrist crease.
6. Insert the needle at an angle of 25–30°. On entering the artery, blood will flow into the syringe/hub.
7. On completion, compress the artery for 5 min using a cotton wool ball to prevent bruising.

Venous lines

PERIPHERAL VENOUS LINE

Ideal sites include the dorsal surface of the foot and hand. If the baby is likely to need a Silastic long line then avoid the long saphenous vein and the veins in the antecubital fossa. Use the temporal veins only if unsuccessful at other sites — the baby's head will need to be shaved and the hair can take many months to regrow.

Equipment
- Alcohol swab
- 24 g IV cannula
- T-piece with luer lock flushed with 0.9% saline.

Procedure
1. Clean site with alcohol swab.
2. A cold light source may facilitate visualisation of the vein.
3. Insert cannula bevel upwards. When blood flows back slowly advance the cannula over the stylet and into the vein.
4. Remove the stylet and attach the cannula to T-piece.
5. Secure cannula in place. Do not cover the skin over tip of cannula as this site must be observed for extravasation. Be careful not to fully encircle a digit or to compress a digit with tape as this can result in ischaemic damage.

NB. Once the stylet has been pulled back, it should not be reinserted into the plastic cannula because of risk of shearing the tip.

LONG LINE

These are inserted when infants require TPN, other concentrated solutions (e.g. 20% glucose solution) or inotropes which are causing venoconstriction when given via a peripheral line. ***Blood cannot be given via a Silastic long line***.

They should not be inserted at the time of suspected or proven septicaemia until 48 h of antibiotic treatment has been given.

Suitable sites include the long saphenous veins either in front of the medial malleolus or below the knee, the veins in the antecubital fossa and the temporal scalp veins. In general, lines in the arm last longer than those in the leg.

Equipment
- Sterile pack
- 0.5% chlorhexidine gluconate solution
- Silastic long line (23 or 27g — the 27g should only be used in the smallest infants <750 g when insertion of a 23 g line is not possible)
- If no introducer is available in the pack, use a 19 g butterfly needle or 20 g IV cannula.

Procedure

1. An aseptic technique should be employed.
2. Choose the access site and measure the distance to the right atrium.
3. Expose the area and clean with chlorhexidine gluconate solution.
4. Use sterile towels to achieve a large sterile area.
5. Prime the line with heparinised saline (1 IU/mL).
6. Ask the assistant to squeeze the limb above the sterile area.
7. Use one of two techniques to cannulate the vein:
   a. Butterfly needle with plastic extension removed
      (i) Insert the needle until blood flows out freely. Do not attempt to push the needle too far into the vein.
      (ii) Insert the line through the needle. The angle of the butterfly is critical and it may be quite fiddly. The line will pass freely when the position is correct.
   b. IV cannula (Fig. 21.5)
      (i) Use a blade to cut the plastic tubing of the cannula through 360° just below the hub.
      (ii) Leave both the cannula and the hub in situ on the stylet.
      (iii) Insert the complete cannula into the vein until blood flows freely. Advance no more than 0.5–1 cm.
      (iv) Remove stylet and hub.
      (v) Introduce the line through the cut cannula to the desired length.
8. Ensure good haemostasis. This is often difficult and a topical haemostat may be needed or compression for up to 20 min.
9. Secure in place using Steristrip and an occlusive sterile dressing.
10. Connect the line to a heparinised saline infusion (1 IU/mL) at 0.5 mL/h.
11. X-ray to check position. **NB.** Not all lines are radio-opaque. If the line is radiolucent, inject 1 mL of contrast in the 5 s prior to X-ray exposure. The tip should lie in the right atrium.
12. Silastic lines must be replaced every 28 days and removed in any baby thought to be septicaemic.

INDWELLING CENTRAL LINE

These should be inserted under sterile conditions and general anaesthesia in theatre.

UMBILICAL VENOUS CATHETER

This is usually used in the emergency situation during resuscitation of the newborn infant. It may be used when peripheral IV access has been unsuccessful, for exchange

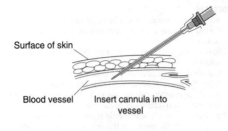

Surface of skin

Blood vessel   Insert cannula into
                 vessel

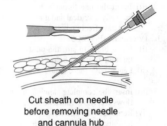

Cut sheath on needle
before removing needle
and cannula hub

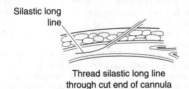

Silastic long
line

Thread silastic long line
through cut end of cannula

Fig. 21.5   Method for insertion of silastic long line (it may be easier to cut the sheath on the needle before insertion of cannula).

transfusion and for venous access in the first few days of life for the extremely preterm baby where minimal handling is required. A UVC can be inserted up to 1 week of age.

Equipment
● 0.5% chlorhexidine gluconate solution or alcohol swab
● Umbilical tape

- 5 or 6FG UV catheter
- 5 mL syringe containing 0.9% saline or heparinised saline (1 IU/mL).

Procedure

1. An aseptic technique should be employed.
2. Loosely tie umbilical tape around the base of the cord in case of excessive bleeding.
3. Identify the vein — there are two arteries and one vein; the vein has a thin wall and a large lumen when compared with the artery.
4. Prime the catheter with saline. Do not leave the catheter open to the atmosphere because negative intrathoracic pressure could cause an air embolus.
5. Insert the catheter until blood flows easily. Occasionally the umbilical vein is kinked and advance of the catheter is blocked at 1–2 cm beyond the abdominal wall. Gentle traction on the cord usually relieves this. If obstruction occurs at more than 2 cm and only partly gives way to pressure, the catheter is probably either wedged in the portal system or coiled up in the portal sinus. Withdraw the catheter partway and reinsert.
6. Aim to place the UVC within the right atrium measured as the distance between the umbilical stump and the mid-sternum. During resuscitation, if difficulties arise in advancing the UVC, withdraw to approximately 2 cm beyond the umbilical stump.
7. During resuscitation, tighten the tape around the umbilical cord to keep the UVC in place. For longer use, enclose the catheter immediately distal to the umbilical stump in two 2 cm square pieces of sleek tape. Secure the tape to the umbilical stump using two separate sutures.

MANAGEMENT OF CENTRAL LINES, LONG LINES AND UVCS

- The tips of these lines lie in the right atrium. They should therefore be handled in a sterile manner and breakage into the lines kept to a minimum.
- Risk of bacteraemia may be related to the frequency with which the line is broken into.
- Do not use Silastic long lines for bolus drugs unless no other access is obtainable. There is a high risk of breakage to these lines when small-volume syringes (which can generate very high pressures) are used.
- Do not use UVCs except during resuscitation for any drugs, dextrose concentrations of >15% or TPN unless the tip lies in the inferior vena cava or the right atrium.
- Central lines and UVCs should never be left open to the atmosphere because of the risk of air embolus.

Arterial lines

Arterial access should be obtained in any baby requiring inspired oxygen concentrations of >40% in the first few hours after birth or in any baby in whom frequent blood gas analysis is anticipated.

PERIPHERAL ARTERIAL LINES

The radial and posterior tibial arteries may be cannulated (for location see p. 357). The femoral and brachial arteries are end arteries and should not be used. Catheterisation of the temporal artery has been associated with cerebral infarction.

Equipment
- Alcohol swab
- 24 g intravenous cannula
- T-piece with luer lock flushed with heparinised saline (1 IU/mL)
- 2 mL syringe containing heparinised saline (1 IU/mL).

Procedure
1. Clean site with alcohol swab.
2. Visualise the artery (see arterial blood sampling, p. 357) using a cold light source or palpate for arterial pulsation.
3. Insert cannula bevel uppermost at 25–30°.
4. When blood flushes back into the hub, advance the cannula over the stylet and into the artery.
5. Remove the needle and immediately occlude the end of the cannula with a bung. Fixate securely. Make sure the fingers or toes can be clearly visualised to look for signs of ischaemia. Remove the bung from the cannula and attach the luer lock T-piece.
6. Attach the line to an infusion of heparinised saline (1 IU/mL) and run at 1 mL /h. An invasive BP monitoring system may also be attached if required.

UMBILICAL ARTERIAL CATHETER

The umbilical arteries constrict within a few minutes of birth. Closure is delayed with hypoxia and acidosis. Successful catheterisation is most likely in the first hour. By 4 days of age it is usually not possible to insert a UAC.

Equipment
- 0.5% chlorhexidine gluconate solution
- UAC pack containing fine non-toothed forceps and a blunt ended dilator

- Umbilical tape
- 3.5 /5FG UAC or 4/5FG Searle catheter (which allows continuous measurement of P_aO_2)
- Three-way tap
- 5 mL syringe containing heparinised saline (1 IU/mL).

Procedure

1. A full sterile technique should be employed.
2. Inspect the baby's legs and buttocks for discoloration.
3. Measure the distance between the shoulder tip and the umbilical stump to determine how far the UAC will need to be inserted (Fig. 21.6).
4. Attach three-way tap to UAC and flush with heparinised saline.
5. Tie a loose ligature around the base of the cord in case of excessive bleeding.
6. Cut the cord horizontally 1–1.5 cm from the stump using a scalpel blade.
7. Identify the arteries — there are two arteries and one vein; the arteries have relatively thick walls and a small lumen when compared with the vein.
8. Using fine forceps and a blunt-ended dilator, gently tease open the artery.
9. Gently insert the UAC into the artery to the required length. Blood should flow back freely.
10. Obstruction may be encountered at :
    a. 1–2 cm: This is where the vessels turn downwards. Try turning the umbilical stump towards the baby's head
    b. 4–5 cm: This is probably due to spasm and kinking of the artery at the origin of the iliac vessels. The use of gentle sustained pressure should overcome this.
11. Enclose the catheter immediately distal to its insertion into the umbilical stump in two 2 cm square pieces of sleek tape. Secure the tape to the umbilical stump using two separate sutures.
12. Inspect the baby's legs for any new discoloration. If the leg or toes are blue or white, remove the catheter.
13. X-ray the chest and abdomen to confirm the UAC position. If the UAC is in the artery, the catheter will dip down first towards the pelvic bone then turn upwards as it enters the iliac artery, finally lying to the left of the spine. A high UAC should lie at the level of the diaphragm (T4–T8 vertebrae on CXR) and a low UAC between L3 and L5. Never leave a UAC at the level of L1, i.e. opposite the origin of the renal arteries.
14. Attach the UAC to an infusion of heparinised saline (1 IU/mL) run at 0.5 mL/h. An invasive BP monitoring system may also be attached if required.

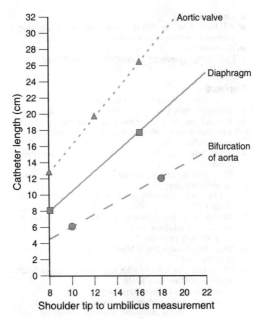

Fig. 21.6 Length of UAC.

INVASIVE BP MONITORING

This should be considered in:

- an infant during acute phase of RDS and requiring ventilation
- an infant in whom indirect methods of BP measurements suggest significant hypo- or hypertension
- any infant on inotropic drugs

Equipment
- Arterial line in situ
- BP transducer
- Heparinised saline (1 IU/mL) to flush and as continuous infusion.

Procedure
1. Secure the arterial line firmly and attach to a long extension line with a luer lock

2. Flush transducer with heparinised saline (1 IU/mL).
3. Ensure you know how to zero and calibrate the BP transducer and how to connect this to a continuous monitor.
4. Place the transducer at mid-axillary level.
5. Switch the line to the arterial cannula off and open the transducer to the atmosphere to zero it. **NB.** Do not open the arterial cannula to the atmosphere!
6. Close the transducer to the atmosphere and open to the arterial line. A continuous BP waveform should now be visible on the monitor.
7. Re-zero every 24 h.
8. If there is doubt about the authenticity of the readings:
   - check there is no air or blood in line or dome
   - re-zero
   - check against a non-invasive technique (but beware that oscillatory methods over-read when there is significant hypotension; invasive BP is always likely to be more accurate than non-invasive.)
   - consider replacing transducer.

Intraosseous access

Equipment
- Alcohol swab
- 18FG IO needle with trocar
- 5 mL syringe.

Procedure
1. Identify insertion site. Ideally use the anterio-medial surface of the tibia 1–2 cm below the tibial tuberosity. Alternatively, use the anterolateral surface of the femur 2–3 cm above the lateral condyle.
2. Clean skin with alcohol swab.
3. Insert the needle at 90° to the skin.
4. Advance the needle until a give is felt as the bone cortex is penetrated.
5. Remove the trochar, attach a 5 mL syringe and aspirate to confirm position. This bone marrow can be used to obtain a blood gas, FBC and blood sugar.
6. Give drugs as bolus injections. If the infant requires volume expanders, these must be pushed in via a syringe as fluid will not flow in rapidly enough via an IO needle.

Intracardiac injection

This should only be used in extreme circumstances when attempts at UVC or IO insertion have failed.

Equipment

- Alcohol swab
- 21 g needle or butterfly needle flushed with 0.9% saline
- Syringe containing drug (usually adrenaline).

Procedure

1. Attach the syringe to the needle.
2. Clean site with alcohol swab.
3. Insert the needle immediately lateral to the left sternal edge in the fourth intercostal space, i.e. immediately below a line joining the nipples.
4. Aspirate the syringe as the needle is being inserted.
5. When a flashback of blood is obtained, inject the drug.

CSF collection

LUMBAR PUNCTURE

This is usually performed as part of an infection screen when CSF should be sent for microscopy, culture, protein and glucose estimation. Occasionally, CSF is required as part of the work-up in a child thought to have a metabolic disorder. A LP may also be used to remove CSF in babies with post haemorrhagic ventricular dilatation whilst the high CSF protein prevents shunt insertion. The L4/L5 space is usually used. If this is unsuccessful consider the L3/L4 space. Never insert the needle above this as the spinal cord extends to L3 in the newborn. Never use a needle without a stylet as it may become blocked and there is a risk of implantation dermoid cyst in later life.

Equipment

- 0.5% chlorhexidine gluconate solution
- Sterile dressing pack
- 24 g 1.5 inch spinal needle with stylet
- Pressure manometer
- Plastic dressing aerosol spray.

Procedure

1. A full aseptic technique should be employed.
2. The infant should be laid on one side and held by an experienced nurse at the shoulders and hips. Gently flex the shoulder and hips so that the spine is softly curved but remains horizontal. Overflexion of the neck may result in apnoea.
3. Locate the space between the L4 and L5 vertebrae which is immediately below a line joining both iliac crests.

4. Insert the LP needle into the midline until a give is felt as the needle enters the subarachnoid space, approximately 5–7 mm in a preterm infant and 10 mm in a term infant.
5. If LP is being undertaken for post haemorrhagic ventricular dilatation, measure the opening pressure, (normal values <7 cm H_2O).
6. Place 10 drops of CSF in three sterile bottles for microscopy, culture and protein examination, and some in a fluoride oxalate bottle for glucose estimation.
7. Withdraw the needle
8. Cover the insertion site with aerosol plastic dressing.

VENTRICULAR TAP

This is usually performed in post haemorrhagic hydrocephalus where insufficient CSF can be removed via a LP. Always confirm by USS that the ventricles are dilated. This procedure should never be performed without prior discussion with a consultant as it may result in significant complications, e.g. ventriculitis.

Equipment
- Sterile dressing pack
- 22 g 2.5 inch spinal needle with stylet
- Safety razor
- Plastic dressing aerosol spray.

Procedure
1. *A full aseptic technique* should be employed
2. If necessary shave a small area of the scalp. Try not to remove an excessive area of hair as it may take many months to grow back, causing considerable distress to parents.
3. The infant should be laid supine.
4. Palpate the lateral corners of the anterior fontanelle.
5. Insert the needle into the lateral corner of the anterior fontanelle using a 'Z' track technique and angle it forwards and inwards towards the inner canthus of the ipsilateral eye. The lateral ventricle is usually entered at a depth of 2–4 cm (earlier if there is gross ventricular dilatation). Remove the stylus. If the ventricle has been entered, CSF will well up in the needle.
6. Never attach a syringe to the cannula. Always allow the CSF to drip out spontaneously.
7. Remove the needle and seal with aerosol plastic dressing.

Urine collection

SUPRAPUBIC ASPIRATION OF URINE

This is the preferred method for obtaining a urine sample for microscopy, culture and sensitivity as part of an infection screen in a sick infant where antibiotics are to be commenced immediately following screening. It should also be used where an equivocal result has been obtained from a bag specimen. Ideally, perform 1–2 h following the last episode of urination and confirm the presence of urine in the bladder using USS.

Equipment
- Alcohol swab
- 23 g needle
- 5 mL syringe
- Elastoplast.

Procedure
1. Clean the skin with an alcohol swab.
2. Attach needle to syringe and insert into the abdomen 1 cm above the pubic bone perpendicular to the skin. Aspirate continuously until urine is obtained. Do not insert the needle more than 2 cm in a preterm infant and 3 cm in a term infant.
3. Withdraw the needle and cover the puncture site with an Elastoplast.

BLADDER CATHETERISATION

This is usually performed when there is bladder distension which cannot be reduced by manual expression or in acute renal failure where accurate urinary output measurements are required.

Equipment
- Sterile pack
- 0.5% chlorhexidine gluconate solution
- Analgesic lubricating jelly (0.1% xylocaine gel)
- 3–5FG urinary catheter or 5FG feeding tube.

Procedure
1. A full aseptic technique should be employed.
2. Abduct the thighs and identify the urethral meatus.
3. Clean the perineum, swabbing away from the meatus.
4. Liberally apply the analgesic lubricating gel to the urethral orifice and the end of the catheter.
5. Insert catheter — usually some urine will be obtained when in the correct position. Secure the catheter to the thigh with adhesive tape.

Thoracentesis

NEEDLING OF THE CHEST

This is used as a therapeutic and diagnostic procedure in the critically ill infant with respiratory and/or haemodynamic compromise, or both due to a pneumothorax or pleural effusion.

Equipment
- Alcohol swab
- 23 g butterfly needle
- Three-way tap
- 10 mL syringe
- Bottle of sterile water.

Procedure
1. Either attach the butterfly needle to the three-way tap and syringe or place the end in a bottle of sterile water.
2. Insert the needle into the second intercostal space in the mid-clavicular line. If using a syringe apply continuous suction — a rapid flow of air will occur when the pneumothorax is entered. Rotate the three-way tap to waste the air and then repeat the aspiration/waste cycle.
3. If the air leak is continuous, the butterfly tubing may be left underwater and allowed to bubble whilst a chest drain is inserted.

CHEST DRAIN INSERTION

Equipment
- Sterile dressing pack
- 0.5% chlorhexidine gluconate solution
- 1% lignocaine
- 8, 10 or 12FG chest drain depending on size of infant — use largest possible
- Scalpel and fine straight blade
- Fine blunt forceps
- Underwater seal chest drainage bottle and tubing
- Silk suture
- Steristrips
- Opsite dressing.

Procedure
1. A full aseptic technique should be employed.
2. Except in a dire emergency, sedation with diamorphine should be given prior to insertion.
3. For a lateral chest drain, using a roll under the shoulder, lie the baby on its side at 45° with the side requiring the chest drain uppermost. Stretch the arm out and raise above the head.
4. Clean the skin over the insertion site and infuse a small amount of 1% lignocaine through the tissues down to the parietal pleura, wait 1–2 mins for anaesthesia to work.
5. Make a small incision through the skin parallel to and immediately above the rib (the intercostal vessels lie immediately below the ribs).
6. With a pair of forceps, bluntly dissect through the intercostal muscle down to and including the parietal pleura.

7. Using an appropriately sized drain, remove the trocar and grasp the tip of the drain with a pair of forceps. Push the drain and forceps through the chest wall. Release the forceps and advance the drain, aiming anteriorly. The use of a trocar during insertion risks impaling/penetrating the lung therefore only use it if there are difficulties with insertion of drain. If a trocar is used, apply a clamp 2 cm distal to the tip.

8. The drain should be inserted into either:
   — *lateral* : third to fifth intercostal space just posterior to the anterior axillary line, well away from breast tissue; the lateral route is preferred
   — *anterior* : second to third intercostal space in the mid clavicular line, direct the tip anteriorly. The nipple and breast bud must be avoided.

9. Connect the drain to an underwater seal and observe for air bubbles and swinging on respiration. If necessary, connect the drain to low suction pressure 5–10 cm H_2O.

10. Fixate the drain using single sutures, Steristrips and an Opsite dressing. *Do not use a purse-string suture as this will result in a permanent, disfiguring scar.*

11. Perform CXR to check the position of the drain.

12. If a pneumothorax does not resolve following insertion of a chest drain, consider whether the drain is working correctly before inserting another drain. The maximum number of drains required should be two on each side.

Pericardial puncture

Used for drainage of a pericardial effusion. In babies, pericardial effusion is rarely seen except following cardiac surgery. Ideally a tap should be performed under echocardiographic control. The ECG must be monitored throughout the procedure. ST segment changes or widening of the QRS interval indicates ventricular damage by the needle.

Equipment
- Sterile dressing pack
- 0.5% chlorhexidine gluconate solution
- 18g over the needle cannula
- 5 mL syringe.

Procedure
1. Confirm the ECG monitor is working.
2. A full aseptic technique should be employed.
3. Clean the xiphoid and subxiphoid areas with chlorhexidine gluconate solution.
4. Attach the cannula to the syringe.

5. Puncture the skin immediately inferior to the left side of the xiphisternum.
6. Advance the cannula slowly towards the tip of the left scapula, aspirating continuously until fluid is obtained. Remove the needle and aspirate the fluid to dryness.
7. If a constant flow of blood is obtained, the ventricle has been entered and the cannula should be withdrawn
8. If fluid is obtained, the cannula can be left in situ for further taps at a later date.

Abnormal paracentesis

This is usually done in the emergency situation to remove ascites where ventilation is being compromised. It can also be undertaken for diagnostic purposes. Conditions which result in ascites often have organomegaly; palpate the abdomen carefully before inserting the needle.

Equipment
- Alcohol swab
- 1% lignocaine
- 18 g cannula
- Three-way tap
- 10 or 20 mL syringe.

Procedure
1. Clean skin with alcohol swab.
2. Except in the emergency situation, infiltrate the skin with local anaesthetic.
3. Insert the cannula in the left lower quadrant midway along a line joining the umbilicus to the anterior iliac spine. A give is felt as the peritoneum is punctured.
4. Aspirate slowly.
5. If a large volume of fluid is present, aspirate slowly and intermittently to prevent shock.

Exchange transfusion

Indications
- Severe anaemia (Hb <10 g/dL) with normal or increased blood volume in a newborn infant
- Severe Rhesus disease or other blood group incompatibility with one of the following:
  — cord Hb <10 g/dL
  — cord Hb 10–12 g/dL and cord bilirubin >80 μmol/L.
  — cord Hb >10 g/dL and SBR increasing by >10 μmol/h or likely to cross exchange transfusion line

- Bilirubin above exchange transfusion line (Fig. 9.4)
- Clinical evidence of kernicterus with jaundice whatever the level of serum bilirubin
- Acute poisoning
- Severe septicaemia
- Polycythaemia (*venous* haematocrit (>70% and symptomatic). Do not rely on a capillary haematocrit. Measure on a free-flowing venous sample which has been spun at 3000 rpm for 10 min.

Volume of blood to be exchanged

- *Anaemia*: severe anaemia with hydrops — a single volume exchange i.e. 85 mL/kg, should be performed.
- *Removal of toxins*, e.g. hyperbilirubinaemia — a two-volume exchange, i.e. 170 mL/kg should be performed. This should remove approximately 90% of the infant's RBCs and, in hyperbilirubinaemia, decrease the serum bilirubin by 55%.
- Polycythaemia — the infant's blood is exchanged with either HAS or 0.9% saline. The aim is to reduce the haematocrit to 0.5–0.55. The following formula calculates the volume to be exchanged (in mL) usually about 20 mL/kg:

$$\text{(baby's Hct} - \text{desired Hct)} \times \text{weight (kg)} \times 85$$

Type of blood

Blood should be cross-matched against mother's and baby's blood. In an emergency, use O-negative blood. Although blood is leucodepleted it should also be CMV-negative and, if the infant is preterm, irradiated. The blood should be less than 72 h old. The blood should be partially packed, i.e. have a haematocrit of 50–55%, and be warmed via a heating coil.

Venous/arterial access

Baby < 7 days of age

- No catheters in situ — insert a UVC and use an in/out technique The ideal site for a UVC in exchange transfusion is with the tip passed through the ductus venosus so that it lies just above the diaphragm. This may not be possible and a low UVC may have to be used. Do not use the UVC if on AXR the tip is lying in a branch of the portal vein or appears impacted within the liver (Fig. 21.7) as it may cause damage.
- If UAC is in situ, give blood continuously via an IVI while removing aliquots at the same rate from the UAC every 5 min.
- If peripheral arterial line in situ and sampling properly, give blood via IVI while removing aliquots at the same rate from the arterial line every 5 min.

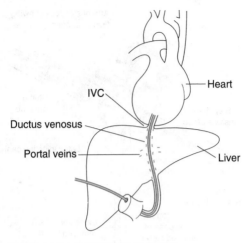

Fig. 21.7 Location of catheter tip when inserting UVC.

Baby > 7 days of age
- If UAC in situ, give blood continuously via an IVI while removing aliquots at the same rate from the UAC every 5 min.
- If UAC not present, attempt to insert peripheral arterial line. If this is unsuccessful attempt to insert UVC. If this is unsuccessful, the help of an anaesthetist, surgeon or paediatrician skilled in the insertion of central neck or femoral lines, for in/out technique, must be requested.

Equipment
- Catheterisation pack
- Exchange transfusion set which contains
  — four-way stopcock
  — umbilical catheter (5FG)
  — two 20 mL syringes
  — calibrated waste blood container
- Blood administration set
- Exchange transfusion record
- Blood warmer
- ECG and BP monitoring.

Procedure
1. A full aseptic technique should be employed.

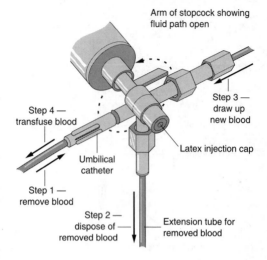

Fig. 21.8 Exchange transfusion.

2. If using an in/out technique, insert the catheter and obtain an X-ray to confirm position. Connect the four-way stopcock (or two three-way taps if not available) to the catheter. Attach in a clockwise direction from the port attached to the catheter (Fig. 21.8):
   — the waste blood container
   — the fresh blood supply
   — a 20 mL syringe.
   A closed circuit must be used at all times to prevent air embolus. During each cycle, withdraw blood from the baby and inject into the waste blood container. Refill the syringe with the fresh donated blood and very slowly inject into the baby. Each cycle should take 5 min, giving blood over no less than 2.5 min.
3. If blood is going to be given continuously via a peripheral line, use a volumetric pump which delivers at the same rate that blood is being withdrawn. Exchange of each aliquot (see below) should take place over 5 min.
4. If indication for exchange is jaundice; immediately prior to starting, re-check SBR and confirm that exchange is still necessary.

5. Take an umbilical swab for microbiology. Send blood for Hb, PCV, glucose, blood gas and culture.
6. Use: 5 mL aliquots for <28 weeks
   — 10 mL aliquots for 28–32 weeks
   — 15 mL aliquots for 33–36 weeks
   — 20 mL aliquots for >36 weeks.
   If not well tolerated reduce the aliquot. The whole exchange should take approximately 1.25–1.5 h.
7. After every 100 mL exchanged give 1 mL of 10% calcium gluconate mixed with the next aliquot of blood. Monitor the ECG closely and stop if the HR falls to <100 bpm.
8. At the end, take blood for Hb, PCV, SB, calcium, glucose, blood gas, coagulation screen and blood culture. Culture catheter tip if catheter is removed. Restart phototherapy if indication for exchange is jaundice.
9. If a UVC has been used, leave in situ until it is clear that a second exchange is unlikely within the next 24 h.
10. Check blood sugar hourly for 4 h after the exchange as rebound hypoglycaemia may occur (secondary to hyper-insulinism in response to the high dextrose content of the infused blood).
11. Do not feed for 2–4 h post-exchange, to decrease the incidence of NEC.

Monitoring

An observer must record constantly the amount of blood being withdrawn and replaced and the time taken for each cycle. HR, ECG, BP and temperature should be recorded regularly and blood sugar and blood gases checked every 30 min. Warning signs to watch for during an exchange and their management are described in Table 21.1. Complications of exchange are shown in Table 21.2.

Imaging

CRANIAL ULTRASOUND (see Ch. 12)

Table 21.1 Warning signs during exchange transfusion

- Vomiting or crying during injection of blood
  — infusion too rapid. Stop until condition improves
- Cyanosis or pallor
  — Check temperature, ECG, pH, $P_a\text{co}_2$
  — Consider too rapid infusion, blood balance error causing hypo/hyper volaemia, metabolic acidosis
- Aspirated blood becomes dark
  — catheter tip may be in branch of portal vein; readjust until brighter blood appears. If readjustment makes no difference, consider deterioration in baby's condition and check temperature, ECG, pH, $P_a\text{co}_2$
- Tachycardia >160/min and bradycardia <100/min
  — consider blood volume disturbance, metabolic acidosis and hyperkalaemia
- ECG abnormalities
  — Circulatory overload may lead to peaked P waves
  — Signs of hyperkalaemia: Stop transfusion. Do not use donor blood. Check K⁺ levels in donor blood. Refer to chapter 8 for management of hyperkalaemia.
  — Arrhythmias: mostly caused by cold blood or hyperkalaemia
- Cardiac arrest
  — cold blood, hyperkalaemia, too rapid injection of calcium gluconate, air embolism
- Convulsion
  — check blood pH, glucose and calcium

Table 21.2 Complications of exchange transfusion

- *Vascular*
  Embolisation with air or clot
  Thrombosis
  Haemorrrhagic infarction of the gut
- *Cardiac*
  Arrhythmias
  Volume overload
  Hypovolaemia
  Arrest
- *Metabolic*
  Hypokalaemia
  Hypocalcaemia
  Hypomagnesaemia
  Acidosis
  Hypoglycaemia
- *Respiratory*
  Oxygen affinity is reduced because the donor blood usually has an oxygen dissociation curve displaced to the right of fetal haemoglobin
- *Haematological problems*
  Thrombocytopenia
  Coagulopathy
- *Infection*
  Bacteraemia
  HIV, CMV, hepatitis B from infected donor blood
- *Hypothermia*

APPENDIX 1

Haematological values in the newborn

Table A1.1   Mean haematological values during the first 2 postnatal weeks in term infants

Haem value	Cord blood	Day 1	Day 7	Day 14
Hb (g/dl)	16.8	18.4	17.0	16.8
HCT	0.53	0.58	0.54	0.52
Red cells (x10^{12}/l)	5.25	5.8	5.2	5.1
MCV (fl)	107	108	98.0	96.0
MCH (pg)	34	35	32.5	31.5
MCHC (%)	31.7	32.5	33	33
Retics (%)	3–7	3–7	0–1	0–1
Nuc RBC (mm^3)	500	200	0	0
Plats (x10^9/l)	290	192	248	252

Table A1.2   Mean red cell values on Day 1 from 24 weeks gestational age

Gestational age (wks)	24	26	28	30	32	34	36	Term
Hb (g/dl)	19.4	19.0	19.3	19.1	18.5	19.6	19.2	19.3
HCT	0.63	0.62	0.60	0.60	0.60	0.61	0.64	0.61
RBC (x10^{12}/l)	4.65	4.73	4.62	4.79	5.0	5.09	5.27	5.14
MCV (fl)	135	132	131	127	123	122	121	119
Retics (%)	6.0	9.6	7.5	5.8	5.0	3.9	4.2	3.2

Table A1.3 Differential white cell counts in term infants (10³ cells/mm³)

Age (days)	Total WBC	Neutrophils	Lymphocytes	Monocytes %	Eosinophils %
0	9–30	6.0–26.0	2.0–11.0	6	2
1	9.4–34	5.0–21.0	2.0–11.5	6	2
7	5.0–21.0	1.5–10.0	2.0–17.0	9	4
14	5.0–20.0	1.0–9.5	2.0–17.0	9	3
28	5.0–19.5	1.0–9.0	2.5–16.5	7	3

Note: An artefactual high neonatal WBC may be reported because automatic cell counters may wrongly include normoblasts (red cell precursors) in the WBC.

Table A1.4 Serum immunoglobulin levels

Age	IgG (g/l)	IgA (g/l)	IgM (g/l)
Cord blood	5.2–18.0	<0.02	0.02–0.2
0–2 weeks	5.0–17.0	0.01–0.08	0.05–0.2
2–6 weeks	3.9–13.0	0.02–0.15	0.08–0.4

APPENDIX 2

Normal values — clinical chemistry

These values are offered as a guide only. Local laboratories may differ. Check normal values with your local laboratory. For less common tests check with your local laboratory to ensure blood is collected in the correct bottles.

Acid base balance
See Chapter 7 for target ranges of pH, PO_2, PCO_2, during evolution of respiratory illness.
Bicarbonate: Term: 18–25 mmol/l
Preterm: 11–25 mmol/l
Base excess: -4 to +3 mmol/l

Alanine amino transferase (ALT)
Newborn to 1 month: up to 70 IU/l

Albumin
Preterm: 21–36 g/l
Term: 25–50 g/l

Alkaline phosphatase
Preterm: up to 600 U/l
Term: up to 300 U/l
Levels above 1000 suggest treatment of metabolic bone disease is necessary.

α1 antitrypsin
0.9–2.2 g/l.
Check genotype in prolonged jaundice.

Ammonia
Term: <100 µmol/l
Preterm: <200 µmol/l

Anion gap
$((Na^+ + K^+) - (HCO_3^- + Cl^-)) =$ Less than 16

Aspartate aminotransferase (AST)
<45 IU/l

Bilirubin
See Chapter 9

Calcium (total)	Preterm: 2.14–2.65 mmol/l Term: 2.18–2.69 mmol/l Correction for protein binding = Measured Ca^{2+} + $\frac{(40 - \text{albumin g/dl})}{40}$ mmol/l
Chloride	95–105 mmol/l
Cortisol	200–700 nanomol/l
Creatine kinase CPK	Less than 600 IU/l. There is a rapid rise and fall in the first 3 days of life.
Creatinine	Week 1: up to 110 μmol/l Week 4: up to 50 μmol/l
CRP	Less than 5 μg/ml
Ferritin	Birth: 65–400 μmol/l 1 week: 90–650 μmol/l
Gammaglutaryl transferase (γGT)	0–250 IU/l
Glucose	2.6–8.0 mmol/l. Measure in laboratory or using new generation glucose oxidase stick test. Treat *hypoglycaemia* if blood glucose <2.6 mmol/l Treat *hyperglycaemia* if blood glucose >10.0 mmol/l and persistent glycosuria (≥+++)
17-hydroxy-progesterone	0–36 hours < 50 nmol/l, thereafter < 18 nmol/l
Lactate	1.4–2.8 mmol/l
Magnesium	0.7–1.0 mmol/l
Osmolality	275–295 mosmol/l Calculate = $(2(Na^+ + K^+) + \text{glucose} + \text{urea})$
Phosphate	1.2–2.8 mmol/l
Potassium	3.2–6.0 mmol/ in plasma; capillary samples higher Consider treatment if K$^+$ >7.0 mmol/l

Protein	54–70 g/l
Sodium	133–145 mmol/l
Thyroxine (Free T$_4$)	4–30 days: 6.2–22.9 pmol/l
TSH	>7 days: 0.3–5.0 mU/l. There is a rapid rise in TSH in the first 24 hours followed by a fall over the next few days; it is difficult to interpret TSH levels in the first week
Triglycerides	1.1–2.7 mmol/l
Urea	0.7–6.7 mmol/l
Zinc	9.2–29 μmol/l

APPENDIX 3

Maternal medication and breast feeding

There are a small number of drugs which are contraindicated during breast feeding due to the risk of toxicity to the infant. A complete list of drugs is available in the British National Formulary (BNF). Drugs commonly encountered that are CONTRAINDICATED include:

Amiloride	Gold
Amiodarone	Indomethacin
Amphetamines	Iodine
Bromocriptine	Lithium
Chloramphenicol	Nitrofurantoin (avoid in G6PD
Cimetadine	deficient infants)
Ciprofloxacin	Oestrogens
Cisapride	Phenindione
Clemastine	Sulfasalazine (avoid in G6PD
Cyclosporin	deficient infants)
Cytotoxic drugs	Tetracyclines
Dapsone	Vitamins A and D in high doses
Ergotamine	Zidovudine (breast feeding usually
Ganciclovir	contraindicated in HIV infection)

Many drugs are excreted in small amounts into breast milk. Usually there are no harmful effects. However, caution is advised if breast feeding mothers are taking the following drugs:

Anticoagulants   Warfarin and heparin appear safe. Give IM Vit K prophylactically to infant to prevent haemorrhage.

Beta-blockers   Monitor infant for beta-blockade and hypoglycaemia.

Corticosteroids   Monitor infant's adrenal function if maternal dose is >40 mg prednisolone daily (or equivalent).

Sedative drugs   e.g., analgesics, anticonvulsants and anti-histamines. These may suppress establishment of breast feeding. Monitor infant for signs of dehydration or failure to thrive.

Note: the above lists are not exhaustive. It is good practice in every case to carefully note the name and dose of a drug prescribed to a breast feeding mother and consult the pharmacist for advice. A suitable alternative drug can usually be suggested.

APPENDIX 4

Neonatal formulary

Prescribing on the Neonatal Unit

The potential for error in calculating small drug doses to be administered to newborn infants is great. We recommend the following tips as a guide to safe practice.

1. Always write in black indelible ink.
2. Always write in block capitals.
3. Doses are prescribed using only:
   g (grams)
   mg (mg)
   micrograms (write in full)
   units (write in full)
4. Indicate dose/kg required on chart to enable your dose calculation to be checked.
5. Carry forward original starting date when rewriting charts.
6. Prescribing should be limited to a single chart per patient. If this is not possible, staple charts together and number them, e.g. 1 of 2.
7. Always rewrite prescription when dose or timing altered.
8. **Always use a calculator**. A decimal point in the wrong place may lead to a fatal dose being administrated.
9. Always refer to your local Drug Administration manual, policy files or Hospital Codes of Practice.
10. Do not be rushed — take time and check your calculation with an experienced colleague whenever possible.

For further information regarding side effects, drug incompatibilities, therapeutic monitoring and the doses of drugs not listed here please consult a pharmacist or reference source, (e.g. Medicines for Children (1999) London; RCPCH).

Therapeutic Drug Monitoring

Serum drug concentrations may be measured to ensure that therapeutic levels are being achieved and/or to exclude toxicity.

When requesting levels, always state:

- time blood was taken
- time last dose of drug was given
- route of administration
- other drugs the patient is receiving.

Usually samples should be taken only when a steady state has been achieved (equivalent to approximately 5 times the drug half-life).

Individual Drug Doses

Aciclovir. *Treatment dose* for systemic herpes simplex: 10 mg/kg IV 8 hourly. *Prophylactic dose*: 5 mg/kg IV 8 hourly. See Chapter 13.

Adenosine. 50 micrograms/kg IV initially. Increase by increments of 50 micrograms/kg at 2 minute intervals until sinus rhythm restored. Maximum single dose = 300 micrograms/kg.

Adrenaline. See Epinephrine

Albumin 20% solution salt poor. 1G/kg IV over 3 hours (1G/kg = 5ml/kg)

Albumin 4.5% solution. 10 ml/kg IV over 20 minutes.

Aluminium hydroxide. 20 mg/kg PO 8 hourly in hyperphosphataemia.

Aminophylline. *Loading dose*: 6 mg/kg IV. *Maintenance dose*: 2.5 mg/kg IV 12 hourly or 5 mg/kg PR 12 hourly. Target level = 8–12 mg/L.

Amphotericin B lipid complex. *Test dose*: 100 micrograms/kg IV infused over 1 hour. Observe for anaphylaxis for 1 hour then continue *treatment* at a dose of 250 micrograms/kg IV per 24 hours. Increase dose by 250 micrograms/kg per 24 hours to maximum dose of 1 mg/kg per 24 hours in severe infection. Check renal function daily.

Amphotericin liposomal (Ambisone). *Test dose* as for Amphotericin B infused over 10–15 minutes. Observe for anaphylaxis for 1 hour then continue *treatment* at a dose of 1 mg/kg IV per 24 hours increasing by 1 mg/kg/day to maximum of 5 mg/kg per 24 hours in proven systemic fungal infection. Check renal function daily.

Ampicillin. *0–7 days*: 75 mg/kg IV 12 hourly, dose suitable for septicaemia and meningitis. *>7 days*: 50 mg/kg IV 6 hourly, dose suitable for septicaemia and meningitis.

Atracurium. *Loading dose*: 0.5 mg/kg IV. *IV infusion* 0.3–0.6 mg/kg/hr. *Infusion for 0.5–5.0 kg baby*: place 60 mg/kg atracurium in 50 mls of 0.9% saline/dextrose 5%. 1 ml/hr of solution = 1.2 mg/kg/hr.

Benzyl penicillin. 60 mg/kg IV 12 hourly. *Meningitis dose*: 60 mg/kg 6 hourly.

Bicarbonate (sodium).

Acidosis: IV dose for half correction in mmol =

$$\frac{\text{weight (kg)} \times \text{base deficit (mmol/l)}}{3} \times \frac{1}{2}$$

Hyperkalaemia: 2.0 mmol/kg IV

Cardiac arrest: 1 mmol/kg IV

We recommend 4.2% sodium bicarbonate = 0.5 mmol/ml as less likely to cause extravasation burns.

Beclamethasone. 200–400 micrograms by inhaler 12 hourly via spacer.

Beractant (Survanta). 100 mg/kg ET. Up to 3 further doses may be given 8 hourly.

Breast Milk Fortifier. e.g. Nutriprem BMF, add 1×1.5 gram sachet to 50 mls breast milk.

Budesonide. 200–400 micrograms by metered dose inhaler 12 hourly via spacer.

Caffeine base. Initial loading dose: 12.5 mg/kg PO/IV. *2nd loading dose*: 12.5 mg/kg PO/IV. 2 hours p.o./1 hour IV later. *Maintenance dose*: 6 mg/kg PO/IV per 24 hours. Target caffeine levels — up to 55 micrograms/ml.

Calcium carbonate. 20–50 mg/kg PO per 24 hours in *hyperphosphataemia*

Calcium Gluconate 10%.

- 0.5 ml/kg IV in *hyperkalaemia*
- 1 ml of 10% solution IV after every 100 ml blood exchanged in *exchange transfusion*.
- 1 ml/kg by slow infusion IV for *symptomatic hypocalcaemia*.

Calcium Resonium. 1 g/kg/per 24 hours PO or PR.

Captopril. 0–1 month: *Test dose*: 10–50 micrograms/kg PO single dose. Monitor blood pressure every 15 minutes for 2 hours. *Maintenance dose*: 10–50 micrograms/kg PO 8 hourly. Age 1 month–2 years: *Test dose*: 100 micrograms/kg PO. *Maintenance dose*: 100 micrograms–2 mg/kg PO 8 hourly. See Table 10.15.

Carbimazole. 250 micrograms/kg PO 8 hourly.

Carnitine. 100 mg/kg PO or IV.

Carob seed flour (Carobel). Used to thicken milk feeds. See manufacturers instructions.

Cefotaxime. Age 0–7 days: 50 mg/kg IV 12 hourly. *Meningitis dose*: 50 mg/kg IV 6 hourly. *Age >7 days*: 50 mg/kg IV 8 hourly. *Meningitis dose*: 50 mg/kg IV 6 hourly.

Ceftazidime. Age 0–7 days: 75 mg/kg IV 12 hourly. *Meningitis dose*: also 75 mg/kg IV 12 hourly. *Age >7 days*: 50 mg/kg IV 8 hourly. *Meningitis dose*: also 50 mg/kg IV 8 hourly.

Cephradine. *Prophylaxis for MCUG*: 25 mg/kg PO 12 hourly from 24 hours before procedure until 48 hours afterwards. *Regular prophylaxis*: 25 mg/kg PO at night.

Chloral hydrate. 20–30 mg/kg PO/PR. Give maximum of 4 doses in 24 hours for *continuous sedation*. 25–50 mg/kg PO/PR single dose as *sedation for procedures*.

Chloramphenicol drops 0.5%. 1 drop each eye 4 hourly, or use ointment sparingly 6–8 hourly.

Chlorothiazide. *Diuretic dose*: 10–17.5 mg/kg PO 12 hourly. *In hyperglycaemia*: 10 mg/kg PO 12 hourly.

Chlorpromazine. 750 micrograms/kg/PO 6 hourly. Increase dose if symptoms are severe to maximum of 1.5 mg/kg 6 hourly. Used for treatment of opiate withdrawal to reduce threshold for seizures.

Chlortetracycline ointment 1%. To eyes 6 hourly for 1 month.

Cimetadine. 5 mg/kg IV/PO 6 hourly. *NB*: enzyme inhibitions may cause elevated caffeine levels.

Ciprofloxacin. 7.5 mg/kg PO 12 hourly or 5 mg/kg IV 12 hourly.

Cisapride. 200 micrograms/kg PO 6–8 hourly, or 1 mg/kg PR 12 hourly. **Caution:** may cause prolonged Q-T interval. Not currently recommended in preterm babies <3 months of age.

Clonazepam. 100–200 micrograms/kg IV bolus dose over 30 minutes. or, 10–30 micrograms/kg/hr IV infusion. *Maintenance*: 25–50 micrograms/kg PO daily.

Colfosceril palmitate (Exosurf). 67.5 mg/kg ET. Repeat after 12 hours if still ventilated.

Cotrimoxazole. *Prophylaxis* against PCP: 480 mg/m^2 PO 12 hourly for 3 days each week, e.g., M, W, F.

Curosurf. See poractant alfa.

Cyclopentolate 0.5%. 1 drop each eye for cycloplegia.

Dexamethasone. *In CLD*: 0.5 mg/kg IV daily × 7 doses, or 0.2 mg/kg IV 8 hourly for 3 days (or 7 days if effect delayed) followed by 0.1 mg/kg 8 hourly for 3 days followed by 0.1 mg/kg daily for 3 days then stop. Doses may be given PO if on full feeds. Give single daily doses in early morning.

In cases of post intubation laryngeal oedema: 0.2 mg/kg IV 8 hourly — up to 3 doses. Commence 4 hours pre-extubation.

Dextrose 40% gel (Hypostop). 0.5 ml/kg. Rub into buccal mucosa. Use only until IV access obtained in hypoglycaemia.

Diamorphine. *Loading dose*: 50 micrograms/kg IV followed by 15–30 micrograms/kg/hr infusion. *Infusion* for 0.5–5.0 kg baby: place 1.5 mg/kg diamorphine in 50 mls of 5%/10% dextrose. 1 ml/hr of solution = 30 micrograms/kg/hr. **NB:** dose may be increased to 60 micrograms/kg/hr in post-operative ventilated babies for analgesia.

Diazepam. 300–400 micrograms/kg IV bolus for seizures. May cause sedation and prolonged respiratory suppression. Used in suppression of symptoms of benzodiazepine withdrawal syndrome. (May require up to 1–2 mg/kg PO 8 hourly).

Diazoxide. *Hypertension*: 1–3 mg/kg IV slowly. Can repeat hourly. *Hyperglycaemia*: 1.7–5.0 mg/kg PO 8 hourly.

Digoxin. 5 micrograms/kg PO 12 hourly. If child is acutely ill, give 5 micrograms/kg IM 6 hourly for 24 hours then 5 micrograms/kg 12 hourly IV or IM.

Dobutamine. 5–15 micrograms/kg/min IV infusion. *Infusion for baby weighing 0.5–5.0 kgs*: place 30 mg/kg dobutamine in 50 mls of 0.9% saline/5% dextrose/10% dextrose.

1 ml/hr of solution = 10 micrograms/kg/min.

Dopamine. 2–5 micrograms/kg/min IV infusion for renal vasodilatation. 10–20 micrograms/kg/min IV infusion for inotropic support. *Infusion for baby weighing 0.5–5.0 kg*: place 30 mg/kg dopamine in 50 mls of 0.9% saline/5% dextrose/10% dextrose.

1ml/1hr of solution = 10 micrograms/kg/minute. Infuse centrally.

Duocal. Fat and carbohydrate supplement. Add to formula milk according to dietician's instructions.

Epinephrine. *Cardiac arrest*: initial dose 10 micrograms/kg IV/IO, or 20 micrograms/kg ET Subsequent doses 100 micrograms/kg IV/IO. 10 micrograms = 0.1 ml of 1 in 10,000 epinephrine solution. 100 micrograms = 1 ml of 1 in 10,000 epinephrine solution.

Epoprostenol. 5–40 nanograms/kg/min IV. Start at 5 nanograms/kg/min IV, increase in steps of 5–10 nanograms/kg/min to maximum dose of 40 nanograms/kg/min.

Erythromycin. 12 mg/kg PO 8 hourly.

Exosurf. See colfosceril palmitate.

Flecainide. 2 mg/kg IV over 15 mins.

Flucloxacillin. 0–7 days: 50 mg/kg IV 12 hourly. *Meningitis dose*: 75 mg/kg 12 hourly. >7 days: 50 mg/kg IV 8 hourly. *Meningitis dose*: 66 mg/kg 8 hourly. Oral dose in superficial infection: 25–50 mg/kg PO 6 hourly.

Fluconazole. *IV/PO Age <14 days*: 6–12 mg/kg every 72 hours. Age 14–28 days: 6–12 mg/kg every 48 hours. *Age >1 month*: 6–12 mg/kg every 24 hours.

5 flucytosine. Use in conjunction with amphotericin B. *Up to 7 days*: 25 mg/kg IV/PO 6 hourly. *Over 7 days*: 25–50 mg/kg IV/PO 6 hourly.

Fludrocortisone acetate. 2–5 micrograms/kg PO per 24 hours.

Folic acid. *Haemolytic anaemia*: 0.25 mg/kg PO per 24 hours for 6 months. *Dietary supplementation in preterm infants <33 weeks gestational age*: See Chapter 15.

Fresh frozen plasma. 10–20 ml/kg single dose IV.

Frusemide. See furosemide.

Furosemide. 1–2 mg/kg IV or PO 12 hourly *diuretic dose*. Up to 5 mg/kg IV with *fluid challenge in pre-renal failure*. See Chapter 10.

Fusidic acid. 25 mg/kg 12 hourly PO.

Gaviscon. Infant Gaviscon is manufactured in twin sachets. One dose = one single sachet. Add to milk feeds. <2.5 kg half dose, 2.5–5 kg — one dose, >5 kg — 2 doses.

Gentamicin. Unit dose is 2.5 mg/kg IV. The interval between doses is varied according to gestational age.

≤ 28 weeks:	24 hours
29–35 weeks:	18 hours
36–40 weeks:	12 hours

41 weeks and older: 8 hours

Levels must be assayed around the 4th dose. (Pre-dose = 5 minutes before the dose, post dose = 1 hour after the dose).
Target gentamicin levels:
   pre-dose — less than 2.0 mg/l
   post dose — 6 - 10 mg/l.

Glucagon. 20 micrograms/kg IM single dose. May be repeated 6–12 hourly.

Glucose 10%. 5 ml/kg IV/PO for hypoglycaemia.

Glyceryl trinitrate GTN. 200 nanograms–10 micrograms/kg/min IV infusion.

Hepatitis B immunoglobulin (HBIG). 200 IU IM within 24 hours of birth at a different site to VZIG.

Homatropine 1%. 1 drop each eye for cycloplegia.

Hydralazine. 0.2–0.5 mg/kg IV every 4–8 hours. Can be given hourly in emergency or 0.25–2.5 mg/kg PO 8 hourly. Start at low dose and increase gradually. See tables 10.14 and 10.15.

Hydrochlorothiazide. 2–4 mg/kg PO 12 hourly.

Hydrocortisone. 2.5–5 mg/kg IV 12 hourly (used in management of hypoglycaemia Chapter 11). Maintenance for CAH: 6.6 mg/m^2 PO 8 hourly.

Hydrocortisone 1% ointment. Top. 6 hourly for nappy rash. Use sparingly 12 hourly for eczema.

Immunoglobulin. 0.4 grams/kg per 24 hours IV for 5 days for isoimmune thrombocytopenia.

Indomethacin. 0.2 mg/kg IV/PO 12–24 hourly × 3 doses, or, 0.1 mg/kg IV/PO 24 hourly × 6 doses, or 0.2 mg/kg IV followed by 0.1 mg/kg × 4 doses 24 hourly.

Insulin. 0.1 units/kg IV + 25% dextrose 4 ml/kg IV in *hyperkalaemia*.
IV infusion: 0.05–0.1 units/kg/hour. Titrate to blood sugar on a sliding scale. *Infusion for baby weighing 0.5–5.0 kg*: place 10 units/kg insulin in 50 mls dextrose 5%/0.9% saline. 1 ml/hour of solution = 0.2 units/kg/hour for treatment of persistent *hyperglycaemia*.

Iodine. See Lugol's iodine

Ipratropium bromide. 125 micrograms by nebuliser 6 hourly, or, 120 micrograms by inhaler using spacer 6 hourly.

Iron (elemental). 0.6 mg/kg PO 8 hourly for 3 months for iron deficiency anaemia.

Iron supplements. Prophylaxis in preterm infants. See Sytron.

Isoniazid. 5 mg/kg PO daily.

Konakion MM. 2 mg PO at birth. Repeat at 4–7 days. Breast fed babies receive third dose at 1 month.

Lidocaine. *Anticonvulsant dose*: loading dose 2 mg/kg IV over 5 minutes (monitor heart rate) followed by 2–6 mg/kg/hr IV infusion. Avoid if phenytoin has been given. *Local anaesthetic*: infiltrate up to 3 mg/kg 1% Lidocaine (1% solution = 10 mg in 1 ml).

Lignocaine. See lidocaine.

Lugol's iodine. (5% iodine and 10% potassium iodide) 0.1 ml (1 drop) PO 8 hourly.

Magnesium sulphate. *In PPHN*: 200 mg/kg IV over 30 minutes followed by 20–60 mg/kg/hr by infusion adjusted to maintain serum magnesium 3.5–5.5 mmol/l. **NB:** magnesium sulphate supplied as 50% solution: dilute to 10% solution for IV infusion. If fluid restriction essential, maximum concentration to be used is 20%. *For hypomagnesaemia*: 50% solution 0.1 ml/kg (50 mg/kg hydrated magnesium sulphate) IM.

Maize starch (Thixo D). Used to thicken milk feeds.

Mannitol 20%. 0.5 gram/kg IV over 20 minutes.

Methylene blue 1% solution in normal saline. 1 mg/kg IV.

Metronidazole. 7.5 mg/kg IV/PO/PR 8 hourly.

Miconazole 2% cream. Apply twice daily to skin.

Miconazole oral gel. 1 ml 6 hourly topically.

Midazolam. For neonatal seizures when ventilated. *Loading dose*: 50 micrograms/kg IV. *Maintenance dose*: 50–150 micrograms/kg/hour.

Morphine. *Loading dose*: 100 micrograms/kg IV, followed by 10 micrograms/kg/hr infusion for sedation or analgesia. 40 micrograms/kg PO 4 hourly initially for treatment of opiate withdrawal.

Naloxone (usually as Narcan Neonatal 20 micrograms/ml). 10 micrograms/kg IM/IV. Some units use adult Naloxone (400 micrograms/ml) at a dose of 100 micrograms/kg IM

Neomycin 0.5% eye ointment. Apply 6 hourly.

Nifedipine. 0.125–0.5 mg/kg PO 12 hourly. See table 10.15.

Nitric oxide. See Chapter 6.

Nystatin cream. Apply topically 6 hourly to skin.

Nystatin suspension 100,000 units in 1 ml. 1 ml PO 6 hourly after feeds.

Octreotide (somatostatin analogue). 1 microgram/kg SC 4 hourly.

Omeprazole. 700 micrograms/kg PO per 24 hours. Dose may be increased to 3 mg/kg per 24 hours. *Note*: enteric coated granules may be added to bicarbonate 8.4% solution to form a suspension if administered by NGT (**consult pharmacist for advice**).

Pancuronium. *Loading dose*: 100 micrograms/kg IV followed by 50 micrograms/kg every 4–6 hours.

Paracetamol. 15 mg/kg PO/PR 4–6 hourly. Maximum of 4 doses in 24 hours.

Paraldehyde. 0.3 ml/kg PR. Dilute in equal volume of olive oil, or 5% solution at 0.5–2.0ml/kg/hr IV infusion.

Phenobarbitone. *Convulsions: Loading dose*: 20 mg/kg IV followed by further 10 mg/kg IV if seizures continue. *Maintenance dose*: 6 mg/kg IV/PO per 24 hours. Target levels of phenobarbitone 20–40 micrograms/ml. *Liver enzyme inducing dose*: 2 mg/kg per 24 hours.

Phenylephrine 2.5%. 1 drop in each eye for cycloplegia.

Platelets. 20 ml/kg IV.

Poractant alpha (Curosurf). 100–200 mg/kg ET initial dose, followed by up to 2 further doses of 100 mg/kg ET at 12 and 24 hours.

Potassium acid phosphate. 1 mmol/kg PO 24 hourly.

Potassium chloride. 1 mmol/kg 12 hourly with feeds PO, or, 0.2 mmol/kg/hour IV infusion for acute depletion until K^+ in normal range.

Prednisolone. 2 mg/kg PO per 24 hours for 5 days for isoimmune thrombocytopenia.

Propranolol. *Neonatal thyrotoxicosis*: 250–750 micrograms/kg PO 8 hourly. *Hypertension*: 300 micrograms–2.0 mg/kg PO 8 hourly.

Prostacyclin. See epoprostenol.

Prostaglandin E2. *To maintain patency of PDA*: 3–20 nanograms/kg/min. Start at low dose and increase until clinical response achieved. *Suggested administration*: make up 1 microgram in 1 ml solution. Rate of infusion (ml/hr) = 0.06 × wt(kg) × dose required (nanograms/kg/min).

Pyridoxine. 50 mg (*NB*: **not** per kg) single dose IV.

Pyrimethamine. *Treatment of congenital toxoplasmosis*: 1 mg/kg PO per 24 hours. See under spiramycin for schedule.

Ranitidine. 1.5 mg/kg IV 12 hourly, or, 1–2 mg/kg PO 8 hourly.

Rifampicin. 5 mg/kg PO 12 hourly for 2 days. *Prophylaxis* in meningococcal contacts.

Salbutamol. *For wheeze*: 1.25 mg by nebuliser up to 4 hourly, or, 100–200 micrograms by inhaler using spacer 6 hourly. *For renal hyperkalaemia*: 2.5 mg by nebuliser single dose.

Sodium benzoate. 250 mg/kg bolus IV followed by 250 mg/kg/day infusion if ammonia >180 mmol/l.

Sodium bicarbonate. See bicarbonate (sodium)

Sodium nitroprusside. Commence at 500 nanograms/kg/min IV infusion, increase to a maximum of 8 micrograms/kg/min in hypertension. See Table 10.14.

Sodium valproate. 20 mg/kg PO per 24 hours starting dose, increase up to 30 mg/kg PO 12 hourly.

Somatostatin. See octreotide.

Spiramycin. *Treatment of congenital toxoplasmosis*: 100 mg/kg PO per 24 hours for 6 weeks, alternating with 3 weeks of sulphadiazine and pyrimethamine. Continue 9 week regime for 1 year.

Spironolactone. 1–2 mg/kg PO 12 hourly.

Sucralfate. 30 mg/kg 6 hourly PO.

Sulphadiazine. *Treatment of congenital toxoplasmosis*: 50 mg/kg per 24 hours PO. See under spiramycin for schedule.

Survanta. See Beractant.

Sytron. *Prophylactic dose in preterm infants*: Commence on day 28. 0.5 ml (2.75 mg iron) PO daily until 1.5 kg then 1.0 ml PO per 24 hours until 1 year.

THAM 3.6%.
Calculate dose for half correction in mmol alkali required

$$= \frac{\text{wt (kg)} \times \text{base deficit (mmol/L)}}{6}$$

1 ml is approximately equal to 0.5 mmol of bicarbonate.

Theophylline. *Loading dose*: 5–6 mg/kg PO. *Maintenance dose*: 1–2 mg/kg PO 12 hourly. Target level = 8–12 mg/L.

Thyroxine. 8–10 micrograms/kg per 24 hours PO preterm infants. 5–8 micrograms/kg per 24 hours PO term infants. Give as crushed tablets.

Thixo D. See manufacturers instructions.

Tolazoline. 1 mg/kg IV bolus over 5 mins followed by 0.1 mg/kg/hour infusion.

Trimethoprim. *Treatment dose*: 4 mg/kg PO 12 hourly. *Prophylactic dose*: 2 mg/kg PO at night. *Prophylaxis for MCUG*: 4 mg/kg 12 hourly from 24 hours before MCUG until 48 hours afterwards. *NB*: in preterm infants use cephradine instead of trimethoprim.

Vancomycin. IV unit dose and interval vary with gestational age: Infuse over 1 hour:

<27 weeks:	27 mg/kg every 36 hours
27–30 weeks:	24 mg/kg every 24 hours
31–36 weeks:	27 mg/kg every 18 hours
37 weeks and older:	22.5 mg/kg every 12 hours

Levels must be assayed around the 4th dose (pre-dose = 5 minutes before dose).

Target levels: pre-dose: 6.0–10 mg/l.

Our microbiology department suggests monitoring pre-dose levels only.

Varicella–zoster immunoglobulin (VZIG). 250 mg IM.

Vitamins (DOH). 5 drops PO daily (660 IU Vitamin A, 280 IU Vitamin D, 20 mg Vitamin C).

Vitamin D. For MBD use 1000 IU/day PO.

Vitamin K. IM 1 mg if birthweight >1.5 kg, 0.5 mg if birthweight <1.5 kg,

- or PO   1 mg at birth, followed by 0.5 mg at 1 week and 1 month (breast fed babies)
- or, p.o.   1 mg at birth single dose (formula fed babies). See also under Konakion MM.

APPENDIX 5

Growth centiles

The following growth charts are modified with permission from the Child Growth Foundation. The original charts can be obtained from Harlow Printing Limited, Maxwell Street, South Shields, Tyne and Wear, NE33 4PU (Tel: 0191-455-4286; Fax: 0191-427-0195).

Girls: preterm 23 weeks to term: head circumference and weight.

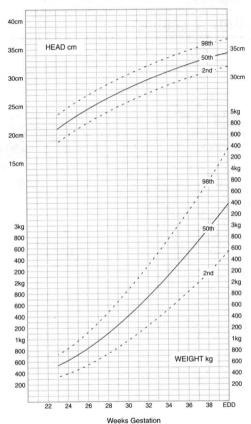

Weeks Gestation

Fig. A5.1

Girls: preterm 30 weeks to 52 weeks: head circumference, length and weight

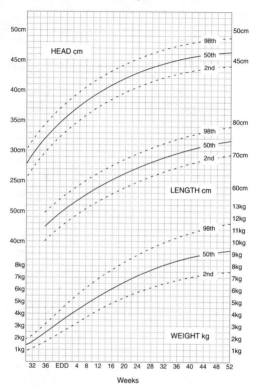

Weeks

Fig. A5.2

Boys: preterm 23 weeks to term: head circumference and weight

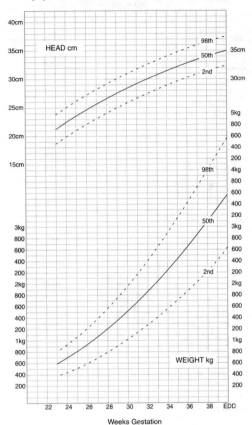

Fig. A5.3

Boys: preterm 30 weeks to 52 weeks: head circumference, length and weight

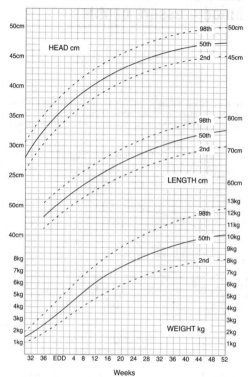

Fig. A5.4

APPENDIX 6

Blood pressure centiles

Invasive blood pressure monitoring should be used where possible in infants receiving intensive care. Centiles for intra-arterial mean blood pressure in preterm infants are given below.

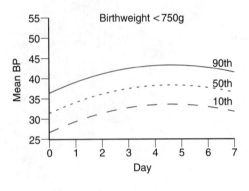

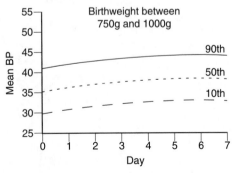

The gestational age in weeks approximates to the 10th centile for mean blood pressure on the first day and is a useful aide memoire. See Chapter 6 for guidelines to the management of blood pressure.

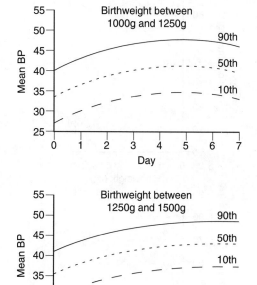

Fig. A6.1   Mean blood pressure changes within first 7 days in preterm infants. (Redrawn from p157 Early Human Development. C. Sunningham et al. 56 (1999) 151-165.)

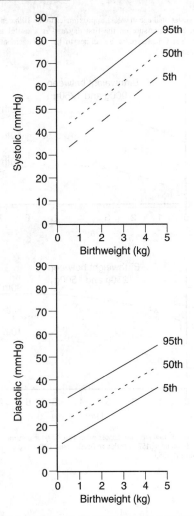

Fig. A6.2 Centiles for neonatal systolic and diastolic blood pressure by birthweight (boys and girls).

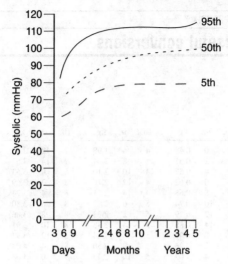

Fig. A6.3   Centiles for systolic blood pressure from birth to 5 years.

APPENDIX 7

Useful conversions

lb.	oz.	kg	lb.	oz.	kg	lb.	oz.	kg
1	0	0.45	4	6	1.98	7	12	3.52
1	2	0.51	4	8	2.04	7	14	3.57
1	4	0.57	4	10	2.10	8	0	3.63
1	6	0.62	4	12	2.16	8	2	3.69
1	8	0.68	4	14	2.21	8	4	3.74
1	10	0.74	5	0	2.27	8	6	3.80
1	12	0.79	5	2	2.33	8	8	3.86
1	14	0.85	5	4	2.38	8	10	3.91
2	0	0.91	5	6	2.44	8	12	3.97
2	2	0.96	5	8	2.50	8	14	4.03
2	4	1.02	5	10	2.55	9	0	4.08
2	6	1.08	5	12	2.61	9	2	4.14
2	8	1.13	5	14	2.67	9	4	4.20
2	10	1.19	6	0	2.72	9	6	4.25
2	12	1.25	6	2	2.78	9	8	4.31
2	14	1.30	6	4	2.84	9	10	4.37
3	0	1.36	6	6	2.89	9	12	4.42
3	2	1.42	6	8	2.95	9	14	4.48
3	4	1.47	6	10	3.01	10	0	4.54
3	6	1.53	6	12	3.06	10	2	4.59
3	8	1.59	6	14	3.12	10	4	4.65
3	10	1.64	7	0	3.18	10	6	4.71
3	12	1.70	7	2	3.23	10	8	4.76
3	14	1.76	7	4	3.29	10	10	4.82
4	0	1.81	7	6	3.35	10	12	4.88
4	2	1.87	7	8	3.40	10	14	4.93
4	4	1.93	7	10	3.46	11	0	4.99

Fig. A7.1 Conversion of lbs to kg.

kPa to mmHg		mmHg to kPa	
2.0	15	15	2.0
2.5	19	20	2.7
3.0	23	25	3.3
3.5	26	30	4.0
4.0	30	35	4.7
4.5	34	40	5.3
5.0	38	45	6.0
5.5	41	50	6.7
6.0	45	55	7.3
6.5	49	60	8.0
7.0	53	65	8.7
7.5	56	70	9.3
8.0	60	75	10.0
8.5	64	80	10.7
9.0	68	85	11.3
9.5	71	90	12.0
10.0	75	95	12.7
10.5	79	100	13.3
11.0	83		
11.5	86		
12.0	90		

Fig. A7.2 Conversion of kPa to mmHg.

INDEX